MW01196783

Physician Communication with Patients

Physician Communication with Patients

RESEARCH FINDINGS AND CHALLENGES

Jon B. Christianson, PhD, Louise H. Warrick, DrPH,
Michael Finch, PhD, and Wayne Jonas, MD

THE UNIVERSITY OF MICHIGAN PRESS | ANN ARBOR

Published in the United States of America by
The University of Michigan Press
Manufactured in the United States of America
♾ Printed on acid-free paper

2015   2014   2013   2012   4 3 2 1

A CIP catalog record for this book is available from the British Library.

Library of Congress Cataloging-in-Publication Data

Physician communication with patients : research findings and
   challenges / Jon B. Christianson ... [et al.].
      p. ; cm.
   Includes bibliographical references and index.
   ISBN 978-0-472-11828-1 (cloth : alk. paper)— ISBN 978-0-472-
02836-8 (e-book)
   I. Christianson, Jon B.
[DNLM: 1. Communication.   2. Physician-Patient Relations.   W 62]
610.696—dc23   2012005029

Contents

Figures and Tables

Abbreviations

ACE	angiotension-converting enzyme
ACS	acute coronary syndrome
AHRQ	Agency for Healthcare Policy and Research
AHT	adjuvant hormonal therapy
ALS	amyotrophic lateral sclerosis
AOR	adjusted odds ratio
ARD	adjusted risk difference
BP	blood pressure
CAHPS	Consumer Assessment of Healthcare Providers and Systems
CANCODE	computerized interaction analysis system with established reliability and validity
CAM	complementary and alternative medicine
CARE	consultation and relational empathy measure
CHD	coronary heart disease
CI	confidence interval
CME	continuing medical education
COPD	chronic obstructive pulmonary disease
CPR	cardiopulmonary resuscitation
CRC	colorectal cancer
CST	communication skills training
DA	decision aid
dB	database
DM	diabetes mellitus
DNR	do not resuscitate
ED	emergency department
EMR	electronic medical record
EOC	Expected Outcome of Communication
EOV	educational outreach visits
ES	effect size
FFS	fee for service
FP	family practice
GATHA-ESP	instrument for interview assessment of family medicine trainees
GHHOS	Glasgow Homeopathic Hospital Outcome Score
GlyHb	glycosolated hemoglobin
GP	general practitioner

HbA1c	hemoglobin A1c
H-CAHPS	Hospital Consumer Assessment of Healthcare Providers and Systems
HCV	hepatitis C virus
HHS	U.S. Department of Health and Human Services
HIV	human immunodeficiency virus
HRQL	health-related quality of life
HRS	Health and Retirement Study
HTN	hypertension
ICU	intensive care unit
IDM	individual decision making
IQR	interquartile range
IRR	adjusted incidence rate ratio
KCS	Kalamazoo Consensus Statement
MBI	Maslach Burnout Inventory
MCO	managed care organization
MD	physician
MEP	Medical Expenditure Panel Survey
MPCC	Measure of Patient-Centered Communication
MPS	member patient satisfaction
MSA	metropolitian statistical area
MYMOP	Measure Yourself Medical Outcome Profile
NS	nonsignificant
OBSE	Objective Structured Clinical Examination, an evaluation method that uses simulated MD-patient encounters in a standardized setting
OR	odds ratio
PA	physician assistant
PACE	Presenting, Asking, Checking, Expressing (patient education system)
PAUSE	Personal connection, Allow for questions, Understandable, Sit down, and Educate
PBS	physician belief system
PCAS	Primary Care Assessment Survey
PCOM	physician communication-provision of information
PCP	primary care physician
PDM	participatory decision making
PN	practice nurse
PPRI	Physician-Patient Relationship Inventory
PSA	prostate-specific antigen
PSS	psychosocial spiritual
QOC	Quality of Communication questionnaire
QoL	quality of life
RCT	randomized control trial
RD	risk difference

RIAS	Roter Interaction Analysis System, method of coding doctor-patient interaction using frequency count of communication "utterances"
RR	relative risk
RT	randomized trial
RWJF	Robert Wood Johnson Foundation
SCCS	Self-Confidence in Communication Skills
SDM	shared decision making
SEGUE	Set the stage, Elicit information, Give information, Understand the patient's perspective, End the encounter
SIG	significant(ly)
SLE	systemic lupus erythematosus
SPIKES protocol	Setting, patient Perception, request for Invitation to deliver the news, Knowledge provision, Empathy, Strategy with patient
STAK	satisfaction, trust, autonomy, knowledge
STI	sexually transmitted infection
UK	United Kingdom
US	United States
VA	Veterans Affairs

1 | Introduction

What Do We Want in a Physician Visit?
What Should We Expect?

We all have a good idea of how we want things to go when we visit a physician. We expect—count on—being able to talk to the physician about why we are there. This means telling him or her what feels wrong, explaining why we think prior treatment recommendations are not working, and even suggesting what we think the problem could be or recommending something new to try. We hope that the physician will listen, possibly ask questions that help us clarify our thoughts, and provide new information that could be useful. Most of us hope for some expression of empathy for whatever the problem is that led us to seek attention. We then expect the physician to combine our information with more information collected through tests or an examination and tell us what he or she thinks is wrong. We hope that the explanation is relatively clear and nontechnical, so that we can remember it and respond to the inevitable questions from family members, friends, and coworkers. Finally, we expect that the physician will explain our options and elicit our input about what to do next. That could mean more tests, a scheduled visit with a specialist, a change in lifestyle, or even the news that there is nothing more that can be done at the present time. Again, we hope that the physician will describe these "next steps" or "treatment options" in a way that is easy to understand, with some sympathy for the fact that we may still be thinking about the diagnostic discussion and not listening as closely as we should be. Certainly, we would appreciate it if the physician asked us about our ability to follow the recommendations, given the other demands in our lives, and gave us some sense of what it will all cost. But is this way too much to ask of our physicians? Are these typical patient "expectations"—or perhaps it would be more accurate to call them "hopes"—too high? Are they unreasonable?

Have our physicians been trained to understand and meet these expectations? Do they have enough time to do so?

Some experts would say they that these expectations are not only reasonable but are even necessary if patients are to get the care that they need and the outcomes that they should expect. In 1999, representatives from academic institutions, providers of physician continuing education programs, and leaders of physician organizations met to discuss what they called the "essential elements in physician-patient communication." They developed a list of these essential elements, which formed the basis for a document called the Kalamazoo Consensus Statement (Makoul 2001). Their consensus statement likely would resonate strongly with most patients today and certainly is consistent with many of the current recommendations for health care reform that are being discussed in the medical community and the public political arena: "The group endorses a patient-centered, or relationship-centered, approach to care, which emphasizes both the patient's disease and his or her illness experience" (Makoul 2001, 391). The consensus statement described a sequence of "tasks" that the authors believed should characterize physician communication during the physician-patient "encounter" and that, when carried out with competence and empathy, could be expected to improve patient health. They include allowing the patient to complete an "opening statement," eliciting concerns and establishing a rapport with the patient; using open- and closed-ended questions to gather and clarify information, along with different listening techniques to solicit information; identifying and responding to the patient's personal situation, beliefs, and values; using language the patient can understand to explain the diagnosis and treatment plan; checking for patient understanding; encouraging patients to participate in decisions and exploring the patient's willingness and ability to follow the care plan; and asking for other concerns the patient might have and discussing follow-up activities expected of the patient, before closing the visit (Makoul 2001, 391).

What Are We Likely to Experience?

While these observations about what constitutes exemplary physician communication are sensible and are likely to be intuitively appealing to most patients, numerous anecdotes in the popular media and a growing body of research suggest that the reality of physician communication with patients can fall considerably short of the ideal. Concerns in the health care field about shortcomings in physician communication certainly are not new. Studies of physician communication have been carried out and critiqued through review articles at an impressive rate over the past three decades. It is striking that concerns persist despite ongoing, often creative efforts to address them. There is no shortage of ideas and programs for improving physician communication, but there also seems to be no shortage of relatively recent studies, anecdotal reports, and media coverage suggesting that physician communication remains a serious issue in American medicine.

In a *Los Angeles Times* article about physician communication, it was observed that a physician expression of empathy "not only reassures patients that they are in good hands, but it also helps them process the information provided . . . That feeling from a doctor can cement the trust necessary for good care" (Ulene 2009). Articles in the *New York Times* and *Boston Globe* (Dunham 2008; Chen 2008) summarized an analysis of conversations that occurred between physicians and their patients with lung cancer (Morse, Edwardsen, et al. 2008). While the number of conversations analyzed in the study was relatively small (20), the results were striking. Given 384 opportunities to express empathy toward their patients, physicians did so only 10 percent of the time. Physician commentators on this study suggested that while these physicians may have been concerned about extending the length of the visit, it was their experience that expressing empathy early in the encounter actually shortens visit length; patients who quickly perceive that their physicians have some empathy for their situations make fewer attempts to solicit empathetic physician responses throughout the visit. The author of another *New York Times* article (Grady 2008) described results from a study of the communication behaviors of physicians while treating patients with advanced cancer. Physicians were unlikely to pursue opportunities presented by patients to discuss negative emotions such as fear, anger, or sadness, although female physicians were much more likely than male physicians to pursue such opportunities. A leader of an ongoing university-based program to teach physicians to demonstrate greater empathy when communicating with patients, described in the *Washington Post* (Boodman 2007), observed, "Doctors don't know how to listen to, or talk to, patients . . . They know how to diagnose."

Physicians seem particularly challenged in circumstances that require them to convey bad news to patients. This happens frequently in the area of cancer treatment, when physicians must communicate to patients that their illnesses are terminal. In a *New York Times* article that described a new program to train physicians to convey bad news more effectively and with more empathy, the author states that "the stilted, jargon-ridden, information-packed sentences in which most doctors encase bad news are pointless. Patients remember nothing about them except the fact that the doctor clearly has not a clue what they are experiencing" (Zuger 2006).

The *Los Angeles Times* article noted previously (Ulene 2009) observes that "communication skills are glossed over in medical school and residency training, and most physicians are never taught how to deliver bad news—although it's a regular part of doctors' jobs."

WebMD Health News (Boyles 2008) reported on a commentary published in the *American Journal of Medicine* relating to studies on the frequency of physician diagnostic errors. The physician commentator suggested that patients could assist physicians in avoiding diagnostic errors if physicians "communicate to patients more about what diagnoses they are considering rather than just telling patients what tests to get or what medications to take."

Reuters news service (Harding 2009) used the lead-in sentence "Doctor-patient communication can be fraught with misunderstanding . . ." in reporting the results of a study that assessed agreement between patients and their physicians about the seriousness of the patients' osteoarthritis of the knee and physician recommendations regarding the need for surgery. The most compelling finding of the study was that in 18 percent of the physician-patient encounters there was disagreement between patients and physicians regarding whether the physician had recommended knee replacement surgery. One important implication of this finding, according to a physician commentator, is that physicians should not assume that patients have understood their recommendations. Instead, they should ask patients for their understanding of what has been recommended.

An article in the *New York Times* (Tarkan 2008) described findings of a study in the *Annals of Emergency Medicine* that addressed communication with patients in emergency departments. Patient understanding was measured with respect to their diagnosis, treatment, instructions for care once discharged, and indications suggesting they should return to the hospital. A striking finding was that "78 percent of patients did not understand at least one area and about half did not understand two or more areas. The greatest confusion surrounded home care—instructions about things like medications, rest, wound care and when to have a follow-up visit with the doctor." While emergency rooms can be difficult environments in which to communicate effectively with patients, similar findings from studies based in other settings were described in a 2004 *New York Times* article (Levine 2004): "Research shows that only 15 percent of patients fully understand what their doctors tell them, and that 50 percent leave the doctors' offices uncertain of what they are supposed to do to take care of themselves."

In 2007, the *New York Times* (Murphy 2007) published a discussion of the pros and cons of establishing a new medical specialty in the area of "lifestyle medicine." Advocates suggested that physicians too often overlook opportunities to include lifestyle changes in the treatment plans for their patients, even when such changes clearly have scientific support. It was observed that "doctors may vaguely recommend that patients lose weight or get more sleep." They may resist entering into lifestyle conversations, because they do not have healthy lifestyles themselves, are not knowledgeable in this area, or fear that offering lifestyle advice would extend the length of the patient visit.

Media reports such as these suggest that issues surrounding physician communication are not of interest solely to the health care community— they have great salience for the general public as well. The accounts also underscore the many different dimensions to physician communication and the ways in which breakdowns in communication between physicians and patients can manifest themselves. In the remainder of this chapter, we discuss these different dimensions in the context of the framework that we used to organize the book.

Physician Communication in Context

Researchers who study physician communication, as well as organizations and individuals that seek to improve it, are guided by mental models, sometimes stated, but often implicit. These models influence the organization of literature reviews, the formulation of research questions, and the structure and targeting of educational efforts. For instance, Kreps, O'Hair, et al. (1994) describe a transformation model of communication and health outcomes, while Ong, de Haes, et al. (1995) suggest a three-part model that relates "background variables" to content of physician communication and subsequently to patient outcomes. Arora (2003) discusses logical connections between physician communication and patient outcomes. Beck, Daughtridge, et al. (2002) present a schematic that links physician communication behaviors to patient outcomes, using it to structure their literature review of observational studies of physician-patient interactions. Weiner, Barnet, et al. (2005), in their discussion of "whole person" primary care, include a graphical "conceptual framework for communication with and without the obstacles to whole person, integrated care," which includes environmental and physician characteristics. Feldman-Stewart, Brundage, et al. (2005) develop a relatively complete conceptual framework—"a tool for organizing and summarizing relevant research" (801)—which they use to discuss findings related to physician communication in cancer treatment. Our logic model (displayed in fig. 1.1) draws from all of these past efforts to various degrees (especially Ong, de Haes, et al. 1995), as well as from logic models used in other health services research studies (e.g., Scanlon, Christianson, et al. 2008).

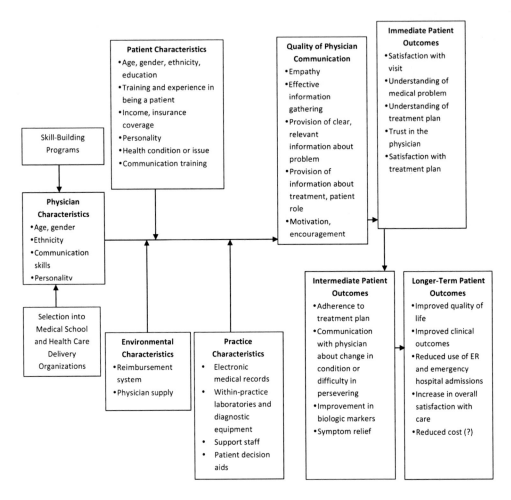

Fig. 1.1. The role of physician communication: a logic model

Physician Characteristics and Physician Communication

The literature on physician communication emphasizes the relationship between physician characteristics and physician communication (see table 1.1). Physicians come to their profession with different personalities, as well as different experiences during their lives and their medical school training. Any of these can influence the quality of their communication with patients. For instance, physicians who have "outgoing" or "warm" personalities—who are "people persons"—may naturally show empathy for their patients and be skillful in identifying patient concerns. They may instinctively assume the appropriate posture or ask questions in an appropriate way to elicit information from the patient. Physicians who are the products of a specific medical school culture may place either more or less importance on communication with patients in comparison to physicians who trained at a different medical school. Physicians who possess a personality type that is excessively task oriented may be more concerned with "getting through the visit" than with taking the time to demonstrate empathy toward patients or to gather information about the patient's social environment that could affect treatment planning.

Irrespective of these characteristics, it is assumed that physicians can be taught skills that can make them more effective in communicating with patients. These skills include how to elicit information from patients using verbal and nonverbal cues, how to detect the "covert" reasons for a visit, how to secure patient commitment to treatment plans, and how to demonstrate empathy toward patients. Physicians bring their "skill sets" to each physician-patient encounter. In figure 1.1, physician communication skills are included as physician characteristics. Over time, the average quality of physician communication with patients can be improved by placing more emphasis on evaluating innate personality characteristics as part of the medical school admissions process. However, improving the communication between a specific physician and her or his patients requires improving the communication skills of the physician through targeted educational and other interventions. As we discuss in subsequent chapters, there is mixed evidence concerning the effectiveness of these initiatives when directed at medical school students, residents, or practicing physicians.

Mediating Factors

In our logic model, we hypothesize that the impact physician characteristics have on how physicians communicate with their patients and, as a re-

TABLE 1.1.   Assumptions about the Problem

Physician communication is affected by the personal characteristics of physicians, but the impact of physician characteristics is mediated by other factors, such as patient characteristics, practice characteristics, and environmental characteristics. It is the combination of these factors that affects the quality of physician communication in the physician/patient encounter. This suggests that the quality of communication will vary across patients and practice environments, for any single physician, as well as across physicians.

- Physician characteristics directly affect the quality of physician communication.
- Practice, environmental, and patient characteristics mediate the impact of physician characteristics on physician communication in the physician-patient encounter.

sult, on the quality of physician communication is mediated or influenced by several factors. We categorize those factors as patient characteristics, practice characteristics, and environmental characteristics (see fig. 1.1).

Patient Characteristics.   Patient characteristics may influence the way in which physicians approach the physician-patient encounter and how comfortable the physician is during the encounter. For example, physicians may experience considerable anxiety in meetings with patients who have terminal illnesses requiring that physicians convey the "bad news" that further treatment is not recommended. This anxiety can inhibit communication with patients. The gender of the patient also can be important, especially regarding issues relating to sexual health. Physicians may feel more inhibited discussing sexual health with patients of the opposite gender and may therefore fail to communicate important information to them. Also, physicians may stereotype patients from specific socioeconomic or ethnic groups or by age and physical appearance, making inappropriate assumptions about their ability to understand information about their conditions or treatment plans. This could lead to the incomplete provision of information by physicians or to the inappropriate simplification of treatment plans. While patient characteristics may contribute to or "trigger" physician communication that is deficient, the implication is not that this is the "fault" of the patient. Indeed, not all physicians will respond to patient characteristics in the same way. We have chosen to create a separate category for "patient characteristics" as mediating factors in our conceptual framework to underscore the potential importance of those characteristics for the quality of physician communication in the physician-patient encounter.

Recently, there has been considerable interest in initiatives directed at improving the skills of patients in communicating with their physicians. These initiatives mirror programs designed to improve physician communication skills, with the same goal—improving the quality of physician-patient communication. In these programs, patients are trained to be more systematic and assertive when communicating with physicians during an office visit. Physicians may communicate differently with patients who are more organized and/or assertive in questioning their physicians.

Practice Characteristics. The physical surroundings of the practice also can affect communication. In practice environments that are crowded and noisy, it may be difficult for physicians to focus on communication with their patients, and it may be equally difficult for distracted patients to understand what their physicians are saying. Practice characteristics also can encompass the tools of the physician's practice that may hinder or support effective communication with patients. These tools could include the availability of patient "decision aids" that support collaborative decision making, electronic health records (EHRs) with accessible and up-to-date clinical histories, and in-office laboratories and imaging equipment. With respect to EHRs, advocates have argued that they will "free up" physician time that then can be spent in providing a better explanation of treatment alternatives or developing a more effective treatment plan. However, others have expressed concern that physicians will focus too much on the EHR during the patient visit and that this will detract from their ability to establish empathy with their patients or will reduce the time available to listen carefully to patients.

Environmental Characteristics.   It is often argued that in the broad environment in which medical care is delivered, the financial realities of a typical physician's practice can be a barrier to effective physician communication. When primary care physicians are reimbursed on a fee-for-service basis and when reimbursement rates are relatively low in comparison to practice costs, physicians may feel pressure to see more patients in their practice day, reducing visit length to do so. This could have a detrimental impact on the quality of communication with patients along multiple dimensions, such as the collection of information about the patient's problem and the development of a mutually acceptable treatment plan. Similarly, when specialists are reimbursed more for carrying out procedures than for collecting the information from patients that is needed to make an adequate diagnosis, physician-patient communication may suffer. These problems can be compounded, especially in the treatment of patients with multiple conditions, by pressures on physicians to follow an increasing number of evidence-based treatment guidelines (an environmental characteristic), which can create significant time management problems for physician practices (Ostbye, Yarnall, et al. 2005). Feeling increased time pressures, physicians may believe that following recommended guidelines regarding effective communication with patients is not feasible. Recently, concern also has been expressed that new physician pay-for-performance incentives and performance reporting initiatives, although intended to improve quality of care, could focus physicians' attention on completing specific tasks for which they receive financial rewards, rather than treating the "whole patient." By rewarding physicians for "checking the box" to indicate that a specific care process was carried out during a visit, they could reduce the time spent in the kind of empathetic questioning that could lead to a broader, more complete understanding of patient problems and concerns.

These mediating factors, individually or in combination, are assumed to influence the relationship between physician characteristics and the quality of physician communication in the physician-patient encounter. To varying degrees, they are amenable to change, but accomplishing change in each case likely requires initiatives structured in different ways with very different resource requirements. For instance, changing payment policies is a political as well as a technical challenge. Improving communication through installation of EHRs requires substantial funds and training, and government subsidies may be needed to accelerate the adoption process.

For any given physician at any point in time (i.e., given the personal qualities and communication skill set possessed by the physician), the logic model suggests that the quality of physician communication can vary with the presence, absence, or intensity of the mediating factors. In chapter 4 of this book, we discuss the empirical evidence regarding how specific mediating factors in all three areas affect physician communication. However, discussions of variation in physician communication behaviors and of possible interventions to improve physician communication typically focus exclusively on the role of physician characteristics and give relatively little attention to mediating factors related to practice setting or patient characteristics. By doing so, they risk overlooking potentially important variation in physician communication "across practices"; that is, physicians with identical characteristics might perform differently in their communication with patients depending on practice characteristics and the characteristics of the patients in their practices. Consequently, observed differences across practicing physicians in the quality of physician-patient communication may not entirely reflect differences in physician personalities or skills. Focusing on physician characteristics as determinants of poor physician-patient communication risks overlooking potentially fruitful interventions to improve communication that could be directed at altering mediating factors.

Aspects of Physician Communication

How is the quality of physician communication best understood? The Kalamazoo Consensus Statement provides a reasonable starting point for addressing this question. The relative quality of physician communication can be described, if not measured, by the degree to which the different "essential elements of communication in the medical encounter" are present or absent and by how well they are carried out (see table 1.2). As noted already, these elements include eliciting the patient's concerns; gathering information using various different approaches, including appropriate verbal and nonverbal cues; developing a treatment approach in consultation with the patients; discussing patient beliefs and values that could affect the diagnosis or the feasibility of the treatment plan; and encouraging feedback from the patient regarding the patient's understanding of the diagnosis, the treatment plan, and the patient's responsibilities going forward.

In addition to the approach proposed in the Kalamazoo Consensus Statement, frameworks proposed by other researchers for discussing the nature of physician communication also are widely used. One such framework was developed by researchers to categorize observed physician communication behaviors. As summarized by Ong, Visser, et al. (2000), "these systems identify instrumental behaviours (cure-oriented) on the one hand and socio-emotional (care-oriented) on the other. The first type belongs to the cognitive domain and includes behaviours such as giving information and asking questions. The second type belongs to the emotional domain and involves behaviours such as showing empathy or concern and making personal remarks" (146).

This conceptual discussion clearly raises issues concerning measurement of the quality of physician communication. In particular, if the quality of physician communication cannot be assessed accurately and reliably, it is not possible to determine the relative influence of deviations in any of the elements of communication (see table 1.2) on quality of care and patient health outcomes. Designing sensible, cost-effective programs to improve physician communication depends on understanding these relationships. Measuring the impact of interventions to improve physician communication requires measures that are relatively sensitive to changes in physician, patient, practice, and environmental characteristics.

Researchers have taken two different approaches to measuring the quality of physician communication (Arora 2003). The most common approach is to ask patients for their perceptions. These data are relatively easy to collect, and using the patient as the "reporter" of the quality of physician communication has considerable intuitive appeal (Ong, de Haes, et al.

TABLE 1.2.   Assumptions about Important Aspects of Physician Communication

Physician communication is multifaceted, and the importance of different aspects of physician communication can vary with patient needs.
- Different elements of physician communication are important, including demonstration of empathy, education about illness, education about treatment, and creation of expectations about patient roles in treatment.
- Elements of physician communication vary in importance depending on patient needs: palliative care, chronic illness management, lifestyle modification, decision making regarding treatment options.

1995). Because one presumably is interested in how physician communication ultimately affects patient health, patient assessments of the quality of that communication would seem worthwhile. Sometimes, instead of or in addition to reporting their perceptions, patients are asked to report the presence or absence of particular physician behaviors thought to be indicators of quality in physician communication. However, the useful knowledge that can be gained from this approach may be limited. For instance, it may be unreasonable to expect patients to assess whether relatively nuanced aspects of a physician's demeanor elicited responses from them that, in turn, contributed to more accurate diagnoses or better treatment plans. Also, the accuracy of the patient as "reporter" of objective behaviors could be influenced by a variety of considerations, including the patient's medical condition. (This is true as well for patient perceptions of the quality of the communication.) These issues do not rule out the use of patient perceptions or patient reports as a basis for constructing measures of the quality of physician communication, but they do suggest caution in the interpretation of findings based solely on these measures.

The second approach to measuring quality of physician communication involves observation by researchers using unobtrusive techniques. This fly-on-the-wall approach has several strengths. Most important, by coding video or audio records, researchers can construct measures of all aspects of physician communication, except patient perceptions. A drawback of this approach, from a research standpoint, is that it can be expensive. It also requires the consent of the physician and patient, who then know that they are being observed. Moreover, there is research suggesting that when data are collected from patients and by observers as part of the same study, patient perceptions are better predictors of near-term patient outcomes, such as satisfaction with the visit (Arora 2003). In general, at this juncture, a conservative conclusion is that there are ongoing issues relating to the measurement of the quality of physician communication that need to be addressed and that this complicates attempts to determine if specific efforts to improve physician communication are successful.

Effects of the Quality of Physician Communication on Patients and Patient Health

The remainder of the logic model in figure 1.1 depicts the cascade of effects that the quality of physician communication is presumed to have on patients (see table 1.3). These include immediate, intermediate, and longer-term patient outcomes.

Immediate Patient Outcomes. Immediately after the physician-patient encounter, the patient is likely to have formed an opinion regarding the encounter, and that opinion is likely to be influenced by the quality of physician communication. Also, the patient's immediate recall of important aspects of the encounter, such as the diagnosis and the details of the treatment plan, is assumed to be affected by physician communication.

Intermediate Patient Outcomes. Subsequent to the physician-patient encounter, the patient typically has several responsibilities relating to execution of the care plan. Here it is assumed that the willingness and ability of the patient to carry out the care plan will be influenced by physician communication. For example, the more effectively the physician communicates the importance of the care plan and gains patient commitment to it, the more likely it is that the patient will adhere to the plan. When the physician has established a trusting relationship with the patient by demonstrating empathy, integrity, and understanding, the patient will be more likely to contact the physician with concerns or with questions relating to the care plan and its execution. Therefore, better physician communication is assumed to lead to greater satisfaction with the care plan, better adherence, more timely revisions to the plan, and possibly improvement in biologic markers of disease.

Longer-Term Patient Outcomes. Adherence to the care plan and timely revision of it are assumed to lead to improved long-term patient quality of life and health, less frequent use of inappropriate care settings (e.g., less use of the emergency department and fewer emergency hospital admissions), greater satisfaction with overall medical treatment, and (possibly)

TABLE 1.3. Assumptions about the Impact of Physician Communication on Patients and Patient Health

Physician communication can affect patient knowledge and attitudes, care management behaviors, and health outcomes.

- Physician communication can have immediate effects on patients that relate to satisfaction with the visit, comprehension of the diagnosis and treatment, and trust in the physician.
- Satisfaction with the physician visit, trust in the physician, and an understanding of the diagnosis and treatment plan will enhance adherence to the plan, improve the likelihood that patients will contact physicians when problems with the plan or unexpected outcomes occur, and possibly improve biologic markers of disease.
- Adherence to the treatment plans, supported by timely physician consultations, will improve patient outcomes related to quality of life and medical condition, reduce unnecessary or inappropriate utilization of services, and possibly reduce costs.

lower patient costs. Clearly, these longer-term outcomes are affected by many things in addition to physician communication, including patient characteristics. The depiction of the logic model in figure 1.1 omits the direct effect of these other factors on longer-term patient outcomes in order to focus attention on the role of physician communication.

Improving the Quality of Physician Communication

On the left part of the logic model in figure 1.1 are factors relating to physician characteristics, patient characteristics, environmental characteristics, and practice characteristics that offer the possibility for intervening to improve physician communication. The first consists of interventions that are designed to change the ways in which physicians communicate with patients. (We discuss the empirical evidence regarding the effectiveness of these types of intervention in chapter 5.) Their goals might include improving physician understanding of the importance of physician communication to quality of care and, ultimately, patient outcomes; improving the abilities of physicians to demonstrate empathy toward patients and gain patient trust; improving the skills needed by physicians to collect information needed to make accurate diagnoses; improving physician abilities to develop care plans collaboratively with patients; and improving physician abilities to communicate diagnosis and treatment options and elicit patient commitment to carrying out the care plan.

Other interventions could be directed at changing the influence of mediating factors as they relate to the relationship between physician characteristics and the quality of communication. For instance, programs that prepare patients for their physician visits by, for example, training them to ask the appropriate questions of their physicians and to confirm that their understanding of the diagnosis and treatment plan is correct before closing the encounter are available and in use in a variety of treatment settings (Boodman 2007). Although they are aimed at making patients better consumers of physician services, better informed, more assertive consumers could alter the communication patterns of physicians and therefore the nature and quality of physician communication. We summarize the empirical evidence of the impact of these types of intervention on physician communication when discussing patient characteristics in chapter 4.

Another set of possible interventions to improve physician communication could be carried out at the system level. Payment reform has been suggested as a key factor in creating a more supportive environment for communication. At the practice level, we previously noted that investment in EHRs has been touted as a way to enhance the availability of comprehensive and timely patient information at the physician's desk, possibly leading physicians to ask better questions of patients and collect patient information in a more systematic manner. Reorganizing office space and staff responsibilities could relieve time pressure on physicians and thereby result in improved physician communication. We discuss the limited evidence on the impact of practice-level interventions in chapter 4.

Organization of the Remaining Chapters

Chapters 2–5 summarize the empirical evidence regarding the different components of the physician communication logic model as displayed in figure 1.1. In chapter 2, we review the evidence that poor physician communication occurs during the physician-patient encounter. If research does not conclusively demonstrate the presence of poor-quality physician communication, the case for devoting resources to improving communication certainly would be in question. In chapter 3, we summarize the evidence regarding whether improvement in physician communication leads to improved patient outcomes. If this evidence is not convincing (even in the presence of evidence suggesting that physician communication is of poor quality), the case for investing in programs to improve physician communication could be questioned. As seems more likely, if there is limited evidence linking some elements of physician communication to patient outcomes but stronger evidence linking others, the research results could play a useful role in making decisions about the design of programs to improve physician communication. In chapter 4, we summarize research that identifies and assesses the importance of factors that are related to the quality of physician communication, including physician characteristics and mediating factors (depicted on the left side

TABLE 1.4.   Assumptions about Efforts to Improve Physician Communication

It is possible to identify aspects of physician communication that can be improved through programmatic efforts and to implement these efforts successfully in existing training programs or practice environments.

- Areas of physician communication that warrant improvement can be identified through observation or patient evaluations.
- Effective programs to improve physician communication can be designed that address areas of deficiency.
- Physician communication improvement programs can be implemented effectively as part of medical curriculums or ongoing practice, as appropriate.
- Physician communication improvement programs can be modified in a timely manner in response to changes in environmental and practice characteristics.

of fig. 1.1). The research findings in this chapter are potentially important for structuring and targeting initiatives to improve physician communication. In chapter 5, we review the results of evaluations of programs that have attempted to improve physician communication. We also discuss the match between the objectives of these programs, the research findings regarding the most important factors related to poor communication (chapter 4), and findings regarding the relationship between physician communication and patient outcomes (chapter 3). In chapter 6, we describe the characteristics of several ongoing programs to improve physician communication. We chose the particular programs included in this chapter to illustrate initiatives being carried out in different settings by different sponsors and especially to highlight the motivations of sponsors in their support of these programs. In the last chapter of the book, we discuss the implications of our findings for public policies aimed at improving health care quality, as well as the challenges and opportunities posed by anticipated changes in the health care delivery system. The appendix supports the discussion in the concluding chapter by summarizing evidence relating to other initiatives designed to change physician behavior with the goal of improving the quality of patient care and patient outcomes. In the appendix, we discuss the strength of evidence regarding interventions to improve physician communication in comparison to the evidence supporting the effectiveness of these other initiatives.

2 | What Is the Evidence That Physician Communication Is Deficient?

Anecdotal evidence, supported by the results of consumer surveys (Blendon, Buhr, et al. 2003), suggests that poor physician communication is pervasive in America and in other countries as well. The need for research to document its existence likely would seem questionable or even mildly amusing to most patients and health care providers. Conventional wisdom also seems to support the notion that poor physician communication can result in patients being dissatisfied with their physician consultations, inadequate care, missed opportunities to improve patient health, and, possibly, poorer health. However, even if true, these general assumptions by themselves provide little guidance in how to improve patient communication.

In this chapter, we review and summarize the published literature on the existence of poor physician communication. (In chapter 3, we address the impacts of poor physician communication on patients.) We here draw conclusions regarding where the research is strongest relating to the existence of physician communication shortcomings; that is, we ask for which of the "essential elements" of physician communication that were described in chapter 1 has poor physician performance been established the most convincingly? This information is critical to the targeting of efforts to improve physician communication. For instance, if there is not a strong research basis for concluding that physicians perform poorly in collecting the information they need to form accurate diagnoses, the case for new efforts to improve physician interviewing skills must rest largely on intuition, rather than evidence. In contrast, if there is strong evidence that physicians are poor at exhibiting empathy toward their patients, implementing programs to train physicians in how to do this more effectively might be warranted.

In this chapter, we summarize research findings related to the aforementioned issues. First, we provide an overview of the existing literature, organized by areas of potential communication deficiencies addressed in individual studies and by practice type or setting in which data collection occurred. Then, we summarize the research evidence regarding the existence and nature of poor physician communication. In summarizing the evidence, we present article findings in the tables at the end of the chapter and discuss selected individual studies in the text to illustrate the nature of the overall findings. In the concluding section of the chapter, we interpret our findings with respect to their implications for improving physician communication.

Identifying Relevant Literature

We searched the literature to identify peer-reviewed papers published in English that were relevant to the research questions in this chapter. We searched Medline, JSTOR, and the databases of the Cochrane Library and the Agency for Healthcare Policy and Research (AHRQ) for review articles and individual studies (not contained in review articles) published from 2000 to 2008. While review articles sometimes were limited to particular aspects of physician communication, the individual articles contained summaries of past work as well. We combined these sources of information to provide a historical perspective on physician communication, as well as more detailed information regarding selected, recently published studies.

We used a combination of such keywords as "physician-patient relations," "communication," "quality of health care," "palliative care," "empathy," "patient participation," "treatment outcome," "patient-centered care," and "outcome assessment (health care)" to identify studies for inclusion in this chapter and in chapter 3. We constructed a database containing the articles identified in the search process. Our search process was designed with broad inclusion criteria. We included studies employing a variety of methodologies, focusing on many different medical conditions, and set in different countries. The initial search yielded over 1,100 references. After eliminating articles not directly related to physician communication, we reviewed over 300 articles or abstracts. In many cases, evidence relating to poor physician communication was found in the context of broader studies of communication in health care. We did not include studies related to poor patient communication or patient health literacy unless they had a substantial component directed at physician communication issues.

What Is the Evidence Regarding the Existence of Poor Physician Communication?

Our search process generated 8 review articles and 58 individual studies (not included in the reviews) that addressed evidence that poor physician communication exists. As indicated in table 2.1, 18 of the 58 individual studies were carried out in clinical settings related to specialty outpatient care, with 8 of these studies focusing on cancer treatment. Another 5 studies combined primary care and specialty care settings. That there is an extensive literature addressing communication issues in physician encounters with cancer patients is understandable. Conveying cancer diagnoses can be both emotionally and technically difficult for physicians, and cancer patients may be especially sensitive to the empathy shown by physicians and to physician knowledge of their personal situations. Both of these considerations focus attention on the quality of physician communication.

Six of the individual studies addressed physician communication in delivering palliative care, 12 in primary care. Relatively few studies ($n = 6$) were conducted in inpatient settings, and two of these related to communication around hospital discharge issues. Eleven studies were not carried out in clinical settings, relying instead on surveys of individuals drawn from the general population (6); the subpopulation of individuals with specific illnesses (3); or individuals with a particular type of insurance coverage, in this case Medicare (2).

Of the 8 review articles, 5 focused exclusively on physician-patient interactions in oncology settings. Two other reviews addressed studies of physician communication relating to end-of-life care (see table 2.2).

In assessing the practice settings for the literature on physician communication problems, two conclusions seem warranted. First, a substantial portion of this literature relates to physician communication with cancer or palliative care patients, and relatively few studies are set in primary care practices. Second, studies that document problems with primary care physician communication rely mostly on survey data collected from the general population or from people with specific medical problems. The relative lack of attention to documenting physician communication problems in primary care settings is unfortunate. A substantial proportion of all physician-patient interactions presumably occurs during primary care visits, and many of the external pressures on physician communication with patients are felt most severely by primary care physicians. If the concepts of patient-centered care and the medical home are widely adopted (as discussed in chapter 7), it seems likely that primary care physicians will assume even greater importance as first-line communicators with patients.

In table 2.3, we display the research studies and reviews organized by type of communication problem or problems addressed. We also link each perceived problem to one or more of the elements of communication specified in the Kalamazoo Consensus Statement. This linkage is unavoidably arbitrary in some instances, as the match is not always exact and because there are cases in which the perceived problem can be related to more than one element. The type of data used to identify the communication problem is indicated in table 2.3 as well.

A relatively large number of studies attempted to measure or otherwise assess communication problems using concepts related to patient understanding; in these studies, the data needed to construct measures were typically collected through patient surveys or interviews. Patient self-reported problems related to "understanding" arguably could be a consequence of physician failure to check for patient understanding of diagnoses, treatment options, treatment plans, or expected patient roles. In a closely related topic, 10 individual studies or reviews assessed patient desire for greater participation in treatment decisions, again using measures constructed from patient responses. There were 11 studies or reviews that documented missed opportunities by physicians to gather information about patient concerns and problems related to health and quality of life. These studies primarily relied on analysis of videotapes or audiotapes.

In summary, table 2.3 suggests that existing research studies address, relatively comprehensively, different aspects of physician communication. However, there are few studies of physician communication related to the personal beliefs, values, and situations of patients. Other elements of physician communication identified in the Kalamazoo Consensus Statement are each addressed to some degree in three or more studies or reviews.

Evidence from Reviews. In table 2.4, we summarize the evidence from review studies that address poor physician communication. This is a reasonable starting point, although, as already noted, most of the reviews focus on cancer patients. In a recent review of this type, Back (2006) describes the literature relating to physician interactions with patients under stressful circumstances. Concluding that physicians lack skills in this area, Back suggests guidelines to assist physicians in acknowledging and responding to patient emotions. Baile and Aaron (2005), in a second review of studies involving cancer patients, report that physicians miss opportunities to respond to patients with empathy, ignore the wishes of patients to discuss health-related quality-of-life issues, and avoid talking about such important topics as patient prognosis. In their 2005 review of 50 studies in the oncology area, Hagerty, Butow, et al. (2005) also found that prognosis often was not discussed with patients or that the discussion lacked sensitivity. Other problems included patients not understanding their disease, the intent of treatment, or the language used by the oncologist. Hack, Degner, et al. (2005), reviewing oncology studies published from 1992 to 2004, found evidence that physicians failed to give enough attention to patient psychosocial and health-related quality-of-life concerns. Physicians also lacked skills needed to convey disease information. As a result, patients reported a variety of unmet communication needs. Thorne, Bultz, et al. (2005), in another review of oncology studies, concluded that physicians lacked skills in breaking bad news. Taken together, these review articles relating to physician communication with cancer patients cite multiple problems, ranging from lack of empathy; to poor collection of information from patients; to poor communication of information about patient diseases, prognoses, and treatment plans. The large number of studies that have addressed physician communication in this setting lends weight to the findings.

In other clinical areas, Curtis, Engleberg, et al. (2005) reviewed communication by physicians in interactions with COPD patients. They concluded that physicians generally did not know patient wishes with respect to end-of-life care, but it is not clear if this was a failure of patient communication, physician communication, or both. Siegler and Levin (2000) also summarized results of studies of physician communication concerning end-of-life care. Three studies documented poor communication by physicians about do-not-resuscitate orders and advance directives.

Evidence from Individual Studies. Table 2.5 contains brief synopses of 59 individual studies of physician communication, arranged in chronological order. These studies, in total, largely confirm findings in the review articles. Individual studies based on patient surveys document that patients want their physicians to provide more information of almost every type—underprovision of information or poor provision of information were frequently mentioned communication problems. As an example, a study by Nelson, Mercado, et al. (2007) found that 78 percent of patients with chronic illness received no information on 9 of 18 items judged to be critical to meeting their needs. Disagreements between patients and physicians about the information the physician conveyed were reported in some studies as well (e.g., Oates, Sloane, et al. 2007).

Other studies addressed the "listening" skills of physicians. Marvel, Epstein, et al. (1999) analyzed audiotapes of physicians in family practice, finding that the average length of time that physicians gave patients to itemize their concerns was 23 seconds. Over the entire visit, patients were given 26 seconds to discuss their problems.

Not all of the individual studies reported inadequate physician communication. For example, Slutsman, Emanuel, et al. (2002) found that a high percentage of patients judged by their physicians to be terminally ill were satisfied with several aspects of physician communication. A small number of other studies reported results that were equivocal, rather than clearly negative, with respect to physician communication performance. It is possible that "publication bias" could explain the few studies with positive results; that is, studies reporting problems with physician communication may be more likely to be submitted to academic journals and subsequently chosen for publication. However, there is no way to explore the validity of this supposition with the information available.

Conclusions

The literature reviewed in this chapter and summarized in tables 2.4 and 2.5 is difficult to summarize succinctly. A relatively large number of studies documents the existence of physician communication problems, and the study findings are striking at times. Physician communication is measured in a variety of ways (depending on the specific objectives of study authors) that provide further support for the conclusion that poor physician communication is commonplace. However, in some ways, the evidence is not as convincing as one would expect, given the attention that this issue has received in the media and by academic researchers. In particular, the preponderance of evidence relates to communication with cancer patients. More information is needed regarding the quality of physician communication in different treatment settings and with different types of patients, in order to have a clearer picture of how pervasive physician communication problems are and how they vary across treatment settings and patient characteristics. In the next chapter, we will address whether and how physician communication affects health.

TABLE 2.1.   Settings for Individual Studies

Setting	Number of Studies	Reference
Clinical Outpatient		
Primary care	12	Kravitz, Callahan, et al. 1996; Marvel, Epstein, et al. 1999; Barry, Bradley, et al. 2000; Britten, Stevenson, et al. 2000; Elkington, White, et al. 2001; Rhoades, McFarland, et al. 2001; Deveugele, Derese, et al. 2002; Jenkins, Britten, et al. 2003; Jerant, von Friederichs-Fitzwater, et al. 2005; Robinson and Heritage 2006; Abdulhadi, Al Shafaee, et al. 2007; Ling, Trauth, et al. 2008
Specialty (surgery, pulmonary, hepatology, neurosurgery, HIV, HTN)	10	Adams, Smith, et al. 2001; McManus and Wheatley 2003; Zickmund, Hillis, et al. 2004; King, Yonas, et al. 2005; Barfod, Hecht, et al. 2006; Bokhour, Berlowitz, et al. 2006; McLafferty, Williams, et al. 2006; Ruiz-Moral, Perez Rodriguez, et al. 2006; Harding, Selman, et al. 2008; Morse, Edwardsen, et al. 2008
Combined primary care and specialty	5	Koning, Maille, et al. 1995; Levinson, Gorawara-Bhat, et al. 2000; Bell, Kravitz, et al. 2002; Tarn, Heritage, et al. 2006; Nelson and Hamilton 2007
Oncology or oncology combined with other specialties (thoracic, radiation)	8	Keating, Weeks, et al. 2003; Koedoot, Oort, et al. 2004; Goncalves, Marques, et al. 2005; Travado, Grassi, et al. 2005; Davidson, Vogel, et al. 2007; Oates, Sloane, et al. 2007; Pollak, Arnold, et al. 2007; Dimoska, Butow, et al. 2008
Palliative or end-of-life care	6	Detmar, Muller, et al. 2001; Farber, Urban, et al. 2004; Knauft, Nielsen, et al. 2005; Morita, Akechi, et al. 2005; Audrey, Abel, et al. 2008; Levin, Li, et al. 2008
Hospital discharge	2	Calkins, Davis, et al. 1997; Makaryus and Friedman 2005
Clinical Inpatient		
ICU	4	Azoulay, Chevret, et al. 2000; Teno, Fisher, et al. 2000; Nelson, Angus, et al. 2006; Nelson, Mercado, et al. 2007
Community (adult ambulatory service)		
Cross section	6	Murphy, Chang, et al. 2001; Davis, Schoenbaum, et al. 2002; Slutsman, Emanuel, et al. 2002; Safran, Karp, et al. 2006; AHRQ 2008; Blendon, Buhr, et al. 2008
Disease-specific (cancer, ALS)	3	Pho, Geller, et al. 2000; McCluskey, Casarett, et al. 2004; Poon, Haas, et al. 2004
Medicare beneficiaries	2	Montgomery, Irish, et al. 2004; Wilson, Schoen, et al. 2007

TABLE 2.2.   Settings for Review Articles

		Reference
Clinical Outpatient		
Oncology	5	Baile and Aaron 2005; Hack, Degner, et al. 2005; Hagerty, Butow, et al. 2005; Thorne, Bultz, et al. 2005; Back 2006
Palliative or end-of-life care	1	Curtis, Engelberg, et al. 2005
Clinical Outpatient		
Obstetrics, pediatrics, trauma, oncology	1	Fallowfield and Jenkins 2004
Palliative or end-of-life care	1	Siegler and Levin 2000

TABLE 2.3.   Aspects of Poor Physician Communication

Evidence of ineffective or poor communcation	Reference	Type of data used to measure physician communication
Information Gathering		
Missed opportunity of physician to elicit patient concerns and health-related quality of life (HRQL) problems	Back 2006	Review of oncology studies
	Baile and Aaron 2005	Review of oncology studies
	Hack, Degner, et al. 2005	Review of oncology communication research
	Marvel, Epstein, et al. 1999	Patient-completed measures
	Ruiz-Moral, Perez Rodriguez, et al. 2006	Consultation videotapes/patient-completed measures
KCS: — Information-gathering techniques	Nelson, Mercado, et al. 2007	Patient-completed measures
— Elicit patient concerns, establish rapport	Nelson and Hamilton 2007	Transcribed audiotapes of consultation
— Identify person's personal situation	Kravitz, Callahan, et al. 1996	Patient-completed measures
	Koedoot, Oort, et al. 2004	Transcribed audiotapes of consultation
	McCluskey, Casarett, et al. 2004	Patient-completed measures
	Travado, Grassi, et al. 2005	Physician-completed measures
Missed opportunity of physician to elicit patient questions and concerns	Back 2006	Review of oncology studies
	Curtis, Engelberg, et al. 2005	Review of oncology studies
	Abdulhadi, Al Shafaee, et al. 2007	Outpatient focus groups
	McLafferty, Williams, et al. 2006	Quality-of-care survey, patient rating of MD behavior
KCS: — Let patient complete opening statement	Barry, Bradley, et al. 2000	Patient interview
	Deveugele, Derese, et al. 2002	Transcribed videotapes of consultation
— Elicit patient concerns, establish rapport	Blendon, Buhr, et al. 2008	Patient-completed measures
	Ling, Trauth, et al. 2008	Transcribed audiotapes of consultation
— Check for patient understanding	Robinson and Heritage 2006	Consultation videotapes/patient-completed measures
— Explore patient willingness and ability to follow care plan	Collins, Clark, et al. 2002	Focus groups
— Other concerns, follow-up activities		
Empathy		
Missed opportunity of physician to demonstrate an understanding of patients' emotions during consultation	Back 2006	Review of oncology studies
	Levinson, Gorawara-Bhat, et al. 2000	Transcribed audiotape of consultation
	Ruiz-Moral, Perez Rodriguez, et al. 2006	Consultation videotapes/patient-completed measures
	Morse, Edwardsen, et al. 2008	Transcribed audiotapes of consultation

TABLE 2.3—*Continued*

Evidence of ineffective or poor communication	Reference	Type of data used to measure physician communication
KCS: — Elicit patient concerns, establish rapport — Identify person's personal situation, values, beliefs	McCluskey, Casarett, et al. 2004 Pollak, Arnold, et al. 2007 Jenkins, Britten, et al. 2003 Dimoska, Butow, et al. 2008 Collins, Clark, et al. 2002	Patient-completed measures Transcribed audiotapes of consultation Patient-completed measures Transcribed audiotapes of consultation Focus groups
Missed opportunity of physician to respond to patients' concerns or emotions during consultation KCS: — Elicit patient concerns, establish rapport — Identify person's personal situation, values, beliefs	Baile and Aaron 2005 Levinson, Gorawara-Bhat, et al. 2000 Morse, Edwardsen, et al. 2008 Travado, Grassi, et al. 2005 Deveugele, Derese, et al. 2002 Dimoska, Butow, et al. 2008 Collins, Clark, et al. 2002	Review of oncology studies Transcribed audiotapes of consultation Transcribed audiotapes of consultation Physician-completed measures Transcribed videotapes of consultation Transcribed audiotapes of consultation Focus groups
Doctor didn't listen KCS: — Let patient complete opening statement — Elicit patient concerns, establish rapport	Davis, Schoenbaum, et al. 2002 Safran, Karp, et al. 2006 Rhoades, McFarland, et al. 2001 Blendon, Buhr, et al. 2008 Collins, Clark, et al. 2002	Telephone interview Patient-completed measures Observed consultation interactions Patient-completed measures Focus groups

Participation in Decision Making

Expressed patient desire for greater participation in treatment decisions KCS: — Explore patient willingness and ability to follow through	Baile and Aaron 2005 Hack, Degner, et al. 2005 Koning, Maille, et al. 1995 Ruiz-Moral, Perez Rodriguez, et al. 2006 Adams, Smith, et al. 2001 Slutsman, Emanuel, et al. 2002 Goncalves, Marques, et al. 2005 McCluskey, Casarett, et al. 2004 Jenkins, Britten, et al. 2003 Harding, Selman, et al. 2008	Review of oncology studies Review of oncology communication research Patient-completed measures Consultation videotapes/patient-completed measures Patient-completed measures Patient-completed measures Patient-completed measures Patient-completed measures Patient-completed measures Transcribed audiotapes of consultation

TABLE 2.3—*Continued*

Evidence of ineffective or poor communciation	Reference	Type of data used to measure physician communication
Treatment Plan		
Unfulfilled information needs or misunder- standing by patients fol- lowing consultation: disease cause, disease severity, diagnosis, di- agnostic tests, medica- tion use, treatment de- cision, risks or side effects of treatment, prognosis, follow-up care	Baile and Aaron 2005	Review of oncology studies
	Hack, Degner, et al. 2005	Review of cancer communication research
	Hagerty, Butow, et al. 2005	Review of communicating progno- sis in cancer
	Thorne, Bultz, et al. 2005	Review of oncology studies
	Koning, Maille, et al. 1995	Patient-completed measures, un- filled needs
	Britten, Stevenson, et al. 2000	Transcribed audiotapes of consul- tation
	Azoulay, Chevret, et al. 2000	Interviews with ICU patient or pa- tient representative
KCS: — Check for patient understanding	Zickmund, Hillis, et al. 2004	Transcribed recorded semistruc- tured patient interview
	King, Yonas, et al. 2005	Patient interview and patient-com- pleted measures
	Makaryus and Friedman 2005	Patient-completed measures
	Jerant, von Friederichs-Fitzwater, et al. 2005	Patient focus groups
	Ruiz-Moral, Perez Rodriguez, et al. 2006	Consultation videotapes/patient- completed measures
	Teno, Fisher, et al. 2000	Patient interview
	Nelson, Mercado, et al. 2007	Patient-completed measures
	Nelson and Hamilton 2007	Transcribed audiotapes of consul- tation
	Oates, Sloane, et al. 2007	Patient-completed measures
	Abdulhadi, Al Shafaee, et al. 2007	Patient focus groups
	McLafferty, Williams, et al. 2006	Patient-completed measures
	Bell, Kravitz, et al. 2002	Patient-completed measures
	Davis, Schoenbaum, et al. 2002	Telephone interview
	Kravitz, Callahan, et al. 1996	Patient-completed measures
	Slutsman, Emanuel, et al. 2002	Patient-completed measures
	Nelson, Angus, et al. 2006	ICU director–completed measures
	Koedoot, Oort, et al. 2004	Transcribed audiotapes of consul- tation
	Safran, Karp, et al. 2006	Patient-completed measures
	Goncalves, Marques, et al. 2005	Patient-completed measures
	McCluskey, Casarett, et al. 2004	Patient-completed measures
	Pho, Geller, et al. 2000	Patient-completed measures
	Keating, Weeks, et al. 2003	Patient- and physician-completed measures
	Poon, Haas, et al. 2004	Patient-completed measures
	Calkins, Davis, et al. 1997	Patient-completed measures
	Barry, Bradley, et al. 2000	Patient interview

TABLE 2.3—*Continued*

Evidence of ineffective or poor communciation	Reference	Type of data used to measure physician communication
	McManus and Wheatley 2003	Physician-completed measures
	Deveugele, Derese, et al. 2002	Transcribed videotapes of consultation
	Harding, Selman, et al. 2008	Transcribed audiotapes of consultation
	Blendon, Buhr, et al. 2008	Patient-completed measures
	Ling, Trauth, et al. 2008	Transcribed audiotapes of consultation
	Elkington, White, et al. 2001	Physician-completed measures
	Collins, Clark, et al. 2002	Focus groups
Patients not knowing purpose or potential side effects of medication. KCS: — Check for patient understanding	Calkins, Davis, et al. 1997 Britten, Stevenson, et al. 2000 Makaryus and Friedman 2005	Patient-completed measures Transcribed audiotapes of consultation Patient-completed measures
Missed opportunity of physician to discuss medication purpose, use, adverse effects, or adherence to medication therapy KCS: — Check for patient understanding — Explore patient willingness and ability to follow care plan	Bokhour, Berlowitz, et al. 2006 Tarn, Heritage, et al. 2006 Davidson, Vogel, et al. 2007 Wilson, Schoen, et al. 2007 Barfod, Hecht, et al. 2006	Transcribed audiotapes Transcribed videotapes and patient-completed measures Transcribed audio- and videotapes Patient-completed measures Notes on observation of consultation and transcribed interviews
Failure of MD to give ICU patient surrogate informational brochure KCS: — Other concerns, follow-up activities	Azoulay, Chevret, et al. 2000	Interviews with patient or patient representative

End of Life

Missed opportunities to talk about prognosis, dying, personal concerns, and spirituality at end-of-life care	Back 2006 Hagerty, Butow, et al. 2005 Siegler and Levin 2000	Review of oncology studies Review of communicating prognosis in cancer Review of end-of-life communication

TABLE 2.3—*Continued*

Evidence of ineffective or poor communciation	Reference	Type of data used to measure physician communication
KCS: — Identify person's personal situation, values, beliefs	Detmar, Muller, et al. 2001	Transcribed audiotape of consultation
	Morita, Akechi, et al. 2005	Bereaved family–completed measures
	Knauft, Nielsen, et al. 2005	Patient-completed measures
	Audrey, Abel, et al. 2008	Transcribed audiotapes/nonparticipant observer
	Levin, Li, et al. 2008	Medical record audit
	Farber, Urban, et al. 2004	Physician-completed measures
Physician insensitivity/difficulty in delivering "bad news"	Back 2006	Review of oncology studies
	Baile and Aaron 2005	Review of oncology studies
	Hagerty, Butow, et al. 2005	Review of communicating prognosis in cancer
KCS: — Identify patient's personal situation, values, beliefs	Fallowfield and Jenkins 2004	Review of delivering sad, bad, and difficult news
	Thorne, Bultz, et al. 2005	Review of costs of poor communication in oncology
	Farber, Urban, et al. 2004	Physician-completed measures
	Slutsman, Emanuel, et al. 2002	Patient-completed measures
	Goncalves, Marques, et al. 2005	Patient-completed measures
	McCluskey, Casarett, et al. 2004	Patient-completed measures

TABLE 2.4. Evidence from Review Studies That Poor or Ineffective Physician Communication Occurs ($n = 8$)

Reference	Review Type (R) Number of Studies (N) Study Setting (S) Review Purpose (P) Review Dates (D)	Key Findings related to poor or ineffective communication by physicans
Siegler and Levin 2000	(R) Selective review (N) Not reported (S) End-of-life (P) Review end-of-life care and provide recommendations to improve communication (D) Not reported	From 1986 to 2001, 6/7 studies conducted in various settings found that although patients often stated that they would like to talk to their MDs about end-of-life care or CPR, a small proportion did so. 3 MD surveys from 1993 and 2000 found that MDs limited the amount of information they provided, controlled communication with patients, and believed they should avoid prognostication. 3 other studies (1992–95) documented poor communication by MDs with hospitalized patients about do-not-resuscitate discussions, removal from the ventilator, and advanced directives; a 1991 study of MD-patient pairs documented a SIG lower rating by MDs on physical, functional, and quality-of-life status, compared to patients. As a result of poor communication about prognosis, patients may make decisions based on overly optimistic views about their prognoses, leading them to choose aggressive treatment that decreases their quality of life and does not substantially increase their life expectancy.
Fallowfield and Jenkins 2004	(R) Systematic review, 4 dB (N) Not reported (S) Pediatrics, obstetrics, trauma, and cancer (P) Assess impact that giving sad, bad, and difficult news has on doctors and patients (D) 1993–2003	Review focuses mainly on problems encountered from 3 areas of research: parents in an obstetric or pediatric setting, people in acute trauma situations such as accident and emergency departments, and patients with cancer. 12 studies are reported on patient views on receiving news related to congenital anomalies (3), pediatric cerebral palsy (1), adult cancers (8), and trauma (1). These studies had a wide range of objectives and ranged in sample size from 13 to 351 patients. Authors found that systematic research is limited by practical and ethical concerns with interviewing patients or the families immediately after having received bad news. Thus, many reports have been based mainly on retrospective recall several months or years after the event, with most specific features of the event from very positive or negative experiences, suggesting that if bad news is communicated badly, it can cause confusion, long-lasting distress, and resentment.

TABLE 2.4—*Continued*

Reference	Review Type (R) Number of Studies (N) Study Setting (S) Review Purpose (P) Review Dates (D)	Key Findings related to poor or ineffective communication by physicans
Baile and Aaron 2005	(R) Selective review (N) Not reported (S) Oncology (P) Emphasize outcomes of communication stud- ies and implications for MD training (D) Not reported	Citing selected references, author states that gaps in communication make it difficult for patients to ob- tain timely information (1999 Canadian oncology nurses study), which may lead to patients being dissatisfied with the information they receive, mis- informed about the status of their illness, or igno- rant about the purpose of their treatment (1997 hospital study of advanced cancer patients; 1988 British study; 1997 survey of doctor-patient com- munication in lung cancer; 1984 study of metasta- tic cancer patients). Patients often do not achieve their desires for participation in decision making (2004 review of empathy ability of medical stu- dents) or understand the purpose of clinical trials (2004 Australian study). MDs miss opportunities to respond empathically to their concerns (2005 case studies report) and ignore patient wishes to discuss HRQL issues (Detmar, Muller, et al. 2001; see table 2.5). Poor communication skills may be associated with the increased likelihood of receiv- ing anticancer treatment at the end of life (1998 survey of pediatric oncologists). Authors find that breaking bad news is stressful for the clinician (1996 review article), which may result in attempts to obfuscate or "cushion" the bad news by avoid- ing discussion of important topics such as progno- sis (1988 Canadian report; 1985 British report on nurse-patient communication; 2004 British report on managing the difficult consultation), falsely re- assuring the patient that things will improve, offer- ing treatment that will not further the goals of care, or burying discussions of prognosis in technical jargon.
Curtis, Engelberg, et al. 2005	(R) Selective review (N) Not reported (S) COPD (P) Summarize recent re- search and suggest a re- search agenda on MD end-of-life communica- tion (D) Not reported	Citing selected references authors state that most COPD patients do not discuss end-of-life issues with their MDs (even though they may wish to) and believe their MDs do not know their preferences for end-of-life care (1996 patient survey; 1997 pa- tient education study; 2004 patient survey). In a British study (2001 survey), while 82% of GPs be- lieve they should discuss COPD prognosis, 41% reported doing so. Patient and MD barriers to end- of-life communication are reviewed. MD identified

TABLE 2.4—*Continued*

Reference	Review Type (R) Number of Studies (N) Study Setting (S) Review Purpose (P) Review Dates (D)	Key Findings related to poor or ineffective communication by physicans
		barriers include lack of time; worry that discussion will interfere with patient hope; patient not sick enough yet; patients don't know what kind of care they want and it changes over time; and the role of the MD is to make a patient feel better.
Hack, Degner, et al. 2005	(R) Systematic review, 2 dB (N) Not reported (S) Oncology (P) Critique the empirical literature on the communication needs and goals of cancer patients (D) 1992–2004	The review focuses on patient communication goals and needs and on the influences of patient, MD, and external factors on these goals. Clinical goals are for MDs to correctly assess and manage disease symptoms and to convey this understanding to patients so that patients feel satisfied and share in decision making. MD factors influencing poor communication are identified as lack of ability to assess levels of patient depression and anxiety; busy patient workload and a lack of familiarity with the patient; tendency to ignore symptom assessment unless clinical information is not clear and to ignore patients' symptom reports when positive clinical information is available; failure to ask and lack of attention to patients' psychosocial and health-related quality-of-life concerns; lack of skills to convey disease information; lack of effort to assess patient information need; falsely assume that good communication occurs when complete patient information given; sometimes believe it is better to withhold, distort, or soften potentially negative and emotionally upsetting information from patients in interest of fostering patient hope. The authors conclude that patient satisfaction and psychological well-being are enhanced when MDs perform caring behaviors and when they attend to the emotional needs of patients; cancer patients continue to have unmet communication needs, a substantial proportion of which pertain to unfulfilled needs for disease- and treatment-related information, including extent of disease, prognosis, treatment alternatives, treatment intent, and treatment side effects; and MDs need to discern what information to impart to patients, the extent to which they will involve patients in treatment decision making, and the degree to which they will communicate with patients about their emotional status and other nonmed-

TABLE 2.4—*Continued*

Reference	Review Type (R) Number of Studies (N) Study Setting (S) Review Purpose (P) Review Dates (D)	Key Findings related to poor or ineffective communication by physicans
		ical aspects of quality of life. A research agenda is presented.
Hagerty, Butow, et al. 2005	(R) Systematic review, 3 dB (N) 50 studies (S) Oncology (P) Identify patient preferences, clinician views, and current practice regarding the communication of prognosis. (D) Up to December 2003	Review focused on evidence obtained from descriptive studies of provider practices, patients' behaviors, knowledge, or attitudes; or a systematic review of the descriptive studies. In 31 studies describing the current practice of delivering prognostic information and on patient understanding and awareness of prognosis, the majority (1973–2003) found that, overall, prognosis is often not discussed. The most recent evidence (1993–2002) is varied, with 15 studies finding that prognosis is more often not discussed or that the discussion lacked clarity or sensitivity and with 4 studies to the contrary. There is a specific lack of evidence in patients with advanced cancer and palliative-stage disease. 19 studies on patient understanding and awareness of prognostic information found that, in all stages of disease, many patients reported not being told their prognosis or misunderstood the status of their disease, treatment intent, and their prognosis; there was lack of information clarity; and they did not understand terminology used by oncologists.
Thorne, Bultz, et al. 2005	(R) Focused review (N) Not reported (S) Oncology (P) Analyze impact of ineffective communication (D) Not reported	Poor communication was defined as verbal and nonverbal aspects of the relationship between the clinician and patient that have the potential to create unfavorable outcomes. While this review focuses on outcomes and costs of poor communication (table 3.1), there is an initial summary on the evidence that poor MD communication occurs: patients are often dissatisfied with the amount and nature of information they receive (11 studies cited, 1993–99); while information needs are necessarily highly individualized, this individualization of information is rarely achieved (2 studies, 1997–2000); and recent research on diagnostic and prognostic information (3 studies, 1993–99), specifically on breaking bad news (5 studies, 1995–2001), has found that MDs lack skills in this area (4 studies, 1992–2000), with resulting misunderstandings among patients about the nature and seriousness of their disease (1 study, 1997).

TABLE 2.4—*Continued*

Reference	Review Type (R) Number of Studies (N) Study Setting (S) Review Purpose (P) Review Dates (D)	Key Findings related to poor or ineffective communication by physicans
		One survey (2002) of health care professionals caring for 1,326 patients at the end of life in 3 countries found severe communication problems as part of team assessments in the care of 40% of these patients. The relationship between patient preferences and existing communication guidelines or principles is not well understood (12 studies, 1996–2003), with much of what is understood about breaking bad news based on clinical judgment rather than empirical evidence (5 studies, 1995–2000).
Back 2006	(R) Selective review (N) Not reported (S) Oncology (P) Produce evidence-based communication guidelines in 6 categories, including how MDs handle medical information and how they deal with patient emotions (D) Not reported	Citing 1 to 3 studies for each conclusion, the author finds there is a gap in eliciting patient concerns during consultation; an MD's caring attitude is a therapeutically important aspect of the relationship; MDs have difficulty and suffer emotional stress in conveying bad news to patients; MDs tend to focus narrowly on technical decisions, fail to elicit patient values, and do not clearly discuss the likelihood that a life-sustaining intervention will meaningfully prolong life. For example, in a 1996 survey of patients with breast cancer or melanoma, 57% wanted to talk about prognosis, yet only 27% actually did; likewise, 63% wanted to talk about the effects of the cancer on other aspects of their life, yet only 35% did. In a 1999 study of patients with advanced cancer in which a research nurse used a checklist to elicit patient concerns after a visit with an oncologist, patients were found to have numerous concerns they had not disclosed to their oncologists, and a larger number of concerns was correlated with poorer adjustment to illness. The author finds that detecting and responding to emotion is a separate communication skill from dealing with informational needs. The author concludes with evidence-based guidelines on handling information and dealing with patient emotions.

COPD = chronic obstructive pulmonary disease
CPR = cardipulmonary resuscitation
dB = database(s)   GP = general practitioner

n = number
SIG = significant(ly)

TABLE 2.5. Evidence from Empirical Studies That Poor or Ineffective Physician Communication Occurs (*n* = 59)

References	Study Design (S) Study Purpose (P) Study Setting (T) Study Date (D) Country (C)	Methods	Final Sample Size	Main Measures	Key Findings
Koning, Maile, et al. 1995	(S) Descriptive (P) Study the need of asthma patients (T) Outpatient (D) Not reported (C) Netherlands	Mail survey of patients referred from GPs and specialists	*n* = 121 asthma patients	111 items on needs in questionnaire rated on a 5-point Likert scale	Unfulfilled MD-patient communication needs of patients: patients wanted more information about causes from general practitioner or medical specialist (43%, 45%); diagnostic tests (47%, 50%); prognosis (31%, 39%); long-term medication use (25%, 41%), and greater participation in treatment decisions (31%, 32%)
Kravitz, Callahan, et al. 1996	(S) Descriptive (P) Identify factors influencing patient expectations (T) Internal medicine clinics (D) 1994 (C) US	Post-visit survey with a subsample of telephone interviews 1–7 days post-visit using transcribed audiotape	*n* = 18 MDs and 4 nurse practitioners *n* = 688 patients	8 questions about perceived omissions of care	18% reported 1 or more omissions of care: With respect to communication, MDs failed to ask about specific medical or lifestyle factors (5%) and questions about prognosis were not answered (3%)
Calkins, Davis, et al. 1997	(S) Descriptive (P) Assess patient and MD perceptions of discharge treatment plan (T) Academic medical center (D) 1991–92 (C) US	Patient and MD surveys	*n* = 83 MD-patient pairs at hospital discharge	(1) Patient understanding of purpose and potential side effects of medications; (2) patient understanding of when to resume normal activities; (3) time discussing post-discharge	MDs reported spending more time discussing post-discharge care than did patients; MDs believed that 89% of patients understood the potential side effects of their medications vs. 57% of patients; MDs believed that 95% of patients understood when to resume normal activities vs. 58% of

TABLE 2.5—Continued

References	Study Design (S) Study Purpose (P) Study Setting (T) Study Date (D) Country (C)	Methods	Final Sample Size	Main Measures	Key Findings
Marvel, Epstein et al. 1999	(S) Observational (P) Examine extent to which family MDs elicit patient concerns (T) Urban and rural family practice offices (D) 1995–July 1996 (C) US and Canada	Transcribed audiotapes with qualitative analysis using Beckman-Frankel methods	$n = 29$ $n = 264$ patient visits	Patient-MD verbal interactions; completion rate of patient responses; length of time for patient responses; and frequency of late-arising patient concerns care	patients MDs solicited patients' concerns in 75.4% of the interviews. Patients completed initial statements of concerns in 28% of the interviews. The most frequent barriers to completion were closed-ended questioning by the MD (28.4%), absence of MD solicitation (24.6%), and MD statement (14.0%). The average length of time given patients to itemize their concerns before the first redirection was 23.1 seconds. Over the entire visit, patients had 26 seconds to present their agenda of concerns.
Azoulay, Chevret, et al. 2000	(S) Descriptive (P) Identify factors associated with poor comprehension by family of the status of ICU patients (T) University affiliated medical ICU (D) June–November 1997 (C) France	Interviews with representatives of patients who were visited by at least one person during their ICU stay	$n = 102$ patients admitted to ICU for >2 days, 76 family/friend patient representatives	(1) Representative comprehension of diagnosis, prognosis, and treatment; (2) ICU staff ability to predict poor comprehension	Failure to comprehend the diagnosis, prognosis, or treatment was found in 54% of representatives: diagnosis, 20%; prognosis, 33%; treatment 40% (OR = 10). MD-related factors were first meeting with representative <10 minutes ($p = .03$) and failure to give the representative an information brochure ($p = .02$). Patient and representative factors associat-

ed with poor comprehension: patient age <50 yrs ($p = .03$), unemployed ($p = .01$), referral from a hematology or oncology ward ($p = .006$), admission for acute respiratory failure ($p = .005$) or coma ($p = .01$), favorable prognosis ($p = .04$), family of foreign descent ($p = .007$), no knowledge of French ($p = .03$), representative not the spouse ($p = .03$), and no healthcare professional in the family ($p = .01$).

Authors conclude that patient information is frequently not communicated effectively to family members by ICU MDs. MDs should strive to identify patients and families who require special attention and to determine how their personal style of interrelating with family members may impair communication.

31/35 (89%) of patients did not voice their complete agendas: symptoms (27%), prescription request (41%), previous self-treatment (33%), request for diagnosis (25%), theories about diagnosis (57%), reporting of side effects (70%), worries about diagnosis or prognosis (70%), not wanting a prescription (66%), social context (63%). In all of the 14 consultations with problem out-

Qualitative analysis of interview data to identify patient agendas. Agendas classed as symptoms, diagnosis theories, illness fears, wanted and unwanted actions, self-treatment, and emotional and social issues.

$n = 20$ MDs
$n = 35$ patients

Patient interviews before visit and 1 week after visit. MDs interviews 1 day after visit. Transcribed recordings of consultations.

(S) Descriptive
(P) Describe current communication practice among general practitioners
(T) Community MD practices
(D) Not reported
(C) UK

Barry, Bradley, et al. 2000

TABLE 2.5—*Continued*

References	Study Design (S) Study Purpose (P) Study Setting (T) Study Date (D) Country (C)	Methods	Final Sample Size	Main Measures	Key Findings
					comes at least one of the problems was related to an unvoiced agenda item.
Britten, Stevenson, et al. 2000	(S) Qualitative (P) Identify misunderstanding between patients and GPs on taking medicines (T) 20 GP practices (D) Not reported (C) UK	Transcribed audiotapes with qualitative analysis	*n* = 20 GPs *n* = 35 patients	Misunderstandings between patients and GPs that have potential or actual adverse consequences for taking medicine	Prescribing misunderstandings occurred in 28 of the 35 (80%) consultations. They arose through lack of exchange of relevant information in both directions; from conflicting information or attributions; patient failure to understand the doctor's diagnostic or treatment decision; and actions taken to preserve the MD-patient relationship.
Levinson, Gorawa-Bhat, et al. 2000	(S) Qualitative (P) Assess patients' clues and how MDs respond to these clues (T) Community PCP and surgery practices (D) 1994 (C) US	Transcribed audiotapes with qualitative analysis	*n* = 54 PCPs and 62 surgeons	(1) Frequency and content of patient clues; (2) nature of MD responses to clues coded as positive or missed opportunity	MDs responded positively to patient emotions in 38% of cases in surgery and 21% in primary care; missed opportunities to adequately acknowledge patients' feelings (79% primary care and 62% surgery). Visits with missed opportunities tended to be longer than visits with a positive response (PCP mean time, 2.1 minutes vs. 17.6 minutes; surgeon 14.0 minutes vs. 12.5 minutes).

Pho, Geller, et al. 2000	(S) Descriptive (P) Assess MD patient communication regarding screening recommendations for at-risk relatives (T) Community (D) 1997 (C) US	Telephone-administered survey	$n = 44$ patients <60 years of age diagnosed with colorectal adenomas	(1) Patient awareness of familial risk; (2) MD recommendations for screening	18/44 patients (41%) were aware that close relatives were at a higher risk of colorectal cancer. 6/18 (33%) learned of the association from MD and 12/18 (67%) from non-MD sources. 4/44 (9%) reported MD recommended screening for family members.
Teno, Fisher, et al. 2000	(S) Descriptive (P) Evaluate decision making and outcomes for seriously ill patients with an ICU stay of at least 14 days (T) 5 medical center ICUs (D) 1989–91 (C) US	Interviews conducted during the second hospital week with patients, their surrogate decision makers, and their MDs	$n = 1,457$ patients with an ICU stay of 14 days or more	(1) Prognosis; (2) patient/surrogate MD communication; (3) goals of medical care	38% of patients (or their surrogates) discussed their prognosis with their MD; 34% had talked with their MDs about their preferred approach to care; 45% preferred care focused on extending life; 36% expressed a preference for palliative care. Among those who preferred extending life, 88% reported medical care was consistent with that preference, 2% that their current care was aimed at comfort, and 10% did not know what the current approach to care was. Among those who preferred a palliative approach, 29% reported care was consistent with that preference, 47% believed that medical care was contrary to preference, and 24% did not know what the current approach to medical care was. Those who discussed their care preferences with an MD were 1.9 times more likely to believe that treatment was in accord

TABLE 2.5—Continued

References	Study Design (S) Study Purpose (P) Study Setting (T) Study Date (D) Country (C)	Methods	Final Sample Size	Main Measures	Key Findings
Adams, Smith, et al. 2001	(S) Descriptive (P) Identify patients' perceptions of their involvement in treatment (T) University pulmonary clinic (D) 1995–97 (C) Australia	Mail survey; data for this analysis come from the 12-month follow-up survey only	n = 128 asthma patients	3 questions on 5-point Likert scale on patient choice, control, and responsibility in treatment	with their preferences for palliation. PDM mean score (range 1–100) was 72. See Adams, Smith, et al., 2001, table 3.2, for effect of PDM on health outcomes and utilization.
Detmar, Mueller, et al. 2001	(S) Descriptive (P) Investigate the content of routine communication regarding 4 specific HRQL issues between oncologists and patients and identify consultation factors (T) Outpatient palliative chemotherapy clinic (D) 1996–98 (C) Netherlands	Survey and audiotapes	n = 10 oncologists n = 240 patients with incurable cancer receiving outpatient palliative chemotherapy	Patient and MD questionnaires (5-point Likert scale) and audiotape analysis of communication regarding daily activities, emotional functioning, pain, and fatigue using the Roter Interaction Analysis System	MDs devoted 64% of their conversation to medical/technical issues and 23% to HRQL issues. Patients' communication behavior of medical/technical issues was 41% and HRQL topics 48%. In 20%–54% of the consultations in which patients were experiencing serious HRQL problems, no time was devoted to discussion of those problems; emotional functioning 54% and fatigue 48%. Patients' emotional problems were SIG more likely to be discussed during

Study	Characteristics	Method	Sample	Focus	Results
					on-time visits than during delayed visits (49% vs. 32%, $p = .05$). More time was devoted to emotional issues during the on-time visits ($p = .05$), although the length of visit was similar (16.4 vs. 15.7 minutes). Length of the visit, interruptions, and the number of prior visits had no SIG effect on HRQL communication.
Elkington, White, et al. 2001	(S) Descriptive (P) Evaluate MD communication in managing COPD (T) Community GP offices (D) 1999 (C) UK	Physician mail survey	$n = 214$ GPs	Role of GP in discussing prognosis; personal practice of discussing prognosis; factors influencing GP discussion with patient	82% agreed that GPs have an important role in prognosis discussions; 41% reported often or always discussing prognosis and 15% reported never discussing prognosis. 48% were undecided, and 16% disagreed that most patients with COPD wanted to know about their prognosis. 15% GPs reported rarely or never discussing prognosis, 59% reported that there was insufficient information in the primary care notes to be able to discuss prognosis, 64% found it hard to start discussions with patients, and 64% believed it was the patient's responsibility to initiate discussions.
Murphy, Chang, et al. 2001	(S) Descriptive (P) Explore quality of MD-patient relationship, 1996–99 (T) 12 health insurance	Longitudinal survey: self-administered mail PCAS administered at baseline and at 3 years	$n = 2,383$ patients who identified a PCP and baseline and	Mean of unadjusted summary scales measuring 2 domains of relationship quality (4 scales) quality and organiza-	SIG declines in 3 of the 4 relationship scales: communication quality (ES = .095), interpersonal treatment (ES = .115), and patient trust (ES = .046). Improvement was observed in MD's

TABLE 2.5—*Continued*

References	Study Design (S) Study Purpose (P) Study Setting (T) Study Date (D) Country (C)	Methods	Final Sample Size	Main Measures	Key Findings
	plans (D) 1996–99 (C) US		remained with MD over 3 years	tional features of care (4 scales)	knowledge of the patient (ES = .051). There was a SIG decline in organizational access (ES = .165) and an increase in visit-based continuity (ES = .060); no SIG changes in financial access and integration of care indexes.
Rhoades, McFarland, et al. 2001	(S) Observational (P) Examine MD-patient communication patterns (T) Primary care (D) Not reported (C) US	Observed interactions using a standardized data collection form	n = 22 FP and internal medicine residents n = 60 routine office visits	(1) Amount of time both the resident and the patient spoke; (2) number and type of verbal and external interruptions; and (3) parts of the physical examination performed	(1) Visit time averaged 11 minutes, with patient speaking for about 4 minutes; (2) patients spoke, uninterrupted, an average of 12 seconds after the MD entered the room; (3) 25% of patients were interrupted before they finished speaking; (4) MDs interrupted patients on average twice during a visit; (5) interruptions included computer use (66%), beepers (8%), knock on the door (15%), and leaving the room and returning (31%), with increased frequency of interruptions associated with less favorable patient satisfaction; (6) gender was associated with the pattern of interruptions with female MDs interrupting patients less often

Author	Study characteristics	Method	Sample	Aim / Measures	Findings
Bell, Kravitz, et al. 2002	(S) Descriptive (P) Examine patient unmet expectations (T) Primary care and specialty clinics (D) 1999 (C) US	Patient pre-/post-visit and 2-week post-visit. MD survey post-visit.	n = 45 MDs n = 909 patients	9 measures of unmet expectations in 3 domains: clinical data collection, allocation of clinical resources, and provision of information and counseling	than male MDs and all MDs interrupting female patients more often than male patients 12% of patients reported 1 or more unmet expectations: 5% believed the MD left important questions unasked, 5% believed that important medical information or counseling was not provided. 2 weeks post-visit, patients with unmet expectations reported SIG less satisfaction with care (p = .001), less symptom improvement (p = .001), and weaker intentions to adhere to MD's advice (p = .001).
Collins, Clark, et al. 2002	(S) Descriptive (P) Explore patients' perceptions of their communication with MDs about cardiac testing and treatment recommendations (T) VA clinics (D) Not reported (C) US	4 focus groups stratified by race (white vs. black)	n = 13 cardiac patients who had (1) undergone stress tests or (2) undergone stress test followed by invasive cardiac procedure	Identify MD-patient communication domains	(1) Substance of the information communicated by providers could be vague, unclear, confusing to patients; (2) some recommendations either were inconsistent with expectations or awakened fears based on distressing previous experiences; (3) patients required convincing of the need for additional, invasive tests and therapeutic procedures; (4) black patients expressed the need for trust before undergoing an invasive cardiac procedure
Davis, Shoenbaum, et al. 2002	(S) Descriptive (P) Identify care issues of concern to patients (T) Community	Commonwealth Fund/Princeton national telephone survey	n = 6,722 adults aged 18 years or over	MD-patient communication among the quality of health care issues queried	19% reported that they had experienced 1 or more communication problems the last time they visited a doctor including: leaving the visit

TABLE 2.5—Continued

References	Study Design (S) Study Purpose (P) Study Setting (T) Study Date (D) Country (C)	Methods	Final Sample Size	Main Measures	Key Findings
	(D) April–November 2001 (C) US				with questions about their care that they had wanted to discuss but did not (12%), reporting that the doctor listened some or only a little to what they had to say (9%), or understanding some or only a little of what the doctor told them (7%)
Deveugele, Derese, et al. 2002	(S) Descriptive (P) Explore if MD patient perceptions affect the communicative behavior in consultations (T) Community primary care (D) Not reported (C) Netherlands	Patient questionnaire, MD logs, transcribed videotapes of encounters, scored for time management and communication scored by RIAS	$n = 20$ GPs $n = 299$ patient encounters	Frequency and predictors of MD affective talk (e.g., social talk, concern, agreement, reassurance) and instrumental talk (e.g., give direction, ask questions)	(1) MDs who perceived more social support to be available for the patient provided less affective and instrumental talk ($p = <.05$); (2) MDs and patients used predominantly task-oriented (instrumental) communication (70% of utterances); (3) MDs gave more information on medical issues but less on lifestyle (13% vs. 8% utterances); (4) MDs and patients seldom asked for clarification, suggesting the possibility of more ambiguities and misunderstanding; (5) MD affective talk limited to social talk (9%) and agreement (9%), with little concern (.5%) and reassurance (2%); (6) MD gender, number of years knowing the

Author	Study	Methods	Sample	Focus	Findings
Slutsman, Emanuel, et al. 2002	(S) Descriptive (P) Evaluate the effect of managed care delivery systems on end-of-life care (T) Community (D) March 1996 and June 1997 (C) US	Multistage, cluster sampling strategy, 6 MSA study sites. Telephone survey using questions on MD-patient communication developed for the study.	$n = 988$ patients whose MDs judged them to be terminally ill	Patient-MD relationship among 6 domains of care measured	patient, and the importance of medical and psychosocial aspects as mentioned by the patient did not influence MD communication No SIG differences between the MCO and FFS in the patient-MD relationship domain measured by: trust (MCO 98.7% vs. FFS 96.7%); receiving clear and adequate information about condition (MCO 84.0% vs. FFS 84.7%); MD advocating for patients for care (MCO 98.2% vs. FFS 98.6%); MD delivering bad news sensitively (MCO 94.3% vs. FFS 93.3%); participating meaningfully in treatment decisions (MCO 97.5% vs. FFS 97.4%); and experiencing difficulty in reaching MD by telephone (MCO 13.8% vs. FFS 12.0%)
Jenkins, Britten, et al. 2003	(S) Descriptive (P) Develop instruments to monitor communication and prescribing (T) GP offices (D) Not reported (C) UK	Compare what patients wanted and received from MD using pre-/post-visit surveys	$n = 167$ patients	MD talk with them, listen, explain, diagnose, reassure, advise on medications, to participate in treatment decisions	Patients had high expectations for communication and participation in the consultation with patients receiving less than what they wanted in participation in treatment decisions (9%); explanation of problem (3%) or treatment (4%); reassurance (13%); and choice of treatment (43%)
Keating, Weeks, et al. 2003	(S) Descriptive (P) Compare patients' and their surgeons'	Postsurgical patient interview and surgeon survey. Sample selected	$n = 166$ surgeons $n = 1,154$	Discussion of treatment alternatives for early stage breast cancer	Among 1,154 women eligible for both breast-conserving surgery and mastectomy, only 71% reported that

TABLE 2.5—*Continued*

References	Study Design (S) Study Purpose (P) Study Setting (T) Study Date (D) Country (C)	Methods	Final Sample Size	Main Measures	Key Findings
	reports of discussing treatment alternatives for early stage breast cancer (T) Community (D) 1993–95 (C) US	from hospital pathology databases.	patients with confirmed stage I or II breast cancer		their surgeon discussed both treatments. Surgeons of 730 women returned surveys and reported discussing both treatments with 82% of the patients. 32% of the time, patients and surgeons disagreed about whether both treatments were discussed; with patients more often reporting (22%) that both treatments were not discussed when surgeons reported they were.
McManus and Wheatley 2003	(S) Descriptive (P) Assess variations in consent practice for laparoscopic cholecystectomy (T) Community (D) 2000 (C) UK	Postal survey	$n = 207$ surgeons	Frequency with which potential complications discussed with patients prior to laparoscopic cholecystectomy	44% of surgeons provided written information to patients and 19% gave patients this information on the ward in the immediate preoperative period. There was wide variability on what risks are significant enough to warrant discussion with patients, e.g.: (1) on average, only 3 of the 9 listed complications were mentioned more than 50% of the time; (2) 25% of surgeons never discussed bile duct injury with patients, and a further 22% mentioned it only rarely; (3) 59% rarely or never informed

patients of the risk of retained calculi and 27% usually or always did so; (4) 25% usually or always mentioned general post-operative complications. 83% always discussed the possibility of conversion to open cholecystectomy.

Study	Design / Purpose	Method	n	Frequency and skill	Results
Farber, Urban, et al. 2004	(S) Descriptive (P) Identify MD-perceived skills in palliative care (T) Palliative care (D) 2000 (C) US	National survey of internal medicine and family practice MDs. Questionnaire on 4-point scale.	n = 462 MDs	Frequency and skill in palliative care: (1) cultural aspects; (2) advance directives; (3) giving bad news; (4) pain management; (5) physical symptoms; (6) psychological and cognitive symptoms; (7) social support; (8) economic demands and caregiver needs; (9) patient expectations/hope; (10) spiritual needs	Except for addressing economic demands and the caregiver needs, patient expectations/hope, and patient spiritual needs, MDs rated themselves as always or frequently performing 7 aspects of palliative care (79%–83%) and in an excellent or good manner (68%–82%). For addressing economic and spiritual needs, and cultural aspects, approximately half of the MDs reported that they always or frequently performed the items. 38%–51% of MDs rated themselves as skilled in these areas.
Koedoot, Oort, et al. 2004	(S) Qualitative (P) Determine content and amount of information when proposing palliative chemotherapy (T) Hospital oncology clinic (D) 1998–2000 (C) Netherlands	Transcribed audiotape	n = 33 MDs n = 95 patients with metastatic cancer	(1) Disease, course of cancer, disease-related symptoms, and prognosis; (2) chemotherapy aims, procedures, and side effects; (3) effects of the disease on quality of life; (4) watchful waiting	Medical oncologists did not mention or explain the disease course (47%), symptoms (62%), and prognosis (59%); absence of cure (16%); survival gain (45%); chemotherapy procedure (18%); various chemotherapy side effects (22%–93%); various chemotherapy quality-of-life effects (96%–100%). Watchful waiting was mentioned to only half of the

TABLE 2.5—*Continued*

References	Study Design (S) Study Purpose (P) Study Setting (T) Study Date (D) Country (C)	Methods	Final Sample Size	Main Measures	Key Findings
McClusky, Casarett, et al. 2004	(S) Descriptive (P) Evaluate MDs' delivery of bad news (T) Community (D) Not reported (C) US	Mail survey of patients and their caregivers from database of regional ALS associations	$n = 94$ patient-caregiver pairs, 50 unpaired patients, and 19 unpaired caregivers	Questions derived from the SPIKES protocol: Setting, patient Perception, request for Invitation to deliver the news, Knowledge provision, Empathy, Strategy with patient	MDs broke the news of ALS in all but one instance. Patients rated MD performance as poor (16%), below average (9%), average (31%), good (19%), or excellent (25%). Compared to MDs rated as good or excellent, MDs grouped as poor, below average, or average was SIG related to lower scores in setting ($p = <.001$), determine patient needs and perception ($p = <.001$), invitation ($p = <.001$), knowledge ($p = <.002$), explore patient feelings ($p = <.001$), and summary strategy ($p = <.001$). 50% uninformed of specialty centers or ALS helping organizations.
Montgomery, Irish, et al. 2004	(S) Descriptive (P) Examine changes in the quality of primary care for Medicare beneficiaries, 1998–2000 (T) 13 states with large,	Self-administered PCAS with telephone follow-up at baseline and at 2 years	$n = 4,173$ Medicare beneficiaries aged 65 and older	(1) 5 measures of MD-patient relationship quality; (2) 4 measures of organizational features of care. Change in each beneficiary's	SIG declines in 3/5 measures of MD-patient interaction quality: communication (ES = .19, $p = <.001$), interpersonal treatment (ES = .12, $p = <.001$), and thoroughness of physical exams (ES = 13, $p = <.001$). MDs'

patients, either in one sentence (23%) or explained more extensively (27%).

	mature Medicare HMO markets (D) 1998–99 (C) US	score (1998 vs. 2000) and standardized effect sizes calculated.		knowledge of patients increased SIG (ES = .12, p = <.001). No change in patient trust. For organizational features of care: SIG declines in financial access (ES = .15, p = <.001), visit-based continuity (ES = .26, p = <.001), and integration of care (ES = .06, p = <.05), while organizational access increased (ES = .06, p = <.05). With the exception of financial access, observed changes did not differ by system (FFS, HMO). There was no change in patients' report of visit time minutes.
Poon, Haas, et al. 2004	(S) Descriptive (P) Identify communication factors associated with appropriate short-term follow-up of abnormal mammograms (T) Community (D) 1996–97 (C) US	Patient interview within 6–8 weeks and at 7–8 months of index abnormal mammogram	n = 126 women	Based on sequence of communication events that should occur for a patient to receive appropriate follow-up care for an abnormal mammogram	Patient given results to take home (33%); MD explained further tests in way patient understood (40%); patient told she needed follow-up (71%). Women told follow-up was needed were SIG more likely to receive the appropriate follow-up care (OR = 4.32; p = .004).
Zickmund, Hillis, et al. 2004	(S) Qualitative (P) Identify patient-perceived prevalence, nature, and potential predictors of communication problems (T) Hepatology clinic at a tertiary referral hospital	Transcribed recorded semistructured interview prior to visit; medical record data; and Hospital Anxiety Depression scale and Sickness Impact Profile post-visit	n = 322 outpatients diagnosed with chronic HCV infection	Patient communication difficulties with MD: (1) communication skills of MD; (2) MD diagnosis and treatment skills; (3) being misdiagnosed, misled, or abandoned; (4) being	131/322 (41%) reported communication difficulties with MDs including poor communication skills of MDs (28%), MD incompetence regarding the diagnosis and treatment of HCV infection (23%), feelings of being misdiagnosed, misled, or abandoned (16%), or being stigmatized

TABLE 2.5—*Continued*

References	Study Design (S) Study Purpose (P) Study Setting (T) Study Date (D) Country (C)	Methods	Final Sample Size	Main Measures	Key Findings
	(D) 1998–2002 (C) US			stigmatized by MD	by their MD (9%). 47% reported difficulties with specialists vs. 17% for generalists. Nonresponse with antiviral therapy correlated with perceived MD conflict even after adjusting for treatment in relation to the time of interview. In a multivariate model, patients' psychosocial problems were the best predictors of communication difficulties (63% discriminant ability).
Goncalves, Marques, et al. 2005	(S) Descriptive (P) Obtain patient preference about cancer diagnosis and prognosis and compare with what actually occurs (T) Palliative care oncology clinic (D) 2002–3 (C) Portugal	Pre-visit patient survey	*n = 47* advanced cancer patients	(1) By whom and where did/ should diagnosis be conveyed; (2) who was/should have been with the patient; (3) patient participation in the treatment decisions; (4) palliative care information provided	72% thought they had been informed of their diagnosis; however not all patients stated the diagnosis in a manner clearly showing that they were aware of the nature of their disease. 83% were informed that they were being referred to the palliative care unit, but 17% had received an explanation of the unit's function. 6% were never informed about treatment, and 32% never participated in decisions regarding treatment. 56% reported information was disclosed in an acceptable manner, clearly and

Study	Design	Method	Sample	Measures/Analysis	Results
Jerant, von Friederichs-Fitzwater, et al. 2005	(S) Qualitative (P) Elicit perceived barriers to patient self-management and to support services and resources (T) 12 university PCP offices (D) 2003 (C) US	10 focus groups	$n = 54$ participants with chronic disease	Analysis of focus groups with coding scheme based on emerging content patterns using the grounded theory method	sensitively; 44% found the disclosure poorly carried out. Ineffective communication identified as 1 of 8 barriers to self-management for patients with chronic disease. Other problems included depression, weight problems, difficulty exercising, fatigue, low family support, pain, and financial.
King, Yonas, et al. 2004	(S) Qualitative (P) Assess communication between vascular neurosurgeons and their patients about treatment options and expected outcomes (T) Medical center outpatient neurosurgery clinic (D) 2001–4 (C) US	Cross-sectional post-visit structured interviews, surveys (6-point Likert scale) of patients and MDs; medical record extractions	$n = 44$ MDs; $n = 44$ patients with unruptured cerebral aneurysms	Level of agreement between 44 patient-neurosurgeon pairs on (1) patient's understanding of treatment options; (2) "best" treatment as agreed upon by the patient and MD; (3) risk of stroke or death from attempted treatment or future risk of death and stroke with no intervention	61% of patient-neurosurgeon pairs agreed on the best treatment plan for the patient's aneurysm ($= .51$, moderate agreement). Neurosurgeons' agreement with their patients ranged from 82% ($= .77$, almost perfect agreement) to 52% ($= .37$, fair agreement). Patients estimated much higher risks of stroke or death from surgical clipping (patient 36% vs. neurosurgeon 13%, $p = .001$); endovascular embolism (patient 35% vs. neurosurgeon 19%, $p = .040$); or no intervention (patient 63% vs. neurosurgeon 25%, $p = .001$). Poor communication results in many patients with cerebral aneurysms having an inaccurate understanding of their aneurysm treatment plan and an exaggerated

TABLE 2.5—*Continued*

References	Study Design (S) Study Purpose (P) Study Setting (T) Study Date (D) Country (C)	Methods	Final Sample Size	Main Measures	Key Findings
					sense of the risks of disease and treatment.
Knauft, Nielsen, et al. 2005	(S) Descriptive (P) Identify occurrence of end-of-life MD communication (T) Pulmonary university, county, VA clinics, and oxygen delivery company (D) Not reported (C) US	In-person patient interviews and mail survey of MDs. MDs completed a separate questionnaire for each patient.	*n* = 56 MDs *n* = 115 patients with oxygen-dependent COPD	(1) Talk with MD about end-of-life care; (2) belief about MD's knowledge of their end-of-life wishes	32% of oxygen-dependent COPD patients had end-of-life discussions with their MD. 70% thought their MD probably or definitely knows the kinds of treatments they would want if they were too sick to speak for themselves.
Makaryus and Friedman 2005	(S) Descriptive (P) Ascertain patient knowledge of their medications at hospital discharge (T) Municipal teaching hospital (D) July–October 1999 (C) US	Survey at hospital discharge	*n* = 43 patients	(1) Knowledge of discharge diagnoses; (2) Treatment plan (medication names); (3) possible side effects	12 patients (27.9%) were able to list all their medications, 16 (37.2%) were able to recount the purpose of all their medications, 6 (14.0%) were able to state the common side effect(s) of all their medications, and 18 (41.9%) were able to state their diagnosis or diagnoses. The mean number of medications prescribed at discharge was 3.89. The authors caution: "Whether lack of communication between MD and patient is actually the cause of

Author, Year	Study details	Design	Sample	Measures	Results
					patient unawareness of discharge instructions or if this even affects patient outcome requires further study."
Morita, Akechi, et al. 2005	(S) Descriptive (P) Describe family's perceptions on timing of MD referral to palliative care units (T) Palliative care (D) 2003 (C) Japan	Cross-sectional anonymous mail survey of 9 palliative care units, using a 5-point scale	$n = 318$ bereaved family members of patients admitted to palliative care and died in 2001	(1) Family-perceived appropriateness of the referral timing to palliative care units; (2) determinants of family-perceived appropriateness of the referral timing	(1) Family members reported timing of referrals as late or very late (49%), appropriate (47%), early or very early (4%); (2) of families who rated the timing of referrals as late: 57% of patients were admitted for less than 2 weeks, 46% for 2 weeks to 3 months admission, and 33% longer than 3 months; (3) family belief before admission that palliative care shortens the patient's life (OR = 1.4, $p = .046$), insufficient in-advance discussion with MD about preferred end-of-life (OR = .26, $p = <.001$), insufficient preparation for changes of patient conditions (OR = 1.35, $p = .007$), and hospital treatment setting prior to admission (OR = 2.67, $p = .001$)
Travado, Grassi, et al. 2005	(S) Descriptive (P) Examine MD self-perceived communication skills, effects on patients, psychosocial orientation, and burnout (T) 2 general and 1 cancer hospital	Personally administered survey	$n = 125$ MDs	Self-Confidence in Communication Skills (SCCS), Expected Outcome of Communication (EOC), MD Belief (PBS), Maslach Burnout Inventory (MBI)	SCCS was 74%, with identifying greater difficulty in evaluating anxiety and depression (70%), promoting family communication (69%), helping with uncertainty (68%), and dealing with denial (64%). Mean score (range 1–9) EOC was 3.41 for positive and 5.85 for negative. MDs rated MDs' role in the psychosocial dimensions

TABLE 2.5—*Continued*

References	Study Design (S) Study Purpose (P) Study Setting (T) Study Date (D) Country (C)	Methods	Final Sample Size	Main Measures	Key Findings
	(D) Not reported (C) Italy, Portugal, and Spain				of patient care (PBS) as high (86%.). On the MBI, MDs reported high scores on Emotional Exhaustion (27%); Depersonalization (27%); and poor personal accomplishment (21%). Low psychosocial orientation and burnout symptoms were SIG (p = ‹.01) associated with lower confidence in communication skills and higher expectations of a negative outcome following MD-patient communication.
Barfod, Hecht, et al. 2006	(S) Observational (P) Explore and conceptualize patterns and difficulties in MDs' work with patients' adherence to HIV medication. (T) HIV clinics (D) December 2001–August 2003 (C) US and Denmark	MDs observed during clinical work and subsequently interviewed with a semistructured interview guide	n = 35 MDs: 16 MDs from San Francisco and 18 from Copenhagen	Using a grounded theory approach, notes on observations and transcribed interviews were coded and conceptualized using NVivo software	In 144 consultations main communication patterns were similar in US and Copenhagen (results not quantified): in-depth discussions between patient and MD were rare; patients rarely brought up the subject of adherence; and when MDs brought up adherence, patients usually gave brief answers that often had low believability. It emerged that MDs had individual communication patterns, which were not only determined by their perceptions about

Study	Design	Data source	Sample	Measures	Results
Bokhour, Berlowitz, et al. 2006	(S) Qualitative (P) Characterize the ways in which providers ask patients about medication taking (T) 3 VA medical center clinics (D) Not reported (C) US	Transcribed audiotapes with qualitative analysis	$n = 9$ PCPs $n = 38$ hypertensive patients	Based on sociolinguistic techniques 23 communication activities related to HTN were referenced	patients' adherence, but also strongly influenced by their perceptions about the awkwardness of discussing adherence with patients and their perceptions about the believability of patients' statements on adherence. 38% with a diagnosis of HTN were not asked at all about how they took their medication, and 33% of these patients had uncontrolled HTN. When providers did ask in some format about medication taking, they often did not follow up by seeking information about barriers to taking medication as prescribed. As a result, providers were less likely to be able to determine whether uncontrolled HTN was due to ineffective medication or poor adherence to potentially effective medications.
McLafferty, Williams, et al. 2006	(S) Descriptive (P) Identify elements of MD communication that lead patients to not recommend surgeons (T) Surgery outpatient (D) 2002–4 (C) US	Post-visit patient survey	$n = 1,514$ surgical patients	7 questions based on Institute for Healthcare Communication acronym PAUSE: Personal connection, Allow for questions, Understandable, Sit down, and Educate	Patients reported surgeon failed to ask whether the patient had questions (7%), failed to sit down (7%), used words patients could not understand (5%), failed to educate about condition (4%), failed to introduce themselves (4%), and showed lack of interest in patients as persons (2%) and inadequacies in answering questions (2%). Encounters where the patient would

TABLE 2.5—*Continued*

References	Study Design (S) Study Purpose (P) Study Setting (T) Study Date (D) Country (C)	Methods	Final Sample Size	Main Measures	Key Findings
					not recommend the surgeon included failure to show interest in the patient as a person (52%), adequately explain medical conditions (52%), invite questions (40%), adequately answer questions (36%), use words the patient could understand (28%), introduce themselves (28%), or sit down (28%).
Nelson, Angus, et al. 2006	(S) Descriptive (P) Elicit the views and experiences of ICU directors regarding barriers to optimal end-of-life care (T) 468 ICUs (D) Study closed in 2003 (C) US	Self-administered national mail survey with expert consensus developed instrument	n = 590 ICU directors: 406 nurse directors and 184 MD directors	1) Patient/family and ICU barriers to care; barriers to end-of-life care measured on a 5-point Likert scale, where 1 = huge and 5 = not at all a barrier	Among patient and MD barriers to end-of-life care, unit directors rated as "huge" barriers: insufficient MD training in communication (37%) and inadequate communication between the ICU MDs and patient/families about appropriate goals of care (29%)
Robinson and Heritage 2006	(S) Descriptive (P) Examine the relationship between MD opening questions and patient evaluations of MD communication (T) Urban and rural MD	Pre-/post-visit patient questionnaire and transcribed videotapes	n = 28 family practice MDs n = 142 patients	(1) Open-ended vs. closed-ended MD opening questions; (2) Socio-emotional Behavior subscale of Medical Interview Satisfaction Scale; (3)	Regression analyses found (1) SIG more positive evaluations of MD listening behavior (p = .02) and positive affective/relational communication (p = .05) with open-ended MD opening questions; (2) patients with longer visits evaluate MDs SIG less

Study	Characteristics	Sample	Measures	Results
	office (D) 2003–4 (C) US		transcripts coded for patient problem presentation, visit length	negatively (p = .04)
Ruiz-Moral, Perez Rodriguez, et al. 2006	(S) Qualitative (P) Explore MD specialist communication, and patients' perception of encounter (T) Outpatient surgical departments of 2 hospitals (D) Not reported (C) Spain	n = 27 specialty MDs; n = 257 patients	Recorded videotapes of clinical encounters through the GATHA-ESP scale, a coding questionnaire of 26 items, and postsurgical patient rating of encounter	(1) Presence or absence of 26 MD communicative behaviors; (2) patients rated quality of the interaction and their satisfaction with it in a questionnaire / Analysis of 26 MD behaviors found that most specialists use a "managerial" style where there is no exploration of their patients' emotions (22%); expectations (28%); or psychosocial aspects (8–20%). Less than one doctor out of every four ever gave the patient an opportunity to participate in any type of decision making at the surgery. MDs did not inform patients of causes or diagnosis (25%) or plan of care (37–57%); show an understanding of patients' feelings/emotions (51%); or verbally show empathy (55%). Patients were more satisfied with those encounters they felt were more patient-centered (p = <.001).
Safran, Karp, et al. 2006	(S) Descriptive (P) Test feasibility and value of measuring patients' experiences with individual PCPs (T) 5 commercial and 1 Medicaid health plan (D) May–August 2002 (C) US	n = 215 MDs; n = 9,625 patients: 9,053 commercial; 572 Medicaid	Ambulatory Care Experiences Survey administered to a statewide sample by mail and telephone, using a 5-stage data collection process	Survey produces 6 summary measures on the quality of PCP interactions including MD communication and interpersonal treatment / No SIG differences in MD communication found between commercial and Medicaid PCPs, with overall communication scoring 88.5% (MD: explain in a way that was easy to understand; listen carefully; clear instructions about problems or symptoms; and clear instructions if symptoms got worse). SIG differences in interpersonal treatment (MD: doctor treat with respect; caring and kind; and

TABLE 2.5—*Continued*

References	Study Design (S) Study Purpose (P) Study Setting (T) Study Date (D) Country (C)	Methods	Final Sample Size	Main Measures	Key Findings
					spend enough time) with overall rating 9.3%; commercial 9.4%; and Medicaid 88.7% ($p = .02$).
Tarn, Heritage, et al. 2006	(S) Descriptive (P) Measure the quality of MD communication when prescribing new medications. (T) 2 health care systems (D) January and November 1999 (C) US	Combination of patient and MD surveys with transcribed audiotaped office visits	$n = 45$ MDs: 16 family MDs, 18 internists, 11 cardiologists $n = 185$ patients receiving newly prescribed medications	5-point Medication Communication Index that gives points for MD communication about (1) medication name; (2) purpose or justification for taking the medication; (3) duration of use; (4) adverse effects; (5) number of tablets or sprays to be taken; (6) frequency or timing	MDs stated the specific medication name for 74% of new prescriptions; explained the purpose of the medication for 87%, duration of intake for 34%, number of tablets or sprays for 55%, frequency or timing of intake for 58%, and adverse effects for 35%. MDs fulfilled a mean of 3.1 of 5 expected elements of communication, 62% of necessary elements of new medication.
Abdulhadi, Shafaee, et al. 2007	(S) Qualitative (P) Identify patient perceptions of quality of MD patient interactions (T) Primary care (D) 2004 (C) Oman	Focus groups of type 2 diabetes patients	$n = 27$ patients	Description of emerging themes	6 themes identified: (1) patient-provider manner of communication, e.g., lack of encouraging the patients to ask questions or express their concerns; and lack of transfer of medical information; (2) inexperienced MDs and nurses; (3) long waiting time; (4) lack of continuity of care; (5) insufficient access to health

Study	Design/Purpose/Setting	Methods	Sample	Measures	Findings
					education; (6) patient barriers to good diabetes management. Authors suggest that improving health outcomes of type 2 diabetes may not be possible without improving MD-patient communication.
Davidson, Vogel, et al. 2007	(S) Qualitative (P) Determine how AHT adherence was addressed and identify areas for improvement (T) Community oncologist offices (D) June–August 2005 (C) US	Transcribed video- and audiotaped patient-oncologist interactions and video- and audio-taped follow-up interviews	$n = 14$ MDs $n = 28$ early-stage breast cancer patients	Conversations that addressed patient adherence to medication or framed the expected duration of therapy identified through linguistic analyses	25% of visit time was spent discussing AHT, but MDs did not address adherence with therapy or engage patient in a discussion of emotional or other barriers to continuing with therapy or taking therapy daily. No discussion took place explicitly linking adherence to "best outcomes" of therapy, and no MD discussed what to do if a dose was missed or asked patients if they foresaw any problems with adhering to therapy. Likely time on therapy (persistence) was mentioned in 43% (12/28) of visits but was usually framed as a discussion of "study results." Conversations did not involve patient views regarding the length of therapy, nor was it mentioned that staying on therapy for 5 years can be challenging for patients.
Nelson, Mercado, et al. 2007	(S) Descriptive (P) Identify information needs of chronic critical illness patients and extent to which needs	Survey using in-person questionnaire (4-point Likert scale) within 3 to 7 days after tracheotomy tapping 6 domains	$n = 2$ patients and 98 surrogates of patients undergoing	(1) Ratings of importance and reports (2) whether this information was communicated by the clinicians	While 78% of respondents rated information as important for decision making, they reported receiving no information for 9 of 18 items, with 95% of respondents reporting not

TABLE 2.5—*Continued*

References	Study Design (S) Study Purpose (P) Study Setting (T) Study Date (D) Country (C)	Methods	Final Sample Size	Main Measures	Key Findings
	are met (T) 5 adult ICUs in university-affiliated hospital (D) 2003 and 2005 (C) US	of information needs	tracheotomy for failure to wean from mechanical ventilation		receiving information for approximately one-quarter of the items. Subjects rated knowing their expected functional status at hospital discharge and prognosis for 1-year survival as important; however 80% reported receiving no information about functional status, and 93% reported receiving no information about prognosis.
Nelson M. and Hamilton 2007	(S) Qualitative (P) Identify best practices and gaps in communication (T) Community MD offices (D) March and April 2004 (C) US	Transcribed audiotapes of 32 MD-patient visits	n = 9 PCPs and 8 pulmonologists n = 32 COPD patients	Using Gumperz sociolinguistic methods, analysis of naturally occurring office interactions, with COPD best practices used as framework for analysis. Comparison to best practices treatment guidelines and identification of communication gaps	MDs used the nonspecific term "breathing" (56%) vs. explicit discussion of COPD; usual visit contained 6.4 MD-initiated, symptom-related questions, of which 57% (117 of 204) were general or about the nature of symptoms; 4 of 204 questions (2%) addressed the long-term frequency of symptoms; 38% of MD-patient pairs were misaligned (>2 points apart on a 1 to 10 scale) on disease severity, and 50% (16 of 29) on patients' level of concern about the disease; 10% (3 patients) reported never having had a smok-

Author, year	Study characteristics	Measures	Sample	Outcomes/purpose measures	Results
					ing-cessation discussion with their MD; spirometry, the "gold standard" for diagnosis and monitoring of respiratory disease, was not discussed by 31% of the MDs; HRQL discussions did not occur in 82% of visits, but 84% (24 of 28) of patients described the impact of COPD in their lives as making them dependent on others and limiting their activities; and 78% (7/9) patients starting inhalers did not receive demonstrations or instructions on how to use them
Oates, Sloane, et al. 2007	(S) Descriptive (P) Identify agreement between oncologists and cancer patients of current cancer status (T) VA outpatient medical oncology and radiation oncology clinics (D) 1999–2000 (C) US	Gero-Oncology Health and Quality of Life Assessment Instruments mailed to patients 2 weeks prior to visit and medical record data	$n = 149$ patients	Agreement between MDs' notation of current disease status and patients' concurrent report of the presence or absence of cancer	75.5% of patients who reported they currently had cancer had "no evidence of disease" by MD report; 95.7% of patients who reported they did not have cancer also had no active disease by MD report ($p = .0003$, $\kappa = .14$, poor agreement). Compared to patients with concordant responses, those who discrepantly reported they had cancer had SIG more co-morbid illnesses ($p = <.001$), medications ($p = .03$), and pain ($p = .03$), and lower levels of social ($p = .04$), emotional ($p = .007$), and physical functioning ($p = .03$).
Pollak, Arnold, et al. 2007	(S) Qualitative (P) Assess the prevalence	Transcribed audiotape conversations coded	$n = 51$ oncologists	Number of empathic opportunities and	In 398 conversations there were 292 empathic opportunities; 68% were

TABLE 2.5—*Continued*

References	Study Design (S) Study Purpose (P) Study Setting (T) Study Date (D) Country (C)	Methods	Final Sample Size	Main Measures	Key Findings
	and nature of empathic communication in cancer care (T) University and VA oncology clinics (D) Not reported (C) US	for presence of empathic opportunities and oncologist responses; physician survey	$n = 270$ patients with advanced cancer	empathic continuer responses	direct, and 33% were indirect. When patients initiated an empathic opportunity, oncologists responded with continuers in 27% of patient cases and terminators 73% of the time.
Wilson, Schoen, et al. 2007	(S) Descriptive (P) Determine the prevalence of MD-patient dialogue about medication use (T) Community (D) July–October 2003 (C) US	Cross-sectional survey, Medicare sampling data 5-stage mail/phone protocol	$n = 17,569$ persons aged 65 years or more	Query: (1) if MDs had asked about medications used; (2) if they had talked with any doctors about the medication cost; (3) or changing medicines because of side effects, efficacy, or cost	41% of seniors reported taking 5 or more prescription medications, and more than half had 2 or more prescribing MDs. 32% overall and 24% of those with 3 or more chronic conditions reported not having talked with their doctor about all their different medicines in the last 12 months. Of seniors reporting skipping doses or stopping a medication because of side effects or perceived nonefficacy, 27% had not talked with an MD about it. Of those reporting cost-related nonadherence, 39% had not talked with an MD about it.
AHRQ 2008	(S) Descriptive (P) Track patients' experiences with care in an	5th annual HHS national report on the state of health care quality	$n = 84,779$ hospital patients	Ambulatory adults: composite measure of percentage of adults	9.6% of adult patients reported poor communication with office or clinic visit in the last 12 months (2004).

	office or clinic and satisfaction with communication during a hospital stay (T) Ambulatory and hospitalized patients (D) 2000–2007 (C) US	using MEP, CAHPS, and H-CAHPS Surveys	n = ambulatory patients not reported	whose health providers sometimes or never listened carefully, explained things, showed respect, and spent enough time with them. Hospitalized patients: composite measure of percentage whose doctors sometimes or never showed courtesy or respect, listened carefully, and explained clearly.	Mean percentage of adults having an MD or clinic visit reporting poor communication decreased for the total population from 11.2%–9.6% (2000–2004). The mean percentages of adults with MD office or clinic visits who reported poor communication was lowest among adults 65 and over 2000–2004. In 2007, 6.1% of adult hospital patients reported poor communication with MDs; 22.9% poor communication about hospital discharge information; 27.1% poor communication about medications.
Audrey, Abel, et al. 2008	(S) Descriptive (P) Examine extent to which survival gain was discussed when patients were offered palliative chemotherapy (T) Oncology (D) Not reported (C) UK	Transcribed audiotapes and a nonparticipant observer to capture nonverbal communication. Transcripts analyzed using grounded theory.	n = 37 cancer patients	Treatment decisions and discussion of survival benefit	Although there was consistency in informing patients that a cure was not being sought, the amount of information given about survival benefit varied considerably. In 26 of 37 consultations discussion of survival benefit was either vague or nonexistent. No pattern was discerned by gender or age of the patient, hospital site, cancer site, treatment decision, or the actual survival of the patient. Authors suggest that to aid decision making and informed consent, oncologists should sensitively describe the benefits and limitations of this treatment, including survival gain.

TABLE 2.5—*Continued*

References	Study Design (S) Study Purpose (P) Study Setting (T) Study Date (D) Country (C)	Methods	Final Sample Size	Main Measures	Key Findings
Blendon, Buhr, et al. 2008	(S) Descriptive (P) Provide evidence for differences in perceived quality of MD care by ethnic minorities (T) Oncology (D) 2007 (C) US	Results from a 2007 Harvard School of Public Health/Robert Wood Johnson Foundation (RWJF) national survey of 14 minority ethnic subgroups	n = 4,334 randomly selected adults age 18 or older categorized into 15 race/ethnic groups	(1) MDs spent enough time; (2) MDs listened carefully; (3) MDs explained in an understandable way; (4) had problems communicating with their MD related to language or cultural differences; and (5) felt uncomfortable asking questions	(1) MD "very often" spent enough time with them, 7 minority groups SIG less likely (43%–56%) vs. white (66%); (2) MD "very often" listened carefully, 6 minority groups SIG (58%–63%) less likely vs. white (77%); (3) MD "very often" explained things, 6 minority groups SIG significantly less likely (55%–69%) vs. white (81%); (4) have had problems communicating, 8 minority groups SIG significantly more likely (21%–34%) vs. white (12%); (5) felt uncomfortable asking questions of MDs, 5 minority groups SIG more likely (15%–28%) vs. white (11%)
Dimoska, Butow, et al. 2008	(S) Qualitative (P) Analyze structure of the initial cancer consultation of medical and radiation oncologists (T) Oncology (D) Not reported	Pre-/post-patient questionnaires and transcribed audiotapes with CANCODE computer interaction analysis system	n = 5 medical oncologists and 4 radiation oncologists n = 155 cancer patients attending	(1) Patient anxiety, psychological adjustment, recall, and satisfaction; (2) duration and content of consultation	(1) Medical oncologists allowed patients/families more input (p = <.001) and were more patient-centered (p = <.001) vs. radiation oncologists; (2) radiation oncologists dominated the consultation vs. medical oncologists (p = <.05), but spent a longer period discussing and were

Study	Method	Sample	Focus	Findings
(C) Australia		their first out-patient con-sultation		more likely to bring up, social support issues with patients ($p = <.001$); (3) there was little psychosocial support offered by either medical (34 seconds) or radiation (43 seconds) MDs; (4) patients spent an average of 12 seconds (<1% of the consultation) expressing feelings or seeking reassurance; (5) multivariate analyses found MDs spoke longer if patient was female ($p = <.01$), greater patient anxiety ($p = <.05$), and higher patient education level ($p = <.001$). Authors conclude that both medical and radiation oncologists do not adequately address the psychosocial and support requirements of cancer patients.
Harding, Selman, et al. 2008	(S) Qualitative (P) Identify patient and caregiver communication needs (T) Cardiology (D) Not reported (C) UK	Transcribed, taped semi-structured interview	$n = 20$ congestive heart failure patients not yet seen by palliative care staff	Patient and caregiver needs	(1) Poor understanding of disease, symptom management, and disease progression; (2) confusion regarding implications of diagnosis; (3) no choices offered for managing future exacerbations; (4) MD lack of honesty about prognosis and clear explanations; (5) unclear about various MD role in providing care
Levin, Li, et al. 2008	(S) Descriptive (P Determine DNR utilization patterns as needs analysis for end-of-life communications train-	Retrospective medical record audit of DNR data 2000–2005	$n = 206{,}437$ patients	Documentation and date of DNR orders	In-hospital DNRs increased from 83% in 2000 to 86% in 2005 ($p = <.001$). There were SIG differences across gender (females > males, $p = .00001$), payer (commercial >

TABLE 2.5—*Continued*

References	Study Design (S) Study Purpose (P) Study Setting (T) Study Date (D) Country (C)	Methods	Final Sample Size	Main Measures	Key Findings
	ing (T) Palliative care (D) 2000–2005 (C) US				Medicaid > Medicare, $p = .00001$), and ethnic groups (Hispanic > Black > White, $p = .00001$). For patients who died out of hospital (e.g., hospice), DNR orders increased from 28% in 2000 to 52% in 2005 ($p = <.00001$). Inpatient adults signed 53% of DNRs, surrogates 34%. 63% had DNR signed on the day of death. The authors conclude that the proximity between signing and death may be a marker of delayed end-of-life palliative care and suboptimal doctor-patient communication.
Ling, Trauth, et al. 2008	(S) Descriptive (P Assess the quality of CRC screening discussions based on an Informed Decision Making Model (T) Primary care, VA hospital outpatient clinic (D) 2001–4 (C) US	Transcribed audiotape of clinic visit	$n = 24$ primary care providers, 9 internal medicine faculty MDs, and 5 nurse practitioners $n = 135$ patients	Discussion of (1) patient's role; (2) patient's role in decision making; (3) nature of the decision to be made; (4) alternatives; (5) pros and cons of the alternatives; (6) uncertainties associated with the decision; assessment of (7)	No information decision making elements addressed (50%); nature of the decision (44%); discussion of uncertainties (6%), pros and cons (17%), assessment of patient understanding (6%), inquiring about input from trusted others (1%), and discussion of the patient's role in the decision making (1%). There was no association between race, age, and education level with the occurrence

| Morse, Edwardsen, et al. 2008 | (S) Qualitative (P) Evaluate empathic opportunities and MD responses (T) VA hospital (D) 2001–4 (C) US | Transcribed audiotapes | n = 9 MDs n = 20 oncology or thoracic surgery patients; 10 black and 10 white | patient's understanding; (8) patient's desire for input from trusted others; (9) patient preference Coding on emerging content patterns using the grounded theory method and thematic analysis | of any particular IDM element. The median number of IDM elements addressed was 1. MDs responded empathically to 39/384 empathic opportunities (10%), often shifting to biomedical questions and statements. When empathy was provided, 50% of these statements occurred in the last one-third of the encounter, whereas patients' concerns were evenly raised throughout the encounter. No SIG difference by race; oncologists SIG more likely than surgeons to respond empathically (p = .02). |

ALS = amyotrophic lateral sclerosis
AHT = adjuvant hormonal therapy
CAHPS = Consumer Assessment of Healthcare Providers and Systems CANCODE = computerized interaction analysis system with established reliability and validity
CRC = colorectal cancer
DNR = Do Not Resuscitate
ES = effect size
GP(s) = general practitioner
MD = physician

H-CAHPS = Hospital Consumer Assessment of Healthcare Providers and Systems
HHS = U.S. Department of Health and Human Services
HRQL = health-related quality of life
HTN = hypertension
ICU = intensive care unit
MEP = Medical Expenditure Panel Survey
MSA = metropolitan statistical area(s)
OR = odds ratio
PCAS = Primary Care Assessment Survey

PDM = physician's participatory decision-making style
QOC = Quality of Communication questionnaire
RIAS = Roter Interaction Analysis System, method of coding doctor-patient interaction using frequency counts of communication "utterances"
SIG = significant(ly)
UK = United Kingdom
VA = Veterans Affairs

3 | How Does Physician Communication Affect Patients?

The research findings described in chapter 2 identified elements of physician communication that appear problematic and, therefore, where there appears to be room for improvement. But by themselves, these findings are not sufficient to support the expenditure of resources on specific improvement efforts. In addition, decision makers need to know if weak physician performance relating to a particular element of communication has significant impacts on patients. In the sense we use it here, the term *significant* means that the relationship is strong (passing conventional statistical significance tests or receiving consistent support in rigorous analyses of qualitative data) and that the effects on patients are large enough, potentially, to merit efforts to improve physician communication skills.

Identifying Relevant Literature

To identify the literature reviewed in this chapter, we used the same search strategy described in chapter 2. We did not include studies related to multifaceted interventions or patient health literacy unless they had a substantial component directed at physician communication issues. We found 11 review articles and 21 individual studies (not included in review articles) specifically relating to the relationship between physician communication and patient outcomes (see tables 3.1 and 3.2). This topic also was addressed selectively in several of the review articles and studies summarized in tables 2.4 and 2.5. We have organized our discussion of findings according to type of patient outcome: immediate, intermediate, and longer-term (see fig. 1.1, logic model). We summarize findings from both review articles and individual studies pertaining to each type of outcome. Because review articles typically address a variety of outcomes, some review articles are cited under more than one category of outcome. In the case of both review and individual articles, we also refer to relevant articles summarized in tables 2.4 and 2.5.

Immediate Outcomes

By "immediate" outcomes, we mean outcomes that occur very soon after the physician-patient encounter. For example, these outcomes include relief of anxiety, satisfaction with the visit, and understanding of the treatment plan. In the literature we reviewed, satisfaction with the visit was the most common measure employed, by a substantial margin.

Evidence from Reviews. Stewart (1995) (see table 3.1) reviewed 21 studies published between 1983 and 1993 where "communication" was classified as history taking, discussion of the management plan, or "other." Stewart found that where physicians asked questions about a patient's anxiety level and feelings and showed support and empathy, patient anxiety levels were reduced. The same was true when patients were encouraged to ask questions and physicians were willing to share decision making. Beck, Daughtridge, et al. (2002) reviewed 22 studies where neutral observers were used to assess physician communication. They reported that 22 verbal behaviors of physicians were positively associated with patient outcomes, while 14 verbal behaviors were negatively associated with outcomes (see table 3.1). Immediate outcomes affected by verbal behaviors included short-term patient recall, trust in the physician, intention to comply with physician recommendations, and satisfaction with the encounter. Nonverbal physician behaviors also were found to affect immediate outcomes, but there was less evidence in this regard. Overall, Beck, Daughtridge, et al. (2002) concluded that there is a relative lack of research that uses researcher observations and links verbal and nonverbal physician behaviors to patient outcomes. Ong, de Haes, et al. (1995) reported that physician information-giving behaviors were significantly related to patient satisfaction. They also found that physician "patient-centeredness," understood as physicians allowing patients to express all of their reasons for visiting the physician, was associated with patient resolution of issues (see table 3.1).

Evidence from Individual Studies In one individual study, Adams, Smith, et al. (2001) (see table 3.2) used surveys of asthma patients conducted at three-month intervals to track health outcomes and relate them to a measure of shared physician-patient decision making. They found that a greater degree of shared decision making was associated with greater patient satisfaction. In a study set in the United Kingdom, Little, Everitt, et al. (2001) surveyed patients in three practices regarding their perceptions of physician "patient centeredness" along with several immediate outcome measures. They found that patients of physicians who exhibited less "patient centeredness" were less satisfied, felt less enabled to carry out the treatment plan, and experienced a greater symptom burden (see table 3.2).

Intermediate Outcomes

The intermediate outcomes most commonly addressed in the studies we reviewed were adherence to treatment plans and biologic markers of disease status (e.g., hemoglobin A1c readings for diabetic patients).

Evidence from Reviews.   Stewart (1995) found a relationship between physician communication and symptom resolution, physiologic measures, and pain control (see table 3.1). Beck, Daughtridge, et al. (2002) reported that physician verbal behaviors were related to intermediate compliance with treatment plans (see table 3.1). However, in their review, Ong, de Haes, et al (1995) concluded that the relationship between physician communication and adherence to treatment plans was weak (see table 3.1).

Evidence from Individual Studies.   Several individual studies (see table 3.2) have addressed the relationship between physician communication and intermediate outcomes. For instance, Heisler, Bouknight, et al. (2002) analyzed patient survey responses for individuals with diabetes, finding that better physician communication was related to more effective self-management of this chronic disease. Little, Everitt, et al. (2001) concluded, based on observations in three general practices in the United Kingdom, that a positive approach on the part of physicians was associated with reduced symptom burden among patients after one month. Safran, Montgomery, et al. (2001) examined the impact of physician communication on an indirect measure of patient satisfaction, disenrollment from a physician's practice. They found that a composite measure of the physician-patient relationship (communication, interpersonal trust, knowledge of patient, and patient trust) was a significant predictor of disenrollment. Schneider, Kaplan, et al. (2004) estimated the association between measures of the physician-patient relationship and adherence to antiretroviral therapies for persons with HIV infections. In multivariate models, they found that six of seven physician-patient relationship variables were associated with the degree of patient medication adherence. They concluded that improving the quality of physician-patient relationships is a promising approach to improving medication adherence. Stewart, Meredith, et al. (2000) found that physician communication was an important factor in explaining adherence to therapy among older patients.

Longer-Term Outcomes

Longer-term outcomes refer, primarily, to measures of patient health status and, secondarily, to measures of utilization and costs that, while important in their own right, also can be interpreted as proxies for health status in some cases (e.g., use of the hospital emergency department).

Evidence from Reviews. In her review, Stewart (1995) found evidence of a relationship between physician communication and emotional health. Di Blasi, Harkness, et al. (2001) concluded, based on their literature review, that positive physician communication about the patient's illness and treatment improved health outcomes (see table 3.1). Ong, de Hayes, et al. (1995) also found relationships between physician communication and patient health status and psychiatric morbidity, but they suggested that little was known (at the time of the review) about the relationship between physician communication and patients' longer-term health outcomes (see table 3.1).

Evidence from Individual Studies. A relatively large number of individual studies (see table 3.2) addressed the relationship between physician communication and a variety of different long-term health outcomes. Among cancer patients, Ong, Visser, et al. (2000) found that global satisfaction was "best predicted by information-giving by their doctor" (152). However, in their study, a physician's "verbal attentiveness" was associated with a lower level of patient global satisfaction—a result they characterize as "peculiar and unexpected" (152)—and physician "patient-centeredness" also was negatively related to global satisfaction. Adams, Smith, et al. (2001), analyzing cross-sectional data for people with asthma, found that the score of physicians on a measure of "participatory decision-making style" was associated with better patient quality of life and less work disability and need for acute care services. Epstein, Franks, et al. (2005) found that overall expenditures were higher for patients of physicians who had lower (worse) scores on a measure of "patient-centered communication." Visit length was higher for these patients, but diagnostic testing expenditures were lower. In a study set in Germany, Neumann, Wirtz, et al. (2007)

found that physicians with greater patient empathy were better at conveying information to patients and that this had a preventive effect on depression and improved patient quality of life. Focusing on patients with depression, van Os, van den Brink, et al. (2005) concluded that an accurate diagnosis and adequate treatment resulted in better patient outcomes, but only when physicians demonstrated good communication skills.

Conclusions

The literature on the link between physician communication and patient outcomes is impressive in its scope. However, there are areas where more evidence clearly would be useful for decision makers. Moreover, there are methodological issues that suggest caution in interpreting study results. For example, in assessing the implications of their analysis combining different types of data, Franks, Jerant, et al. (2006) note that the relationships they found between patient perceptions of their physicians and patient outcomes probably did not reflect physician communication style so much as unmeasured patient characteristics. This is likely a concern in other studies as well. The relatively small number of studies that address the relationship between physician communication and utilization of services or costs also would appear to be an important shortcoming of the published literature. As we discuss in chapter 7, advocates for interventions to improve physician communication skills may increasingly be called on to document the financial "rate of return" for such programs, even though this was not an objective in the studies we reviewed.

TABLE 3.1.   Evidence from Review Studies That Physician Communication Affects Health Outcomes, Utilization, or Costs of Care (*n* = 11)

Reference	Review Type (R) / Number of Studies (N) / Study Setting (S) / Study Purpose (P) / Study Dates (D)	Key Findings
Ong, de Haes, et al. 1995	(R) Focused (N) Not reported (S) Not reported (P) To identify purposes of medical communication, measurement of MD-patient communication, specific communicative behaviors, and effect of MD communication on patient outcomes (D) Not reported	Review of studies related to patient satisfaction, adherence to treatment, patient recall and understanding, and health outcomes found that patients were frequently dissatisfied with the information they received (2 studies) and that this had remained constant over 25 years (3 studies); MD affective behavior (3 studies) and information giving (1 study) was important to patient satisfaction, with an MD dominant, controlling style producing less satisfaction (1 study) while behaviors such as using the patient's first name, attempting to establish privacy during an examination, a series of routine social skills (e.g., sitting down while talking to the patient, not interrupting), identifying future tests/treatments, and discussing plans were associated with higher satisfaction (1 study); patient centeredness, where patients were allowed to express reasons for coming (symptoms, feelings, thoughts, and expectations), was related to patient satisfaction and patients' feeling of being understood, resolution of patient concerns, and the doctor having ascertained patients' reasons for coming (3 studies); patient knowledge about illness and acceptance of a treatment plan were associated with greater compliance (3 studies); patient recall of information was best predicted by MDs' information giving behaviors (eye contact, physical closeness); and more MD information giving was related to better patient health status (1 study), and lack of information played an important role in psychological difficulties that can arise during cancer diagnosis and treatment such as uncertainty, anxiety, depression, and problems with coping (8 studies)
Stewart 1995	(S) Systematic review (N) 21 studies, 11 RCTs and 10 analytic (S) MD offices and hospitals (P) Determine if quality of MD-patient communica-	16 studies found positive results; 4 nonsignificant results; 1 inconclusive. Patient health outcomes were measured by physiologic status, functional status, symptom resolution, and emotional status. Communication classified as relevant either to history taking, discussion of the management plan, or other. **Related to history taking:** 4 RCTs mea-

TABLE 3.1—*Continued*

Reference	Review Type (R) Number of Studies (N) Study Setting (S) Study Purpose (P) Study Dates (D)	Key Findings
	tion makes a significant difference to patient health outcomes (D) 1983–93	sured adult patient outcomes of MD interventions; SIG effects of communication elements: asking questions about patient's understanding of the problem, about concerns and expectations, and about patient perception of problem impact on function (decreased anxiety level $p = <.001$, and symptom resolution $p = <.05$); asking patient about feelings (decrease in psychological stress at 2 weeks $p = <.05$); showing support and empathy (reduced psychological distress $p = <.05$); and symptom resolution ($p = <.05$). **Related to management plan:** In 7 RCTs and 5 analytic studies communication elements found to SIG impact health outcomes included (1) patient is encouraged to ask more questions (less anxiety $p = <.05$; less role limitation and physical limitation in 3 studies $p = <.005$, $p = <.05$, $p = <.05$); (2) patient is successful at obtaining information (improved functional status $p = <.005$, $p = <.02$ and improved physiologic status $p = <.05$ for blood pressure and $p = <.05$ for GlyHb in 2 studies); (3) patient is provided with information programs and packages (less pain $p = <.05$, improved function $p = <.025$, and lower mood and anxiety scores $p = <.05$); MD gives clear information along with emotional support (less psychological distress $p = <.05$, symptom resolution $p = <.05$, and lower blood pressure $p = <.05$); (4) MD is willing to share decision making (lower patient anxiety $p = <.01$); and (5) MD and patient agree about the nature of the problem and the need for follow-up (problem and symptom resolution at 1 month $p = <.001$). **Health outcomes affected:** emotional health, symptom resolution, function, blood pressure and blood sugar level, and pain control.
Stewart, Meredith, et al. 2000	(R) Focused review (N) Not reported (S) Not reported (P) Review process, short-term, intermediate, and long-term outcomes of MD-patient communica-	Article highlights lack of evidence in MD-patient communication outcomes in the older population, especially physical health outcomes. Communication was found to be the most important factor in determining adherence to treatment, with less time spent with the patient discussing issues one of the strongest predictors of lower adherence (1

TABLE 3.1—*Continued*

Reference	Review Type (R) Number of Studies (N) Study Setting (S) Study Purpose (P) Study Dates (D)	Key Findings
	tion in the older adult (D) Not reported	study). Less patient knowledge of a medication and its purpose was SIG associated with lower adherence (1 study) while discussion of shared responsibility and roles between the patient and the MD was positively associated with adherence (1 study). Overall there is extensive evidence to support the notion that when the quality of MD communication is rated highly, patients are more likely to be satisfied with their medical care (1 review of 21 studies and 2 individual studies). Patient satisfaction has been shown to influence patient adherence to a medical regimen (2 studies), especially in older patients (1 study). In this study, MDs' expectations of the older patient were conveyed (verbally or nonverbally) to the patient and this affected both compliance and satisfaction and subsequently adherence to the treatment plan. MDs' interpersonal, affective style is more important with older patients in determining satisfaction than the actual subjects discussed (2 studies). The emotional health of the older patient can be influenced by the attitude of the physician (4 studies). Information giving and discussion, especially in palliative care and counseling on advanced directives, decreases patient negative affect (e.g., anxiety) (2 studies). Reference to Stewart 1995, above, for adult studies on communication and health outcomes.
Di Blasi, Harkness, et al. 2001	(R) Systematic, 11 dB (N) n = 25 RCTs (S) Outpatient medical and dental care (P) Identify aspects of the doctor-patient relationship that impacted objective or subjective health status (D) Not reported	Using the model that when threatened by signs and symptoms of illness, individuals respond with cognitive and emotional reactions, 25 studies were divided into cognitive care (the ways by which practitioners can influence patients' beliefs about the effects of treatment) and emotional care (ways through which health professionals can lower unhelpful emotions such as fear or anxiety by providing support, empathy, reassurance, and warmth). No trial examined the effects of emotional care alone. The most frequently investigated clinical disorders were hypertension (n = 8) and pain (n = 6). No studies included an economic evaluation.

TABLE 3.1—*Continued*

Reference	Review Type (R) Number of Studies (N) Study Setting (S) Study Purpose (P) Study Dates (D)	Key Findings
		12/25 trials found patient-practitioner interactions to have a significant influence on health outcomes. 10/19 trials found that practitioners who attempted to influence patients' beliefs about the effects of therapy (e.g., a firm diagnosis or clear expectations for testing) had a significant impact on patients' health outcomes. 4 trials examined the influence of combining cognitive care (i.e., giving patients a clear diagnosis, a positive prognosis, or raising treatment expectations) with emotional care (i.e., being warm and friendly or firm and reassuring) and were found to be significantly more effective than neutral consultations in decreasing pain and increasing the speed of recovery.
Beck, Daughtridge, et al. 2002	(R) Systematic review of studies using neutral observers, 2 dB (N) *n* = 22 studies (S) PCP office (P) Determine which verbal and nonverbal MD behaviors have been linked in empirical studies with favorable patient outcomes (D) 1975–2000	14 studies of verbal communication and 8 studies of nonverbal communication. Measures included short-term (patient recall, satisfaction, intention to comply, and trust); intermediate (compliance); and long-term (symptom resolution, health status, quality of life, and mortality) outcomes. 22 verbal behaviors found to be positively associated with health outcomes in individual studies: empathy; patient-centered behavior; allowing the patient's point of view to guide the conversation; explaining at conclusion of visit; a predominantly passive MD; patient encouragement; provider laughing and joking as a tension release; addressing problems of daily living, social relations, feelings, and patient emotions; asking about and counseling for psychosocial issues; health education; sharing medical data with the patient; discussing treatment effects; friendliness; courtesy; listening; summarizing, talking at the patient's level, and clarifying statements; a more dominant MD; orienting the patient during the physical examination; increased encounter length; and more time spent on history taking. 14 verbal behaviors found to be negatively associated with health outcomes in individual studies: passive acceptance, negative social-emotional interactions, formal behavior, antagonism and passive rejection; high rates

TABLE 3.1—*Continued*

Reference	Review Type (R) Number of Studies (N) Study Setting (S) Study Purpose (P) Study Dates (D)	Key Findings
		of biomedical questioning; interruptions; a one-way information flow from the patient to the provider; antagonistic behavior; directive behavior; utterances concerning the patient's experience or showing interest in the patient; irritation; nervousness; extensive feedback given in the concluding part of the visit; anxiety or tension; dominance; directiveness; and expression of opinion during the physical examination. Nonverbal behaviors associated with favorable outcomes included less mutual gaze; head nodding of the provider; forward lean; more direct body orientation; uncrossed legs and arms; and arm symmetry. Nonverbal behaviors associated with unfavorable outcomes included more patient gaze; body orientation 45 to 90 degrees away from the patient; indirect body orientation; backward lean; crossed arms; task touch and frequent touch. Authors conclude that existing research is limited because of lack of consensus of what to measure, conflicting findings, and relative lack of empirical studies, especially of nonverbal behavior.
Mead and Bower 2002	(R) Systematic review, 2 dB (N) $n = 9$ studies (S) Primary care (P) Identify definitions and measurement of patient-centered care and its association with outcomes (D) 1969–2000	All studies used nonexperimental designs; 5/9 used univariate analysis; the most frequently reported outcome was patient satisfaction; there was no consistent measure of MD patient-centered behaviors. In univariate studies there was a SIG association between MD patient-centered behaviors and compliance ($p = <.05$) (1 study); and SIG negative associations between MDs' controlling statements and self-reported compliance, between compliance and patients' submissive statements followed by MDs' initiated controlling statements, and between satisfaction and MDs' controlling statements followed by patients' accepting statements (1 study). There was no association between patient rating of MD patient-centered behaviors and patient satisfaction (1 study), a SIG association between observer rating of MD patient

TABLE 3.1—*Continued*

Reference	Review Type (R) Number of Studies (N) Study Setting (S) Study Purpose (P) Study Dates (D)	Key Findings
		centeredness (1 study), and both a SIG and non-SIG association depending on the patient centeredness measure used (1 study). In multivariate analyses, MD patient centeredness was not SIG associated with health or utilization outcomes, but patient perception scores were SIG related to reduced levels of discomfort, concern, better mental health scores, and fewer diagnostic tests and referrals (1 study). There was an association with satisfaction but not with resolution of symptoms or concerns, or functional health status (1 study); no association with satisfaction (2 studies), with one of these studies reporting an association between patient perceptions and reduced level of concern. Authors conclude that the key problem is lack of a theoretical framework linking specific dimensions of patient-centered care with specific outcomes.
Arora 2003	(R) Not reported (N) Not reported (S) Not reported (P) To describe key elements of MD behavior, measurement of MD communication behavior, and relationship of MD communication behavior with cancer patient health outcomes (D) Not reported	9 studies of patients with breast cancer and 3 on patients with mixed cancer diagnoses found a beneficial effect of MD behavior on patient outcomes: patients offered treatment choice and greater decisional control experienced reduced anxiety and depression, improved physical functioning, and higher levels of QoL (6 studies); patients who had their questions answered during the initial consultation showed better psychological adjustment at post-visit follow-up (1 study); patients reported a positive relationship between MD behavior (information exchange and interpersonal skills) during the diagnostic consultation and psychological outcome (1 study); psychological distress in early stage breast cancer was associated with difficulty asking questions, expressing feelings, and understanding imparted information (1 study); a positive relationship between more compassionate MD behavior (e.g., providing reassurance, touching the patient's hand, expressing support) and reduced patient anxiety (1 study); patients whose MD's affective tone was rated as angry or irritated reported greater physical and psychological distress and

TABLE 3.1—*Continued*

Reference	Review Type (R) Number of Studies (N) Study Setting (S) Study Purpose (P) Study Dates (D)	Key Findings
		those whose MD had an anxious or nervous tone reported lower global QoL (1 study); and patient rated MD interpersonal manner, information exchange, and decision-making style, associated with changes in patients' anxiety levels from pre- to post-consultation (1 study).
		Authors conclude with recommendations for future research in the areas of conceptual refinement, measurement, and study design.
Michie, Miles, et al. 2003	(R) Systematic, 5 dB (N) n = 30 studies (S) Chronic illness (P) Examine the relationship between the quality of health care professional–patient communication and outcome in chronic illness (D) 1975–99	In 30 studies of patient-centered consultations (3 RCTs, 2 nonrandomized experimental studies, 4 longitudinal [no control group], 16 cross-sectional, 1 descriptive, and 4 qualitative designs), authors determined whether the distinctive concepts (1) the ability to elicit and discuss patients' beliefs (patient perspective) and (2) the ability to activate the patient to take control in the consultation and/or in the management of their illness (patient activation) are differentially associated with health outcomes in chronically ill patients. Of 20 patient perspective studies, 10 used satisfaction, 8 adherence, 9 a physical health outcome, and 2 quality of life as an outcome. In 10 patient activation studies, 2 used satisfaction, 7 adherence, and 7 physical health as an outcome.
		Patient activation (10 studies) is more consistently associated with good physical health outcomes than is patient perspective (20 studies), although there is no difference between the two styles in their association with patient adherence. The authors suggest that supporting patients' independence to manage their own illnesses may lead to a management treatment plan that is structured around the individual patient's lifestyle and beliefs and therefore more likely to produce good health outcomes.
van Dam, van der Horst, et al. 2003	(R) Systematic, 4 dB (N) n = 8 RCTs (S) Hospital and general practice outpatient dia-	4 studies targeting provider consulting behavior modifications; 4 targeting patient behavior changes. Provider targeted interventions tabled here: Study 1: GP (n = 47) and nurse (n = 60)

TABLE 3.1—*Continued*

Reference	Review Type (R) Number of Studies (N) Study Setting (S) Study Purpose (P) Study Dates (D)	Key Findings
	betes care (P) Identify effective provider consulting behavior on diabetic patient health behavior, self-care, and health outcomes (D) 1980–2001	training for patient-centered consulting style did not improve patient (n = 250) self-care, lifestyle, or diabetes control (GlyHb p = .31); did improve patient reported care process and patient satisfaction; and weight and lipid control and diabetes knowledge scores worsened slightly. Study 2: Trained diabetes nurses in the above study delivered better patient-reported diabetes care and had more satisfied patients, but judged their own results, capacities, and patient satisfaction as more negative vs. control nurses. Study 3: GP (n = 18) and nurse (n = 31) training for patient-centered consulting style, at 2-year follow-up, did not improve patient (n = 252) diabetes control (p = .3), self-care, lifestyle, complications, or satisfaction; 19% of the trained providers sustained behavior change. Study 4: 970 GPs in 311 practices supported to negotiate realistic individual goal setting with patients and to improve follow-up and diabetes treatment by prompting, guidelines, feedback, and education; at 6 years, study found improved quality of diabetes care, risk factor scores (weight, BP, lipids), and diabetes control (GlyHb p = .0001); no change in number of complications, mortality, health behavior, and general health. Authors conclude that MD interventions are hard to sustain, need intensive support, and are not effective in improving patient self-care and health outcomes when executed alone.
Thorne, Bultz, et al. 2005	(R) Not reported (N) Not reported (S) Oncology patients (P) Analysis of the impact of ineffective communication (D) Not reported	(Note Thorne, Bultz, et al. 2005 review of poor communication found in table 2.4) Evidence on the financial costs of poor communication is scant. One study found that unresolved emotional issues were associated with 5 times greater use of health services, complementary medicine, and third and fourth line chemotherapy; and twice the rate of emergency department use. However, cost studies on poor communication associated with unnecessary psychosocial distress have not produced consistent results. Data from 3 intervention studies showed that the measurable benefits were not

TABLE 3.1—*Continued*

Reference	Review Type (R) Number of Studies (N) Study Setting (S) Study Purpose (P) Study Dates (D)	Key Findings
		cost justified. However, a meta-analysis of 91 medical-cost-offset studies related to psychological intervention found a significant reduction in utilization of medical services; and a study of health plan billings found a reduction of over 20% at 2-year follow-up for breast cancer patients receiving a cognitive-behavioral psychosocial group compared to a nonintervention group. Poor communication can be associated with unnecessary treatment (e.g., aggressive late stage treatment and frequent use of futile procedures) as well as increased use of complementary and alternative medicine. One survey of health professionals ($n = 1,326$) found that severe communication problems occurred in the assessment of 40% of late stage cancer patients. In another study, although the use of chemotherapy in advanced cancers accounted for no improvement in survival rates, its use had the potential to produce a 100% overall care cost differential. Indirect costs to the health care system include high stress and burnout levels among cancer clinicians (7 reports). Reports have also suggested clinical communication breakdown is increased as a result of managed care, which shifts the role of health care team members and fragments care, as well as can lead to inadequate resource utilization such as advanced care directives and ethical consultation.
Roter, Frankel, et al. 2006	(R) Focused review (N) Not reported (S) Medical visits (P) Review MD expression of emotion through nonverbal behavior in the medical encounter (D) Not reported	There is little research on MDs' emotional self-awareness and ability to judge patients' emotions accurately (compared to patient ratings) and direct evidence linking physicians' nonverbal communication and health consequences is limited. Patient satisfaction is the outcome most frequently studied related to MD nonverbal behavior. MDs more skilled on the expressive task of emotional encoding were rated by patients as listening more and being more caring and sensitive than other doctors, MDs who were more accurate at de-

TABLE 3.1—*Continued*

Reference	Review Type (R) Number of Studies (N) Study Setting (S) Study Purpose (P) Study Dates (D)	Key Findings
		coding body movements received higher satisfaction ratings from their patients, and patients whose MDs who were better able to decode voice tone cues were less likely to cancel medical appointments (3 studies). Nonverbal MD behaviors also were associated with patient satisfaction (1 review and 3 studies), adherence to treatment (1 study), appointment keeping (1 study), and switching doctors (1 study).

CAM = complementary and alternative medicine
n = number
dB = database(s)

GlyHb = glycosolated hemoglobin
PCP = primary care physician
QoL = quality of life
RCT = randomized control trial

TABLE 3.2. Evidence from Empirical Studies That Physician Communication Affects Health Outcomes, Utilization, or Costs of Care ($n = 22$)

Reference	Study Design (S) Study Purpose (P) Study Setting (T) Study Date (D) Country (C)	Method	Final Sample Size	Main Measures	Key Findings
Ong, Visser, et al. 2000	(S) Qualitative (P) Investigate relationship between MD and patient communication and patient outcomes (T) Oncology, outpatient (D) Not reported (C) Netherlands	Transcribed audiotapes of initial visit coded using computerized RIAS, with outcomes measured by mailed questionnaire at 1 week and 3 months	$n = 11$ MD oncologists $n = 96$ cancer patients	Patient: (1) physical distress; (2) psychological distress; (3) quality of life; (4) visit satisfaction; (5) global satisfaction with communication	Correlates of MD communication with outcomes at 1 week: (1) physical distress, MD anger ($r = .21$, $p = .05$); (2) psychological distress, MD anger ($r = .21$, $p < .05$); (3) quality of life, MD anxiety ($r = .23$, $p < .05$); (4) visit satisfaction, MD friendliness ($r = .24$, $p < .01$); global satisfaction, MD anger ($r = .27$, $p < .01$). Correlates of MD communication with outcomes at 3 months: (1) physical distress, no correlates; (2) psychological distress, no correlates; (3) quality of life, no correlates; (4) visit satisfaction, MD social behavior ($r = .30$, $p < .01$), interest ($r = .23$, $p = <.05$), and friendliness ($r = .27$, $p = <.05$); global satisfaction, MD information giving ($r = .31$, $p = <.01$) and verbal attentiveness ($r = .24$, $p = <.01$). Predictors of MD communication at 1 week: (1) physical distress, MD anger SIG ($p = .05$); (2) psychological distress, MD anger SIG ($p = <.05$); (3) quality of life, MD anxiety

83

TABLE 3.2—*Continued*

Reference	Study Design (S) Study Purpose (P) Study Setting (T) Study Date (D) Country (C)	Method	Final Sample Size	Main Measures	Key Findings
					SIG (p = <.05); (4) visit satisfaction, MD friendliness SIG (p = <.01) and MD anger SIG (p = <.05); global satisfaction, MD anger SIG (p = <.01). Predictors of MD communication at 3 months on (1) physical distress, no effect; (2) psychological distress, no effect; (3) quality of life, patient centeredness SIG (p = <.05); (4) visit satisfaction, MD social behavior SIG (p = <.01); (5) global satisfaction MD information giving SIG (p = <.01). MD communication during visits consisted of almost 2.5 times cure-oriented vs. care-oriented behaviors. Analyses found a moderate negative correlation (r = .24, p = <.05) between MD patient centeredness and global satisfaction at 3 months.
Adams, Smith, et al. 2001	(S) Descriptive (P) Identify factors of MD involvement of asthma patients in care and effect on outcomes (T) Pulmonary clinic, uni-	Mail surveys sent at baseline and subsequently at 3-month intervals Data for analysis come from the 12-month follow-up survey	128 adults with moderate to severe asthma under care for 1 year or more	(1) PDM on 5-point Likert scale; (2) Short Form-36 Health Survey; (3) Marks Asthma Quality of Life Questionnaire	Mean PDM was 72 with higher score indicating greater participatory style. PDM SIG correlated (p = .0001) with longer office visits, longer MD-patient relationship, and patient satisfaction. PDM style SIG

Study	Design/Purpose	Intervention/Measures	Sample	Findings
versity teaching hospital (D) 1995–97 (C) Australia				associated with possession of a written asthma action plan (p = .0001), fewer days absent from work (p = .0001), better clinical asthma status (p = .001), higher self-ratings of health status (p = .001), and need for asthma-related acute health-care services (adjusted OR for any hospitalization 2.0, for rehospitalization 2.5).
Little, Everitt, et al. 2001	(S) Descriptive (P) To measure patients' perceptions of patient centeredness and their relationship to outcomes (D) Not reported (T) 3 GP offices (C) UK	Pre-post visit surveys based on the 5 main domains of the patient-centered model: exploring the disease and illness experience, understanding the whole person, finding common ground, health promotion, and enhancing the GP-patient relationship	n = 661 patients	Patient enablement, satisfaction, and burden of symptoms Factor analysis identified 5 components of patient ratings: communication and partnership; personal relationship; health promotion; positive approach; and interest in effect on patient's life. SIG predictors of satisfaction were patients' perceptions of communication and partnership (p = <.001) and a positive doctor approach (p = <.001). Global rating of satisfaction (on a 7-point Likert scale) also showed communication and partnership is the strongest predictor of satisfaction (p = <.001). SIG predictors of enablement were patients' perceptions of the doctor's interest in the effect of the problem on life (p = .001) and health promotion (p = <.001) and a positive approach (p = <.001). A positive approach was SIG associated with less symptom burden (p = .004) and

TABLE 3.2—Continued

Reference	Study Design (S) Study Purpose (P) Study Setting (T) Study Date (D) Country (C)	Method	Final Sample Size	Main Measures	Key Findings
					a personal approach with greater symptom burden at 1 month (p = .001). Referrals were fewer if patients felt they had a personal relationship with their doctor (OR = .70), and if expectations of a personal relationship were not met, referrals were more likely (OR = 1.41). Authors conclude that patients want a patient centered and positive approach, and if MDs do not provide it, patients are less satisfied, less enabled, may have greater symptom burden and use more health service resources.
Safran, Montgomery, et al. 2001	(S) Descriptive (P) Evaluate interpersonal and structural features of care as predictors of patients' voluntary disenrollment from PCP practice (T) Community (D) 1996, 1999 (C) US	Longitudinal statewide survey	n = 4,108 Massachusetts employees enrolled in one of 12 health plans	(1) 4 measures of the quality of MD-patient relations (communication, interpersonal treatment, MD knowledge of the patient, trust); (2) 4 structural measures of care (access, visit-based continuity, relationship	22% of patients voluntarily left their PCPs during the study period. When tested independently, all 8 scales SIG predicted voluntary disenrollment (p = < .001), with larger effects associated with the 4 relationship quality measures. In multivariable models, a composite relationship quality factor most strongly and SIG predicted voluntary disenrollment

				Measures	Results
				duration, integration of care)	(OR = 1.6, p = <.001); and the 2 continuity scales, visit-based continuity and relationship duration, also SIG predicted disenrollment (OR = 1.1, p = <.05).
Heisler, Bouknight, et al. 2002	(S) Descriptive (P) Assess impact of different patient-MD interaction styles on patients' diabetes self-management (T) 25 VA medical centers (D) Not reported (C) US	Survey 80 patients in each of 25 facilities	n = 1,314 patients having received care for diabetes	Patient ratings of (1) MD's PDM style, 4-item scale; (2) PCOM provider communication, 5-item scale; (3) overall self-management scale, 5-item scale; (4) patient understanding, 6-item scale	Ratings of providers' communication effectiveness were more important than a participatory decision-making style in predicting diabetes self-management. Higher ratings in PDM style and PCOM were each associated with higher self-management assessments (p = <.01 in all models). When modeled together, PCOM remained a significant independent predictor of self-management (standardized beta = .18; p = <.001), but PDM style became nonsignificant. Adding Understanding to the model diminished the unique effect of PCOM in predicting self-management (standardized beta = .10; p = .004). Understanding was strongly and independently associated with self-management (standardized beta = .25; p = <.001).
Mercer, Reilly, et al. 2002	(S) Descriptive (P) Investigate the factors that influence patient enablement (T) Hospital outpatient department	Patient survey and MD rating of two dimensions of the patient consultation	n = 4 MDs n = 200 outpatients	(1) Patient expectation; (2) patient perceived MD empathy scale; (3) patient rated enablement scale; (4) MDs' rating of confidence in	Enablement is a measure of the consultation relating to patients' ability to cope with and understand their health and illness as a result of seeing an MD. 3 SIG and independent factors in enablement were identi-

TABLE 3.2—*Continued*

Reference	Study Design (S) Study Purpose (P) Study Setting (T) Study Date (D) Country (C)	Method	Final Sample Size	Main Measures	Key Findings
	(D) Not reported (C) UK			a therapeutic relationship and in treatment	fied by multiple regression analysis: patient expectation, MD empathy, and MD's own confidence in the therapeutic relationship. Together they accounted for 41% of the variation in enablement scores, with empathy being the single most important factor, explaining 66% of the variation.
Kerr, Engel, et al. 2003	(S) Descriptive (P) Examine effect of communication on breast cancer patients' QoL and investigate the role of age in this relationship (T) Community (D) 1996–2001 (C) Germany	Survey administered at 6 months after the recorded diagnosis date and at regular intervals over 5 years	$n = 990$ breast cancer patients	27 QoL variables in 5 functional scales, global QoL measure, body image scores, lifestyle scores, and other worries (financial, future health) scores	45% reported that some aspect of the communication they received was unclear and 59% wanted to speak with medical staff more. 17 of 27 QoL variables were SIG worse ($p = <.01$), up to 4 years after diagnosis, for those patients reporting unclear or insufficient information. For patients over 50 years, QoL was SIG ($p = <.001$) worse when communication was unsatisfactory. Overall, QoL differed by up to 10 points between those reporting clear and unclear communication.
Zachariae, Pedersen, et	(S) Descriptive (P) Investigate the associ-	Patient and physician surveys	$n = 31$ MDs $n = 500$ cancer	(1) Patient satisfaction with personal contact	Higher PPRI scores of MD attentiveness and empathy were SIG ($p = <.01$)

al. 2003	ation of MD communi-cation with patient sat-isfaction, distress, self-efficacy, and perceived control over disease (T) Cancer outpatient clinic (D) Not reported (C) Denmark		patients	and medical aspects of visit; (2) Physician-Patient Relationship Inventory (PPRI) factors attentiveness (10 items) and empathy (4 items); (3) MD estimate of patient satisfaction	associated with greater patient satisfaction, increased self-efficacy, and reduced emotional distress following the consultation. Lower PPRI scores were associated with reduced ability of the physician to estimate patient satisfaction ($p = <.001$). Satisfaction with personal contact was SIG associated with perceived control prior to the consultation ($OR = .84$, $p = <.05$), attentiveness ($OR = 1.08$, $p = <.05$), and empathy ($OR = 1.06$, $p = <.01$), i.e., less patient control over the disease and the greater MD attentiveness and empathy, the greater the likelihood that the patient would be satisfied with the personal contact with the MD.
Kim, Kaplowitz, et al. 2004	(S) Descriptive (P) Examine the relationships of MD empathy to patient satisfaction and compliance (T) Pharmacy (D) 1999 (C) Korea	Survey	$n = 550$ patients in the pharmacy lobby, waiting to pick up their prescriptions after MD visit	(1) MD communication skills: cognitive and affective empathy, information exchange, partnership, MD expertise, interpersonal trust; (2) satisfaction; (3) compliance	Using structural equation modeling, patient-perceived MD affective and cognitive empathy SIG influenced compliance via the mediating factors of information exchange ($ES = .78$, $p = <.01$), perceived expertise ($ES = .50$, $p = <.05$), interpersonal trust ($ES = .25$, $p = <.05$), and partnership ($ES = .64$, $p = <.05$). Patient satisfaction was influenced via perceived expertise ($ES = .50$, $p = <.001$), interpersonal trust ($ES = .17$, $p = <.01$), and partnership ($ES = .52$, $p = <.001$). Satisfaction did not have a SIG ($p = >$

TABLE 3.2—*Continued*

Reference	Study Design (S) Study Purpose (P) Study Setting (T) Study Date (D) Country (C)	Method	Final Sample Size	Main Measures	Key Findings
Schneider, Kaplan, et al. 2004	(S) Descriptive (P) Determine quality of various dimensions of provider-patient relationships and relation to medication adherence in HIV (T) MD offices (D) 1997–98 (C) US	Postal survey and medical records review	n = 20 MDs and 2 nurse practitioners n = 554 HIV patients in practices of provider sample	(1) Adherence scale; (2) MD-patient relationship, 6 scales; (3) patient rating of MD understanding and problem solving ability	.05) relationship to compliance. Multivariate analyses that accounted for the clustering of patients within practices and adjusted for age, gender, education, race, physical health, and mental health found 6 of the 7 MD-patient relationship quality variables were SIG associated with adherence: general communication (OR = 1.15, p = .0001), HIV-specific information (OR = 1.09, p = .02), overall physician satisfaction (OR = 1.14, p = .004), willingness to recommend (OR = 1.09, p = .009), trust (OR = 1.10, p = .03), and adherence dialogue (OR = 1.20, p = <.0001) were all significantly and independently associated with adherence. The authors conclude that better MD-patient relationships and MD-patient communication produce better adherence with therapies.
Bikker, Mercer, et al. 2005	(S) Longitudinal descriptive (P) Determine effect of	Baseline survey at initial consultation with remeasurement (postal	n = 9 MDs n = 187 new outpatients	(1) Empathy; (2) enablement; (3) Short Form-12; (4) Measure	Univariate analysis found empathy score at first consultation highly predictive of ongoing empathy at 3

MD empathy and patient enablement on self-perceived health changes
(T) Hospital outpatient department
(D) 2002
(C) UK

survey) at 3 and 12 months

completed the initial questionnaire, 117 (63%) completed the 3-month, and 76/187 (41%) completed the 12-month follow-up

Yourself Medical Outcome Profile (MYMOP); (5) Glasgow Homoeopathic Outcome Scale (measure of perceived change in main complaint and well-being in relation to impact on daily living)

months (Spearman's rho = .572; p = <.0001), and correlated SIG with enablement at first consultation (rho = .325; p = <.0001) and overall enablement at 12 months (rho = .281; p = <.05). Controlling for the number of subsequent consultations, initial empathy scores were predictive of change in main complaint, and general well-being, at 3 months (rho = .225, .213, respectively; p = <.05). Enablement score at first consultation predicted enablement at 3 months (rho = .255; p = <.05) and 12 months (rho = .282; p = <.05). Initial enablement predicted GHHOS well-being score at 3 months, controlling for number of consultations (rho = .279; p = <.05). Both empathy and enablement at 3 months predicted overall enablement at 12 months (rho = .327; p = <.01 and rho = .577; p = <.0001, respectively). Empathy at 3 months was not SIG related to GHHOS scores at 12 months, whereas enablement scores at 3 months were highly predictive of both GHHOS main complaint and well-being scores at 12 months (rho = .459 and .507, respectively; p = <.0001). Empathy and enablement scores did not cor-

TABLE 3.2—*Continued*

Reference	Study Design (S) Study Purpose (P) Study Setting (T) Study Date (D) Country (C)	Method	Final Sample Size	Main Measures	Key Findings
					relate SIG with changes in Short Form-12 and MYMOP scores.
Epstein, Franks, et al. 2005	(S) Descriptive (P) Assess relationship between patient-centered communication and diagnostic testing expenditures (T) PCP office (D) 2000–2001 (C) US	Transcribed audiotapes of covert standardized patient visits rated using the MPCC. MCO claims	$n = 100$ PCPs participating in a large MCO	(1) MPCC score; (2) diagnostic testing expenditures; (3) hospital expenditures; (4) total expenditures; (5) visit length	MDs with MPCC scores in the lowest tercile generated 11% greater standardized diagnostic testing expenditures and 3.5% greater total standardized expenditures. No SIG relationship between MPCC score and total expenditures with diagnostic expenditures subtracted out (the effect of patient-centered communication on total standardized expenditures appears to reflect its effect on standardized diagnostic testing expenditures). There was no SIG relationship between MPCC scores and standardized hospital expenditures. MPCC scores correlated with increased visit length ($p = .002$).
Shaw, Zaia, et al. 2005	(S) Descriptive (P) Assess relationship between perceptions of provider communication and treatment satisfaction for acute,	Pre-consultation questionnaire, and 1 and 3 months post-consultation telephone interview	$n = 544$ patients with low back pain	(1) MD takes problem seriously, understands their jobs, explained condition clearly, and advised about ways to prevent reinjury	(1) At 1 month: providers took problem seriously (86.4%), explained condition clearly (82.0%), advised on ways to prevent reinjury (73.9%), and tried to understand job (85.1%). All 4 questions SIG ($p = .01$) corre-

	work-related low-back pain (T) Community occupational health clinic (D) 2000–2002 (C) US		(yes/no); (2) improvement in pain (0–10) and function; (3) satisfaction with medical care (1–4)	lated with improvement in pain and function (.17 to .27). (2) After controlling for improvements in pain and function, multiple regression analysis found positive provider assessment explained 2.4% (all 4 questions with $p = <.01$) of variation in patient satisfaction at 1 month vs. 12.8% at 3 months (took problem seriously and explained clearly, $p = <.01$; understand job, $p = <.05$; prevent reinjury, NS). The authors conclude that patients with work-related low back pain place a high value on provider counseling and education, especially during the acute stage (<1 month) of treatment.
van Os, van den Brink, et al. 2005	(S) Descriptive (P) Examine effect of depression treatment, communicative skills and their interaction on patient outcomes for depression in primary care (T) GP office (D) Not reported (C) Netherlands	Secondary analysis of survey data collected at baseline and 3 and 12 months and medical record abstraction	$n = 18$ GPs $n = 215$ GP patients screened previsit for mental health problems and confirmed at subsequent diagnostic interview	(1) Communicative skillfulness assessed by scale consisting of 5 measures of empathy and 4 of support; (2) treatment measured by duration and dosage of antidepressive medication; (3) patient outcome measured severity and duration of the depression episode using published scales	GP communication skills combined with depression treatment in skillful GPs achieved better results than the less skillful GPs applying the same treatment. Within the group of accurately diagnosed patients, the skillfulness of the GP had an ES = .51 on patient change over 3 months, within those who received treatment, ES = .91 and inadequately treated patients with an antidepressant, ES = 1.13. No effect of GP communicative skills was found among the patients who were inadequately diagnosed, who did not receive

TABLE 3.2—*Continued*

Reference	Study Design (S) Study Purpose (P) Study Setting (T) Study Date (D) Country (C)	Method	Final Sample Size	Main Measures	Key Findings
					treatment, or whose treatment was inadequate. At 12 months, treatment and adequate antidepressant treatment are associated with better patient outcomes if applied by communicatively skillful GPs (ES = .48 and ES = .64, respectively), but if applied by less skillful GPs, they are associated with less patient change (ES = .47 and ES = .84, respectively). Authors conclude that it is not the communicative skillfulness of the GP per se that brings about better patient outcomes, but the combination of good skills and depression-specific treatment.
Yiannako-poulou, Papadopulos, et al. 2005	(S) Descriptive (P) Compare rates of BP control with level of adherence to antihypertensive treatment and factors influencing compliance (T) Hospital (D) 1997–99	Structured patient interview using coded questions prior to surgery	$n = 1,000$ elective surgical patients with diagnosed and treated hypertension	(1) Compliance; (2) adequate counseling: (a) MD visit every 3 months, (b) visit MD personally for drug prescription, and (c) each visit MD measures BP, physical examination, provides instructions	Compliance was more common among people that have been adequately counseled by their doctors (43.9%) vs. among those that had not (3.9%), $p = <.001$.

Citation	Study characteristics	Methods	Sample	Measures	Findings
	(C) Greece			about lifestyle, explains importance of BP control; (3) BP control	
Bennett, Switzer, et al. 2006	(S) Qualitative (P) Assess effect of physician communication on prenatal care utilization (T) Community (D) 2002 (C) US	Cultural domain analysis, focus groups, and interviews	$n = 202$ Medicaid, African American women postpartum patients	Emerging themes	Four clinician characteristics that influence communication effectiveness and promote adequate prenatal care emerged: clarity of medical information, continuity of care, trust, and close patient-physician relationship. Women described poor-quality clinicians as unable to provide health information in a clear, accessible form. Literacy was not associated with prenatal care utilization.
Franks, Jerant, et al. 2006	(S) Descriptive (P) Examine relationships between claims-based quality of care indicators and patient perceptions of physician communication (T) PCP office (D) 2001–2 (C) US	3 data sources linked by PCP: (1) claims data process of care measures; (2) transcripts of 2 encounters of standardized patients to measure PCP interactional style; and (3) survey of patient perceptions of PCP interactional style	$n = 100$ PCPs participating in a large MCO $n = 4,746$ patient surveys	(1) MCPP scores; (2) STAK patient perception score (satisfaction, trust, autonomy, knowledge); (3) process indicators: Pap test, mammogram, diabetic eye examination, GlyHb, cholesterol, avoidable hospitalization	There were no clinically important associations between the objective rating of physician style (MPCC) and any process of care outcome. There were SIG physician effects on cholesterol ($p = <.001$) and GlyHb testing ($p = <.001$) indicators but not on other care indicators; and 1 clinically important association between STAK scores and GlyHb testing (AOR = 1.18). The authors conclude from the scant evidence that physicians' patient centeredness substantially affects process of care indicators and that patient activation may be a more effective strategy for improving patient outcomes.

TABLE 3.2—*Continued*

Reference	Study Design (S) Study Purpose (P) Study Setting (T) Study Date (D) Country (C)	Method	Final Sample Size	Main Measures	Key Findings
Aiarzaguena, Grandes, et al. 2007	(S) RCT (P) Assess the effect of 2 communication techniques delivered by GPs on somatizing patients' self-perceived health (T) GP office (D) 2005 (C) Spain	Patient questionnaire at home, assisted by researcher, baseline, 3, 8, and 12 months after the beginning of the intervention	n = 39 GPs n = 156 patients with 6 or more medically unexplained symptoms for women and 4 or more for men	(1) Health-related quality of life (36-item Short Form); (2) summary utility index	Intervention (trained) GPs used psychosocial communication techniques focused on offering a physical explanation (release of hormones) and querying topics in the patient's experience. Control GPs used the standard Goldberg reattribution technique that emphasizes a link between symptoms and emotions. Patients in both groups improved in all dimensions of the Short Form-36. The time course of the quality of life was SIG better for the intervention group in 5 of 8 Short Form-36 scales: bodily pain (p = <.003), mental health (p = <.063), physical functioning (p = .01), vitality (p = .05), and social functioning (p = .03), and in the utility index (p = <.04). The magnitude of the QoL improvement between groups at 12 months ranged from 2.68 for physical functioning to 9.70 for bodily pain in the multivariate adjusted analysis, and from 1.36 for physical

| Heisler, Cole, et al. 2007 | (S) Descriptive
(P) Assess physician information provision and participatory decision making on diabetic self-management and control in older patients
(T) Community
(D) 2003
(C) US | HRS national cross-sectional survey. Independent associations were examined between patients' ratings of their physician's PCOM and PDM with patients' reported diabetes self-management, adjusted for patient sociodemographics, illness severity, and comorbidities. | $n = 1,588$ older community-dwelling adults with diabetes | (1) PCOM scores (range 0–100); (2) PDM scores (range 0–100); (3) diabetes self-management measures: medication adherence, diet, exercise, blood glucose monitoring, and foot care; (4) GlyHb ($n = 1,233$) | functioning to 9.42 for bodily pain in baseline adjusted longitudinal models. The difference between both groups in the utility index was 3.79 points.

Among these older adults, both their diabetes providers' provision of information and efforts to actively involve them in treatment decision making were associated with better overall diabetes self-management. PCOM and PDM were SIG associated with overall diabetes self-management ($p = <.001$) and with all self-management domains ($p = <.001$ in all models), with the exception of PDM not being associated with medication adherence. In models with both PCOM and PDM, PCOM alone predicted medication adherence ($p = .001$) and foot care ($p = .002$). PDM alone was associated with exercise and blood glucose monitoring (both $p = <.001$) and was a stronger independent predictor than PCOM of diet. Better patient ratings of their diabetes self-management were associated with lower HbA1c values ($p = .005$). Authors conclude that practices need to be structured both to maximize the exchange of information and to encourage patients' |

TABLE 3.2—*Continued*

Reference	Study Design (S) Study Purpose (P) Study Setting (T) Study Date (D) Country (C)	Method	Final Sample Size	Main Measures	Key Findings
Neumann, Wirtz, et al. 2007	(S) Descriptive (P) Explore patient- and physician-specific determinants of physician empathy and its influence on patient-reported long-term outcomes (T) Hospital discharged cancer patients (D) 2005 (C) Germany	Postal survey with 3 survey waves	$n = 323$ cancer patients with mixed diagnoses	(1) CARE measure of MD empathy; (2) depression inventory; (3) QoL	involvement in decision making. Using structural equation modeling, results found MD empathy had a very strong direct impact on "desire for more information from physician: findings and treatment options" (beta = .68, $p = <.001$), a moderate effect on "desire for more information from MD: side effects and medication" (beta = .41, $p = <.001$), and a moderate influence on "desire for more information about health promotion" (beta = .33, $p = <.001$). Empathy had an indirect effect on "depression" (beta = .27) and "socio-emotional-cognitive QoL" (beta = .24), which was mediated by "desire for more information from MD: findings and treatment options." Authors conclude that empathy is an important prerequisite for information giving by MDs and through this pathway has a preventive effect on depression and improving QoL.

| Dimoska, Butow, et al. 2008 | (S) Qualitative
(P) Assess effect of medical and radiation oncologists consultation on patient anxiety, recall, and satisfaction
(T) Oncology
(D) Not reported
(C) Australia | Pre-post patient questionnaires and transcribed audiotapes with CANCODE computer interaction analysis system | $n = 5$ medical oncologists and 4 radiation oncologists
$n = 155$ cancer patients attending their first outpatient consultation | Patient anxiety, psychological adjustment, recall, and satisfaction | (See Dimoska, Butow, et al. 2008 for results on poor communication, table 2.5.) Patients rating oncologists as warmer and having discussed a greater number of psychosocial issues had better psychological adjustment and reduced anxiety after consultation: (1) reduced patient anxiety immediately after consultation was SIG associated with an MD who was more warm ($p = <.01$) and spoke longer about psychosocial issues ($p = <.01$); at 1 week reduced anxiety was SIG associated with an MD who was more warm ($p = <.05$); (2) lower scores on the helpless/hopeless scale were associated with a warmer doctor ($p = .051$); lower anxious preoccupation was associated with a higher psychosocial to biomedical talk ratio ($p = .05$); (3) greater patient information recall was associated with shorter consultations ($p = <.001$); patients seeing a radiation oncologist were more satisfied when the psychosocial to biomedical talk ratio was greater vs. no effect with medical oncologist ($p = <.001$); (4) patients seeing a radiation oncologist were more satisfied when the psychosocial to biomedical talk ratio |

TABLE 3.2—*Continued*

Reference	Study Design (S) Study Purpose (P) Study Setting (T) Study Date (D) Country (C)	Method	Final Sample Size	Main Measures	Key Findings
Ling, Trauth, et al. 2008	(S) Descriptive (P Identify association between communication of specific Informed Decision Making elements and completion of CRC screening (T) Primary care, VA hospital outpatient clinic (D) 2001–4 (C) US	Transcribed audiotape of clinic visit	n = 24 primary care providers, 9 internal medicine faculty MDs, and 5 nurse practitioners n = 135 patients due for CRC screening	Association between completion of CRC screening and 9 elements of informed decision making	was greater vs. a medical oncologist (p = <.001). (See Ling, Trauth, et al. 2008 assessment of communication, table 2.5.) (1) 91 of 135 patients completed screening (67%). (2) Patients whose understanding was assessed during the visit had SIG (p = .002) higher rate of completing CRC screening (100%) vs. understanding not assessed (35%). (3) Negative associations were found: less frequent CRC screening for those discussing "pros and cons" (12% vs. 46%, p = .01) and "patient preferences" (6% vs. 47%, p = .001) compared with those who did not. When stratified by prior CRC screening, the association between screening and the discussion of pros and cons was no longer SIG, while the association with eliciting patient preferences remained SIG (p = .02).

AOR = adjusted odds ratio
BP = blood pressure
CANCODE = computerized interaction analysis system with established reliability and validity
CARE = consultation and relational empathy measure
CRC = colorectal cancer
ES = effect size

GlyHB = glycosolated hemoglobin
GP = general practitioner
HRS = Health and Retirement Study
MCO = managed care organization
MPCC = Measure of Patient-Centered Communication
MD = physician
n = number

OR = odds ratio
QoL = quality of life
PCOM = physician communication-provision of information
PCP = primary care physician
PDM = participatory decision-making style
SIG = significant(ly)

4 | What Factors Are Associated with Deficiencies in Physician Communication?

In chapter 3, we summarized evidence on the relationships between physician communication and patient outcomes. While this literature has some shortcomings, it provides overall support for hypotheses that poor physician communication has important implications for patients. In this chapter, we address the literature on factors related to poor communication. Establishing these linkages is important in assessing the appropriateness and effectiveness of programs designed to improve communication, the topic we address in chapter 5.

In chapter 1, we placed factors that could be related to deficiencies in physician communication into one of four categories: physician characteristics; patient characteristics; practice characteristics; and environmental characteristics, or characteristics of the health care system (see fig. 1.1, logic model). We use this same framework to organize our discussion of the literature we review in this chapter. In specifying these categories, we were guided primarily by findings in the published literature and, to a lesser extent, by theoretical frameworks that guided the designs of some studies.

In general, however, the empirical literature on this topic is not grounded in well-developed theories of physician behavior or theories of communication, and most studies are not designed to test theoretical hypotheses. If they are, the theoretical grounding for the empirical analysis is not explained in any detail in the articles. For the most part, the studies are exploratory in nature. The literature that we review in this chapter consists mostly of studies designed to investigate possible statistical associations between factors that quite plausibly could have an effect on physician communication and specific measures of communication. In summarizing findings from these studies, it generally would not be appropriate to reach conclusions regarding causation—for instance, that physician characteristic A caused physician communication behavior of type B that resulted in patient outcome C (see Hall 2003 and Bensing, van Dulmen, et al. 2003 for further discussion of this point).

As in chapter 2, the studies reviewed in this chapter use a variety of data sources but rely primarily on patient surveys and audiotapes or videotapes of physician-patient encounters to identify and quantify factors that plausibly could be associated with quality of physician communication and to measure elements of physician communication. Most of the studies are "observational" in nature and relatively small in scale, with study settings that can be termed "opportunistic" (Bensing, van Dulmen, et al. 2003). While separate measures are constructed for each individual factor, these factors comingle in practice, and the impact of one could well be mitigated by the presence or absence of another. For instance, the same physician could communicate quite differently if practicing with or without the presence of an electronic medical record or if reimbursed on a salaried, as opposed to fee-for-service, basis; or an elderly male physician could communicate with patients differently than a young male physician. This clearly makes it more difficult to isolate the incremental or marginal association between a particular physician characteristic (e.g., being a male) and a specific aspect of communication. Many of the studies we review in this chapter attempt to address this problem by using statistical methods to control for observable differences, but even in these multivariate analyses, unobservable or unmeasured factors are likely to be present that could affect the relationship between the factor or factors being studied and communication. Very few studies address whether interactions among factors are important in predicting scores on different components of physician communication. As a result, it is important to assess the entire body of evidence relating to specific factors and their association with physician communication, as opposed to emphasizing the findings from a single study.

Identifying Relevant Literature

As in prior chapters, we searched the peer-reviewed literature, published in English, to identify studies that addressed factors that may be related to the quality of patient communication. We identified review articles by searching Medline, JSTOR, and the databases of the Cochrane Library and the Agency for Healthcare Research on Quality (AHRQ). We used the same approach to identify individual articles published from 2000 to 2008, including them in our tables and analysis if they were not already included in review articles. The review articles typically addressed issues beyond factors associated with the quality of physician communication.

Consequently, some review articles are included in tables in other chapters as well. Through our literature search and the reference lists of the articles included in the search, we identified some discussion articles that contained informal summaries of literature findings or discussions of their importance. We have referenced these articles as appropriate to illustrate the views of others concerning the evidence.

We employed a combination of such keywords as "communication barriers," "communication," "physician-patient relations," "time factors," "job satisfaction," "palliative care," "burnout, professional," "health care economics and organization," "attitude of health professional," "cultural diversity," and "cultural competency." We used relatively broad inclusion criteria in our search process, including articles using a variety of methodologies and addressing a wide range of factors. We found 595 references in our initial search. We eliminated articles that did not seem relevant for our purposes, ultimately reviewing 354 articles or abstracts. Even though we used broad search criteria, we are likely to have missed some relevant articles, because research results pertaining to the association of specific factors with physician communication are frequently subsumed in larger studies whose primary objective may not have been assessing the association of these factors. This is especially true regarding the relationship between physician communication and patient characteristics. Nevertheless, we believe that the studies we have identified, taken together, provide a reasonable representation of the evidence regarding factors associated with variation in physician communication.

We identified 31 review articles and 48 individual studies that addressed, to varying degrees, the relationship of one or more factors to physician communication. As table 4.1 indicates, a large portion of these articles reported on the relationship between physician characteristics and physician communication. This is consistent with a general view emphasizing that the primary cause of poor physician communication is personal shortcomings, rather than characteristics of the physician practice or of the health care system more generally; that is, the expectation of study authors, as evidenced by the focus they chose and their study designs, was that poor physician communication was predominately a "human problem," as opposed to a "systems problem." The same focus on "human factors" characterized early research on factors related to medical errors, and only after the 2000 Institute of Medicine report *To Err Is Human* directed attention to system factors as leading causes of medical errors was greater attention given to this topic by both researchers and practitioners. In the literature on physician communication, a frequently mentioned "systems factor" is the perception on the part of physicians that there is insufficient time available in the scheduled physician visit to communicate with patients as empathetically and thoroughly as the physician would like. But the literature even in this area is relatively sparse, as it is with respect to other environmental factors as well.

What Is the Evidence Regarding Factors That Are Associated with the Quality of Physician Communication?

We summarize our findings for review articles (see table 4.2) and for individual studies (see table 4.3) by category of factor. In each case, we discuss the review findings first. We cite some reviews multiple times in our discussion, when they address a variety of different factors. (The same is true, but to a lesser extent, for some individual studies.) After discussing the review findings, we discuss findings from several individual studies that we chose (from the set of 48 studies contained in table 4.3) as illustrative of research approaches or general findings.

Physician Characteristics

The relationship between physician characteristics and physician communication has been addressed extensively in both review articles and individual studies. One area of interest has been the association between sociodemographic characteristics (e.g., age, gender, and culture) and communication. These studies often address "pairing" issues, such as whether female physicians communicate more effectively with female patients than do male physicians. Thus, they combine analysis of both physician and patient characteristics. We consider this evidence under the category of "patient characteristics."

A second area of focus in the literature has been the association between physician communication and skills or knowledge acquired through training. This knowledge could relate to how to better communicate with patients or about particular clinical areas. (This differs from the impact of *specific* training programs on communication, a topic we address in chapter 5.) Third, the literature also addresses the relationship between physician communication and physician personality traits and emotional status.

Evidence from Reviews.   Physicians who do not incorporate all of the components of effective communication in their conversations with patients may feel they lack communications skills and have not been trained adequately to communicate effectively with their patients (Siegler and Levin 2000; Griffin, Nelson, et al. 2003; Fallowfield and Jenkins 2004;

Weiner and Cole 2004; Baile and Aaron 2005; Mystakidou, Tsilika, et al. 2005). This finding from review studies provides support for educational programs aimed at teaching physicians how to be better communicators. In some cases, reviews have documented that physicians either feel they do not have or, based on their responses to questions, actually do not have the clinical knowledge to be effective in communicating diagnoses and treatment options (Gordon 2003; McGorty and Bornstein 2003; Quinn, Vadaparampil, et al. 2008). This occurs most commonly when physicians are communicating with patients who are in the last stages of life. For instance, Gordon (2003) reports that physicians have difficulty estimating when a patient will die and that they give optimistic estimates as a result, and McGorty and Bornstein (2003) observe that physicians lack knowledge of and experience with hospices and the services they provide and that this deficiency is associated with inappropriate inclusion or exclusion of hospices in treatment plans. Hack, Degner, et al. (2005) report that deficiencies in the ability of physicians to assess patient levels of depression are associated with inappropriate communication as well.

In addition to lacking the skills and knowledge necessary for effective communication, a physician's mental state may be associated with effectiveness of communication with patients (Ong, de Haes, et al. 1995; Siegler and Levin 2000; Foster 2001; Griffin, Nelson, et al. 2003; McGorty and Bornstein 2003; Fallowfield and Jenkins 2004; Weiner and Cole 2004; Baile and Aaron 2005). This is likely to be a particularly significant factor when communicating bad news to the patient and/or when conversing with a patient about end-of-life care. Physicians experience anxiety and stress when communicating to patients under these circumstances, which can be associated with inadequate explanations provided to patients and family members, lack of empathy, and expenditure of less effort than might be desirable to determine patient comprehension.

Several reviews addressed whether there were basic physician sociodemographic characteristics (e.g., age, gender, and cultural background) that were associated with communication (Bylund and Makoul 2002; Street 2002; Roter, Hall, et al. 2002; Mystakidou, Tsilika, et al. 2005). The reviews generally found that female physicians were more skilled communicators than males. Roter, Hall et al. note, "Female physicians engage in communication that more broadly relates to the larger life context of the patient's condition by addressing psychosocial issues through related questioning and counseling, through the greater use of emotional talk, more emotional talk, more positive talk, and more active enlistment of patient input" (Roter, Hall, et al. 2002, 761). Bylund and Makoul (2002) found that female physicians asked more questions and used more positive nonverbal communication. They found no differences between male and female physicians in the amount of biological information discussed, the quality of the information given, or the amount of social conversation. Street (2002) reported that female physicians engaged in more partnership building and were more interested in patient input, while male physicians spent more time discussing biomedical issues, offering advice, and expressing opinions. Overall, the review studies are generally consistent in painting a picture of female physicians as more active in the social-emotional, or "care-oriented," domain of communication.

Mystakidou, Tsilika, et al. (2005) reviewed how physician ethnicity and culture were associated with the way in which bad news was transmitted to patients. They found that physicians in eastern and southern Europe were more likely to conceal diagnoses from patients, speaking to family members instead, while northern European physicians disclosed diagnoses to patients and then to family members, with patient permission. However, they attributed this difference to a difference in training regarding communication and to culture.

Along with these major groupings of physician characteristics, some reviews have identified very specific factors associated with communication. Baile and Aaron (2005) noted that there can be a disconnect between physicians and patients regarding how much information patients really want and that this disconnect may be associated with underprovision of information by physicians. Similarly, Irwin and Richardson (2006) found that physicians may underestimate patients' needs for information. Williams and Skinner (2003) reported a relationship between physician job satisfaction and physician communications with patients; physicians with higher levels of job satisfaction tend to be more attentive to social aspects of care and more open with patients.

Evidence from Selected Individual Studies. Several of the studies described in table 4.2 relate to the association of physician characteristics with their communication with patients, but the findings of these studies largely confirm those reported in the reviews previously described. For instance, Dosanjh, Barnes, et al.(2001) reported that a higher level of stress and anxiety on the part of residents was associated with more inhibition in delivering bad news to patients, while Bylund and Makoul (2002) found that female general internists gave more empathetic responses to patients than did male internists.

Patient Characteristics

The second category of factors assumed to be associated with physician communication behaviors consists of patient characteristics. As already noted, many of these studies examined physician-patient dyads to explore whether communication is different for physicians and patients with like characteristics (e.g., both female) versus different characteristics (male physician-female patient). While communication clearly is a "two-way street," one way of framing the question is to ask whether physicians communicate differently with some types of patients than with others, all else being equal.

Evidence from Reviews.   In her review, van Ryn (2002) concluded, based on findings from 19 studies, that patient sociodemographic characteristics are independently associated with physician expectations, perceptions, and "affect" toward patients. Schouten and Meeuwesen (2006) found significant differences in consultation length and verbal behavior for white patients versus patients from ethnic minority groups, with physicians showing less affective behavior to minority patients in all but one study. When treating minority patients, physicians were generally less friendly and concerned and more likely to ignore patient comments.

In addition to responding differently to patients with different demographic characteristics, it is possible that physicians may communicate differently with patients who have been "trained," or prepared, for the physician visit. There have been a variety of studies of the effectiveness of patient training programs, with their results summarized in seven reviews in table 4.2. Studies of the effectiveness of these programs focus predominantly on patient actions, such as patient information giving and question asking during the visit, and find that both are typically higher for "trained" patients. In addition, some studies measure patient satisfaction and knowledge acquisition post-visit, which are common immediate outcome measures used to assess the effectiveness of physician communication (see chapter 3). For example, in their review, Wetzels, Harmsen, et al. (2007) reported on one randomized study where patients who had completed a community workshop were more satisfied with the interpersonal aspects of their visits. In their review, Harrington, Noble, et al. (2004) identified two studies where physician encouragement of patient participation in conversations was measured, with encouragement being more likely for "trained" patients. Several studies also included measures of health outcome similar to the intermediate measures used in studies that assess the impact of physician communication (see chapter 3). Studies that measured length of visit did not find that visits were longer for trained patients. Overall, the reviews of literature on the impact of programs to train patients prior to physician visits suggests that these programs change patient behaviors and have beneficial patient outcomes, but these reviews contain very little evidence regarding whether and to what extent physicians communicate differently with trained patients.

Evidence from Selected Individual Studies. Siminoff, Graham, et al. (2006) examined whether patient characteristics were associated with oncologists' communication with breast cancer patients. They audiotaped initial consultations between 58 oncologists and 405 newly diagnosed patients, combining these data with interview data collected from patients and physicians before and after the consultations. The audiotapes were analyzed using the Roter Interaction Analysis System (RIAS). The authors concluded that "providers communicate differently with patients by age, race, education and income" (355). Their results were the strongest with respect to race, with physicians devoting more effort to "relationship building" with white than with nonwhite patients. However, they observed, "Our data cannot tell us if certain patients are simply less communicative and physicians are merely responding to patient cues or if there is a complicated feedback process taking place as the communication process between doctor and patient unfolds" (360).

Among other studies related to the relationship between patient characteristics and physician communication, Frich, Malterud, et al. (2006) examined barriers to treatment for women who were at risk of coronary heart disease, using semistructured interviews conducted from 2000 to 2002 with 20 women in Norway. They found that women's symptoms were misinterpreted or downplayed by physicians. Dimoska, Butow, et al. (2008) reported that oncologists, in their initial consultations with patients, spoke longer if the patient was female (see table 2.5). Rosenberg, Richard, et al. (2006) used videotapes of encounters involving 12 physicians and 24 ethnically diverse patients experiencing psychological distress, concluding that physicians used ethnic stereotypes to guide their care decisions. Patients who are more assertive may precipitate different communication responses from physicians. Cegala, Street, et al. (2007), in a secondary analyses of data from three studies, concluded that physicians provided more information and made more supportive utterances to patients with a high level of participation. Patient disease state can also affect physician communication. Corke, Stow, et al. (2005) found that physicians communicated poorly with simulated patients who had acute, life-threatening illnesses with serious comorbidities; the physicians focused on describing the medical situation but poorly addressed the patient's functional status, values, and fears.

Individual studies not included in reviews of patient training programs are not consistent in their findings, but this might be expected due to the varying characteristics of the training programs. For example, Li and Lundgren (2005) found that patients trained using a multistep process were more satisfied with communication that took place during the visit, but Wetzels, Wenzing, et al. (2005) found that patients who received an instructional leaflet prior to their visits were not any more involved in or satisfied with visits.

Practice Characteristics

Physician practice characteristics may be associated with the way in which physicians communicate with their patients; these characteristics include how patients are scheduled, the level of clinician and other staff support available in the physician practice, and the level and type of technology and decision supports available to physicians and patients in the context of the visit. Review articles contained relatively little information regarding the relationship between practice characteristics and physician communication. Where this was addressed, the focus was primarily on the impact of time constraints on physician communication. Individual studies have been published recently that examine the relationship between use of computers and physician communication with patients during office visits, as well as the effects on communication of use of patient decision aids as employed in practice settings. However, because the use of electronic medical records and patient decision aids as part of patient visits is relatively new, the literature in these areas is sparse.

Evidence from Reviews. The authors of several reviews observed that physicians self-report time pressures as a factor in the nature and length of their communications with patients (Foster 2001; Baile and Aaron 2005; Hack, Degner, et al. 2005; Irwin and Richardson 2006; Mauksch, Dugdale, et al. 2008; Quinn, Vadaparampil, et al. 2008). Limited visit time may interfere with time needed for discussion of diagnosis and treatment (Quinn, Vadaparampil, et al. 2008), increased time required for diagnosis and treatment of cancer patients may lead to less time available to spend with patients and their family members (Baile and Aaron 2005), and a "busy patient workload" can be a factor in poor communication (Hack, Degner, et al. 2005). However, in their review of studies related to time management in physician practices, Mauksch, Dugdale, et al. (2008) reported that having more time for a physician visit was not necessarily associated with improved physician communication with patients.

In a recent review, Leatherman and Warrick (2008) assessed the findings of evaluations of the impact of the use of decision aids (DAs) by patients. They describe DAs as "standardized, evidenced-based tools intended to facilitate the process of making informed values-based choices about disease management and treatment options, prevention or screening" (80S). DAs are used in a variety of settings, including physician practices. Although the review by Leatherman and Warrick found that most evaluations of DAs measured impact on patient knowledge and decisional conflict (with generally favorable findings in each domain), it is also possible that the use of DAs in physician practices could affect the length of a visit as well as physician communication with patients during the visit. However, only a small number of evaluations of DAs identified by Leatherman and Warrick attempted to address these issues. With respect to the impact of DAs on the length of a visit, Kaner, Heaven, et al. (2007) compared three different types of DA used by atrial fibrillation patients during an office visit. They found significant differences in the length of a visit that were related to the complexity of the DA used, but they also found that all visits took considerably longer than the typical physician visit in primary care. The usefulness of these findings is limited by the absence of a "no DA" control group, as well as by the small number of patients involved ($n = 29$). In contrast to the results of Kaner, Heaven, et al. (2007), Ozanne, Annis, et al. (2007) found that use of a DA for patients at high risk of breast cancer ($n = 30$) did not increase visit time, compared to usual care. In a randomized controlled trial, Whelan, Sawka, et al. (2003) also found no effect on visit consultation time associated with the use of a DA by patients with node-negative breast cancer.

Two of the studies previously described also addressed the impact of DAs on physician communication with patients. Kaner, Heaven, et al. (2007) found that physicians dominated conversations with patients, with no difference across type of DA. Also, physician talk was judged to be 93 percent technical versus 7 percent socio-emotional, while patient talk was only slightly less oriented toward technical issues (85% versus 15%). As noted, there was no "usual care" control group in this study, but the findings suggest the possible value of future studies that explore the relationship between use of DAs in physician practices and physician dominance of physician-patient communication and/or orientation of communication toward technical issues. In their study, Whelan, Sawka, et al. (2003) found that use of DAs did not affect physician satisfaction with the decision-making process, which could be related to satisfaction with communication. Laupacis, O'Connor, et al. (2006) examined the impact of DA use on pre-donation of autologous blood before elective open heart surgery, using a randomized study design. They found that patients in the DA group were significantly more satisfied with how they were treated by their health care providers, another possible indirect indicator of the quality of physician communication.

Overall, the most striking finding of the Leatherman and Warrick (2008) review of evaluations of the impact of DAs was the lack of attention given to their possible influence on physician-patient communication. If the support for use of DAs in physician practices grows, this will become an important and potentially fruitful area for future research.

Evidence from Selected Individual Studies. In the United States, the nature of the office visit is now changing as new ways of organizing care are being introduced (e.g., "team-oriented care") and as the use of electronic health records (EHRs) is becoming more common. The use of EHRs during the office visit is receiving particular attention with regard to its potential to change the nature of physician communication with patients. A recent *New York Times* article states, "Doctors in every specialty struggle to figure out a way to keep the computer from interfering with what should be going on in the exam room—making the crucial connection between doctor and patient" (Armstrong-Coben 2009). Studies now are appearing that address this issue.

Rouf, Whittle, et al. (2007) explored whether the presence of a computer in the examination room is associated with the interpersonal elements of physician communication and, in particular, whether this effect varies for experienced versus relatively inexperienced physicians. To address this question, they studied visits by 155 adults to faculty internists and internal medicine residents in a Veterans Administration medical center, collecting data using patient questionnaires and baseline and post-visit physician questionnaires. The authors found that patients seeing residents for their care were more likely to feel that the computer adversely affected the nature of physician communication. The residents themselves also were more likely to say that use of computers inhibited communication than were the more experienced faculty internists. These findings suggest that more experienced physicians may be able to communicate more effectively when using a computer in the examination room. However, the authors suggested that more studies, in different treatment settings and with more patients, are needed to confirm their results.

Makoul, Curry, et al. (2001) compared communication patterns of three physicians using EHRs and three using paper records, videotaping physician-patient encounters during 1997–98. They found differences in communication that favored the physicians using the EHR. For instance, physicians using EHRs were more likely (25% versus 8%) to encourage patients to ask questions. The authors observed that these differences could reflect practice styles of physicians established prior to their use of EHRs. Frankel, Altschuler, et al. (2005) also examined the relationship between having computers in the examination room and communication with patients in another small-scale study, involving nine clinicians (six physicians) and 54 patients. Physician-patient encounters were videotaped at one month before and one and seven months after computers were introduced. The researchers found that factors associated with physician communication before introduction of the computer remained important after introduction, in some cases increasing in importance.

Environmental Characteristics

Physicians and their practices exist within a larger health care system, and the behavior of physicians, including their communications with patients, may reflect the incentives and constraints imposed by that larger system. We identified very few references to these pressures in the review articles in table 4.2, and there were few recent individual articles that addressed the association of system-level factors with physician communication. Certainly, one explanation for this is that opportunities to study the relationship between system-level pressures and communication are limited and sometimes difficult to identify. To conduct research on this issue, there must be variation in the systems-level factor of interest across different health care systems or organizations and/or a change in the factor over time.

Evidence from Reviews.   Concerns regarding malpractice were identified in one review (Siegler and Levin 2000) as being associated with less effective and less open physician communication with patients. A review by Foster (2001) cited a potential barrier to effective communication as physician concern that the extra time needed to communicate effectively in the treatment of dementia was not reimbursable.

Evidence from Selected Individual Studies.   In the United States, the structure of the current fee-for-service reimbursement system has been identified as a possible barrier to effective physician communication. It is argued that fee-for-service reimbursement encourages short visits and that it is impossible for physicians to accomplish all care recommended by guidelines during a typical visit. The time pressure in physician visits, presumably created by the financial incentives in the payment system, could be associated with poorer physician communication as well.

In a study set in the Netherlands, van Dulmen (2000) observed physician-patient encounters involving pediatricians who were reimbursed by a fee-for-service system versus a salary. (In the Netherlands—in contrast to the United States—at the time of the study, pediatricians did not deliver primary care, and access to a pediatrician required a referral.) Van Dulmen chose to investigate whether this difference was associated with the time that pediatricians spent with patients and also the content of their communications. In 1996, he videotaped 302 outpatient encounters involving 21 pediatricians (14 salaried and 7 in a fee-for-service system), coding the content of those encounters using a revised version of the RIAS. The author also collected post-visit survey data from physicians and parents and used multilevel statistical techniques to control for demographic and visit characteristics when analyzing the data. Visits involving salaried physicians lasted four minutes longer, a difference of approximately 25 percent. Salaried physicians "gave more agreements, reflections and reassurances than the pediatricians working on a fee-for-service basis" (594). Gender accounted for very little of the observed differences in physician communication behavior. In an interesting secondary finding, van Dulmen observed that physician self-reports regarding how they spent their visit time did not match the videotapes, suggesting that researchers should be cautious in drawing conclusions from physician reports regarding the content of their communication with patients. Also, van Dulmen cautioned against drawing firm conclusions based on the specific study findings, given the small number of physicians involved and the author's inability to control for some practice characteristics that might have influenced pediatrician behavior.

Conclusions

The literature on the factors that are associated with the quality of physician communication has focused primarily on physician characteristics. There is relatively strong evidence that female physicians perform better in psychosocial aspects of communication and exhibit more empathy toward patients. Physicians generally communicate better with patients of the same gender and race, and they communicate worse with low-income patients or patients in racial or ethnic minority groups. Physicians themselves identify a lack of training in communication as a barrier to communicating effectively with patients.

There are relatively few studies in the published literature addressing the relationships between practice characteristics or system characteristics and physician communication. There is also a lack of research on how practice characteristics and physician characteristics interact in their relation to physician communication. The small number of studies in this area is noteworthy, given the challenges that practice and system redesign could pose for physician communication in the future.

TABLE 4.1.   Factors Related to Poor or Better Physician Communication

Factor	Reference
Physician	
Sociodemographic (age, gender, ethnicity/culture)	Adams, Smith, et al. 2001; Bylund and Makoul 2002; Roter, Hall, et al. 2002; Street 2002; Verhoeven, Bovijn, et al. 2003; Arber, McKinlay, et al. 2004; Knauft, Nielsen, et al. 2005; Street, Gordon, et al. 2005; Mystakidou, Tsilika, et al. 2005; Burd, Nevadunsky, et al. 2006; Park, Betancourt, et al. 2006; Roter, Frankel, et al. 2006; Cox, Smith, et al. 2007; Frantsve and Kerns 2007; Schmid Mast, Hall, et al. 2007
Communication skills training and ability (verbal and nonverbal skills, knowledge)	Curtis, Patrick, et al. 2000; Siegler and Levin 2000; Adams, Smith, et al. 2001; Foster 2001; Ashton, Haidet, et al. 2003; Griffin, Nelson, et al. 2003; McGorty and Bornstein 2003; Fallowfield and Jenkins 2004; Farber, Urban, et al. 2004; Back, Arnold, et al. 2005; Travado, Grassi, et al. 2005; Irwin and Richardson 2006; Roter, Frankel, et al. 2006; Weiner and Roth 2006; Quinn, Vadaparampil, et al. 2008
Clinical knowledge/medical training/experience/role and responsibility clarity	Adams, Smith, et al. 2001; Foster 2001; Ashton, Haidet, et al. 2003; Griffin, Nelson, et al. 2003; McGorty and Bornstein 2003; McIntosh and Shaw 2003; Verhoeven, Bovijn, et al. 2003; Chibnall, Bennett, et al. 2004; Farber, Urban, et al. 2004; Gott, Galena, et al. 2004; Back, Arnold, et al. 2005; Hack, Degner, et al. 2005; McCauley, Jenckes, et al. 2005; Farmer and Higginson 2006; Irwin and Richardson 2006; Barnhart, Lewis, et al. 2007; Frantsve and Kerns 2007; Kelly and Haidet 2007; Harding, Selman, et al. 2008; Quinn, Vadaparampil, et al. 2008
Personality (attitude, bias and beliefs, communication style, fear, discomfort, lack of self-awareness)	Calam, Far, et al. 2000; Curtis, Patrick, et al. 2000; Siegler and Levin 2000; Adams, Smith, et al. 2001; Dosanjh, Barnes, et al. 2001; Foster 2001; Vegni, Zannini, et al. 2001; van Ryn 2002; Ashton, Haidet, et al. 2003; Griffin, Nelson, et al. 2003; Lukoschek, Fazzari, et al. 2003; Maly, Leake, et al. 2003; McGorty and Bornstein 2003; Verhoeven, Bovijn, et al. 2003; Chibnall, Bennett, et al. 2004; Deveugele, Derese, et al. 2004; Fallowfield and Jenkins 2004; Gott, Galena, et al. 2004; Weiner and Cole 2004; Back, Arnold, et al. 2005; Hack, Degner, et al. 2005; Knauft, Nielsen, et al. 2005; Street, Gordon, et al. 2005; Travado, Grassi, et al. 2005; Burd, Nevadunsky, et al. 2006; Farmer and Higginson 2006; Farmer, Roter, et al. 2006; Schouten and Meeuwesen 2006; Frantsve and Kerns 2007; Harding, Selman, et al. 2008; Kaduszkiewicz, Bachmann, et al. 2008; Mauksch, Dugdale, et al. 2008; Quinn, Vadaparampil, et al. 2008
Cultural competency	Lukoschek, Fazzari, et al. 2003; Shapiro, Hollingshead, et al. 2003; Back, Arnold, et al. 2005; Park, Betancourt, et al. 2005; Farmer and Higginson 2006; Park, Betancourt, et al. 2006; Rosenberg, Richard, et al. 2006; Schouten and Meeuwesen 2006; Wachtler, Brorsson, et al. 2006

TABLE 4.1—*Continued*

Factor	Reference
Clarity of diagnosis/prognosis or patient preferences and values	McIntosh and Shaw 2003; Back, Arnold, et al. 2005; Travado, Grassi, et al. 2005; Deep, Griffith, et al. 2008; Kaduszkiewicz, Bachmann, et al. 2008
Job satisfaction	AHRQ 2008

Patient

Sociodemographic (age, gender, ethnicity/culture)	Ong, de Haes, et al. 1995; Bylund and Makoul 2002; Collins, Clark, et al. 2002; van Ryn 2002; Maly, Leake, et al. 2003; Verhoeven, Bovijn, et al. 2003; Arber, McKinlay, et al. 2004; Gott, Galena, et al. 2004; Street, Gordon, et al. 2005; Burd, Nevadunsky, et al. 2006; Farmer and Higginson 2006; Frich, Malterud, et al. 2006; Siminoff, Graham, et al. 2006; Barnhart, Lewis, et al. 2007; Cox, Smith, et al. 2007
Personality	Street, Gordon, et al. 2005; Ong, de Haes, et al. 1995
Training	Post, Cegala, et al. 2001; Cegala 2003; Wetzels, Wensing, et al. 2005; Wetzels, Harmsen, et al. 2007; Kinnersley, Edwards, et al. 2008; Harrington, Noble, et al. 2004; Li and Lundgren 2005; Parker, Davison, et al. 2005; Haywood, Marshall, et al. 2006; Cegala, Street, et al. 2007; Harrington, Norling, et al. 2007; Haskard, Williams, et al. 2008
Physical appearance/ health condition or issue/sexual orientation	Ong, de Haes, et al. 1995; Gott, Galena, et al. 2004; Farmer and Higginson 2006; Farmer, Roter, et al. 2006; Park, Betancourt, et al. 2006

Environment

Medical-legal concerns	Siegler and Levin 2000; McGorty and Bornstein 2003
Reimbursement system	Chibnall, Bennett, et al. 2004; Back, Arnold, et al. 2005; Quinn, Vadaparampil, et al. 2008
Health care system resources/supportive environment	Dosanjh, Barnes, et al. 2001; Chibnall, Bennett, et al. 2004; McCauley, Jenckes, et al. 2005; Park, Betancourt, et al. 2005; Quinn, Vadaparampil, et al. 2008
Cultural norms	Ong, de Haes, et al. 1995; Mystakidou, Tsilika, et al. 2005

Practice

Office technology (computer, EMR, telemedicine, decision aid)	Makoul, Curry, et al. 2001; Frankel, Altschuler, et al. 2005; Liu, Sawada, et al. 2007; Rosen and Kwoh 2007; Rouf, Whittle, et al. 2007; Johnson, Serwint, et al. 2008; Leatherman and Warrick, 2008
Practice setting	McGorty and Bornstein 2003; Hack, Degner, et al. 2005; Street, Gordon, et al. 2005
Visit or practice time	Curtis, Patrick, et al. 2000; van Dulmen 2000; Dosanjh, Barnes, et al. 2001; Foster 2001; Shapiro, Hollingshead, et al. 2003; Verhoeven, Bovijn, et al. 2003; Deveugele, Derese, et al. 2004; Gott, Galena, et al. 2004; Back, Arnold, et al. 2005; Hack, Degner, et al. 2005; Knauft, Nielsen, et al. 2005; McCauley, Jenckes, et al. 2005; Irwin and Richardson 2006; Barnhart, Lewis, et al. 2007; Harding, Selman, et al. 2008; Mauksch, Dugdale, et al. 2008; Quinn, Vadaparampil, et al. 2008

TABLE 4.2. Evidence from Review Studies Relating to Factors That Lead to Poor or Better Physician Communication ($n = 31$)

Reference	Review Type (R) Number of Studies (N) Study Setting (S) Study Purpose (P) Study Dates (D)	Key Findings
Ong, de Haes, et al. 1995	(R) Focused (N) Not reported (S) Not reported (P) Identify purposes of medical communication, measurement of MD-patient communication, specific communicative behaviors, and effect of MD communication on patient outcomes (D) Not reported	In reviewing MD-patient communication, authors identify background and process factors that play an important role in communication. (1) Background factors: cultural norms and differences e.g., beliefs about the elements of good medical care or patient's appreciation of physician's touch which show contradictory results; MD sociodemographic and personality; how MDs see their relationship with the patient, i.e., a paternalistic role with high MD control or as a partnership; and patient characteristics, e.g., information-seeking behavior, sociodemographic, psychological, and psychosocial variables, their physical appearance and disease characteristics. Patients with different diseases have specific needs and expectations regarding their communication and relationship with the MD depending on the particular stage of their illness, especially with chronic disease. (2) Process factors: how well MDs handle their own anxieties and uncertainties about cancer so that does not hinder the MD-patient communication; MDs' assessment of patients' desire for information; MDs' ability to elicit patients' main concerns without interruption as well as patients' perceptions of the illness and the feelings and expectations associated with the disease; the degree to which MDs encourage patient questions and avoid interruptions; MDs' communication of medical information in everyday language; degree of shared decision making about treatment; and MDs' nonverbal communications such as tone of voice, gaze, posture, laughter, facial expressions, touch, and physical distance.
Siegler and Levin 2000	(R) Selective review (N) Not reported (S) End-of-life (P) Review end-of-life care and provide recommendations to improve communication (D) Not reported	Factors that often stand in the way of effective doctor-patient communication include (1) fear of being the bearer of bad news, (2) anticipated disagreements with the patient or family over futile treatment, (3) lack of education about how to deliver bad news, (4) feelings related to physician vulnerability and fear of death, and (5) medical-legal concerns

TABLE 4.2—*Continued*

Reference	Review Type (R) Number of Studies (N) Study Setting (S) Study Purpose (P) Study Dates (D)	Key Findings
Foster 2001	(R) Selective review (N) Not reported (S) Dementia (P) Identify MD challenges to providing dementia care (D) Not reported	Author uses personal experience supported by review articles to identify MD communication barriers: (1) interviewing a family member/caregiver to obtain collateral information is not an ordinary part of adult medical practice; there are few established guidelines; (2) risks giving patient and caregivers different messages that can promote misunderstanding and conflict within the family; (3) talking alone to family members exaggerates the physician's feelings of uncertain responsibility; (4) fear of causing patient and caregiver distress; (5) diagnosis is uncertain and it is difficult to make prognosis; (6) unfamiliarity with community resources; and (6) visit time required usually exceeds allotted visit time and is not reimbursable
Bylund and Makoul 2002	(R) Selective review (N) 11 studies (S) General clinical (P) Identify key findings in relationship between gender and empathic communication (D) 1985–2002	This literature review is included in a study on communication and gender in the MD-patient encounter (see table 4.3). Gender-specific MD behaviors linked to empathy in studies: (1) female MDs ask more questions and patients of female MDs provide more biomedical and psychosocial information than patients of male MDs; (2) female MDs use more partnership building techniques with their patients vs. male MDs; (3) female MDs more likely to use psychosocial discussion, positive talk, and emotionally focused talk vs. male MDs; (4) female MDs use more positive nonverbal communication and tend to spend longer with their patients than male MDs; (5) no difference between male and female MDs in the amount of biomedical information discussed, quality of information given, or social conversation exchanged; (6) female MDs have more emotionally focused talk; (7) female MDs rated themselves as more empathic in their communication than male MDs; (8) female residents in internal medicine tended to receive higher ratings on humanism vs. male residents.
Post, Cegala, et al. 2002	(R) Systematic, 1 dB (N) 16 RCTs (S) Primary care (P) Review evidence about	Interventions classified as high (6/16 studies), moderate (3/16), or low intensive (7/16), based on time, use of live personnel, and estimated cost. Target population adults in 15/16 studies, with

TABLE 4.2—*Continued*

Reference	Review Type (R) Number of Studies (N) Study Setting (S) Study Purpose (P) Study Dates (D)	Key Findings
	effects of patient communication training (D) 1975–2000	mean age 45 years, education 12.6 years, and representation from minority racial groups. Mean number of MDs = 12 (range 1–56). Outcomes: (1) patient question asking, 10/16 studies with 5/10 SIG effect; (2) amount of patient information, 4/16 studies with 3/4 SIG effect; (3) patient verification of information, 1/16 with no SIG effects; (4) patient knowledge of disease, 3/16 with no SIG effect; (5) MD satisfaction, 3/16 with 1/3 SIG effect; (6) patient satisfaction 8/16 with 2/8 SIG effect; (7) disease states and functional status, 4/16 with 4/4 finding SIG results for varying aspects of disease and functional outcomes; (8) adherence to treatment, 2/16, with 2/2 SIG effects on various adherence outcomes. High intensive interventions produced more SIG effects compared to moderate and low interventions. The authors conclude that training produced positive patient outcomes and changed the nature of the MD-patient interactions, with patients exhibiting greater control in the medical visit. They caution that the wide variation in study design, interventions, and measured outcomes limits the review conclusions.
Roter, Hall, et al. 2002	(R) Systematic, 4 dB (N) 26 studies (S) MDs of all levels of training, primarily primary care (P) Quantify effect of MD gender on communication during medical visits (D) 1967–2001	Findings are based on 23 observational studies and 3 large MD report studies. Results are reported by conceptual groupings of physician communication categories and their estimated pooled gender effects size. (1) Information giving: SIG for female MDs on psychosocial information giving (10 studies, ES = .22, p = <.02) and non SIG gender effects for biomedical, directive, and nondirective information giving, and for quality of information. (2) Question asking/data gathering: non SIG gender effects for general, biomedical, psychosocial, or open-ended questioning and a SIG effect on female MDs for closed-ended questioning (4 studies, ES = .28, p = <.003). (3) Partnership behaviors (defined as MD facilitates patient participation in the medical visit or attempts to equalize status by assuming a less dominating stance within the relationship): non SIG gender effects for passive be-

TABLE 4.2—*Continued*

Reference	Review Type (R) Number of Studies (N) Study Setting (S) Study Purpose (P) Study Dates (D)	Key Findings
		haviors, and a SIG effect on female gender for active behaviors (12 studies, ES = .22, p = <.05). (4) Socio-emotional behavior: non SIG gender effects for social conversation, negative talk, emotionally focused talk, and positive nonverbal talk, and a SIG effect on female gender for positive talk such as agreements, encouragement, and reassurance (14 studies, ES = .36, p = <.001). Length of visit reported in 17 studies found a SIG positive effect for female MDs (ES = .21, p = .02). Medical visits with female physicians are, on average, 2 minutes (10%) longer than those with male physicians. The authors conclude that female primary care MDs engage in more communication that can be considered patient centered and have longer visits than their male colleagues; however obstetrics and gynecology may present a different pattern than that of primary care, with male MDs demonstrating higher levels of emotionally focused talk than their female colleagues.
Street 2002	(R) Selective review (N) Not reported (S) General clinical (P) Examine gender differences in medical encounters (D) Not reported	There are 4 overlapping studies with Bylund and Makoul 2002, above. (1) Female MDs tend to conduct longer consultations, give more information, engage in more partnership building, are less directive, express more interest in psychosocial aspects of health (e.g., emotions, lifestyle, family), and are more explicitly reassuring, encouraging, and sharing than are male MDs (9 studies), but differences are small and female MDs are generally more similar than different in their communication (2 studies); (2) contradictory and inconsistent findings on MD facilitative communication (2 studies) and patient satisfaction with MD gender (5 studies); (3) female MDs are more interpersonally oriented (1 study), more concerned about emotional and social aspects of health (1 study), and more interested in the patient's input and partnership (3 studies); (4) male MDs may spend more time focusing on biomedical issues, offering advice, expressing opinions, and independently making recommendations for the other to accept or reject (1 study); (5) gender bias toward male

TABLE 4.2—*Continued*

Reference	Review Type (R) Number of Studies (N) Study Setting (S) Study Purpose (P) Study Dates (D)	Key Findings
		and female patients may generate MD assumptions about patient capabilities and needs (5 studies) and guide clinical treatment (2 studies). Author cautions that although gender-based perceptions and stereotypes can play a prominent role in the medical encounter, little is known about the scope of these beliefs and their impact. He presents an ecological communication model for medical encounters.
van Ryn 2002	(R) Selective review (N) Not reported (S) General clinical (P) Provide framework for guiding research on provider contributions to race/ethnic disparities in health care (D) Not reported	Race/ethnic disparities in care documented for kidney transplant, cardiac procedures, mental health treatment, and pain treatment with the suggestion that there is some evidence of MD contribution. Evidence is presented that (1) patient sociodemographic characteristics independently influence physician expectations, perceptions, and affect toward patients (19 studies, 1984–2000); (2) MD beliefs about patients influence their interpretation of patients' symptoms (4 studies, 1990–2001); (3) MD beliefs about patients' social and behavioral characteristics directly influence their clinical decision making and diagnostic accuracy (7 studies, 1996–2001), especially in mental health (10 studies, 1993–2001); (4) MD conscious beliefs and unconscious stereotypes about patients influence their interpersonal behaviors and communication style (6 studies, 1982–99); and (5) patient sociodemographic characteristics influence the content of encounters (10 studies, 1988–2001). Authors propose a causal model for studying patient race/ethnicity disparities in care and MD behavior.
Cegala 2003	(R) Descriptive (N) 18 studies (S) Primary care (P) Identify the potential of communication skills training for cancer patients; identify research issues (D) 1985–2004	Article divides the review into discourse and health outcomes and identifies the research needed in these 2 areas. 9/18 studies were addressed previously in the author's 2002 review (Post, Cegala, et al. 2002) and conclusions are not substantially different from that review. Discourse outcomes research is needed in training and assessing patient information provision and verifying skills. Author noted that approximately one-half of the studies report SIG more question asking among trained

TABLE 4.2—*Continued*

Reference	Review Type (R) Number of Studies (N) Study Setting (S) Study Purpose (P) Study Dates (D)	Key Findings
		patients than untrained patients, and the studies that do not result in increased question asking are those with less developed interventions. 6 health outcome studies (4 clinical, 2 compliance) were noted, all with SIG effect. More research is needed to examine the relationship between training and health outcomes. Overall, "the largest communication training effects were produced by interventions that involved modeling and/or practice." The challenge is to find the most effective and cost-efficient ways to deliver CST.
Gordon 2003	(R) Focused review (N) Not reported (S) Palliative care (P) Highlight some challenges to effective communication at transitions to palliative care (D) Not reported	MD factors related to poor communication: MDs (1) have trouble estimating when a patient will die (1 study); (2) give a falsely optimistic prognosis to dying patients (1 study); (3) introduce bias when explaining probabilities (2 studies); and (4) define hope in terms of disease response or improved survival and experience treatment failure as "taking away the patient's hope" (4 studies)
Griffin, Nelson, et al. 2003	(R) Focused review (N) Not reported (S) Lung cancer patients (P) Establish evidence-based recommendations for supportive end-of-life care for lung cancer patients (D) Not reported	MD factors related to poor communication: (1) MDs have their own personal fears and a death anxiety (1 study); (2) MDs lack training, knowledge, and experience in giving bad news (7 studies)
McGorty and Bornstein 2003	(R) Focused review (N) Not reported (S) Palliative care (P) Review factors that affect MDs' decisions to discuss hospice options that MDs have control over (D) Not reported	Barriers to hospice use that stem from MD perceptions and priorities: (1) lack of knowledge and negative perceptions of hospice (6 studies) based on perceptions that hospice is inflexible and a last resort, and lack of knowledge about and experience with hospice; (2) discomfort communicating poor prognoses, characterized by deficient MD explanations of terminal illness to patients, insufficient MD education about palliative care, MD discomfort with death and the hospice concept, difficulty admitting limitations when dealing with terminal illness, and fear of diminished stature in the eyes of patients and families (6 studies); (3) instrumentalist perspective, characterized by fear

TABLE 4.2—*Continued*

Reference	Review Type (R) Number of Studies (N) Study Setting (S) Study Purpose (P) Study Dates (D)	Key Findings
		of losing control of patients (3 studies), affiliation with a teaching hospital and fear of malpractice (1 study), pressure from cure-oriented profession and fear of defeat (2 studies), and an effort to appear consistent (1 study); and (4) timing of hospice discussions based upon being wary of suggesting hospice, and waiting until patient has no other options or is too fragile to transfer
Williams and Skinner 2003	(R) Systematic review, 4 dB (N) Not reported (S) Primary care and specialist MDs (P) Explore outcomes of MD job satisfaction (D) Through mid-2002	This review considers a broad range of outcomes related to MD job satisfaction. There are 4 studies that support the idea that MD job satisfaction affects patient relationships. (1) 57 Netherlands MDs with positive work feelings were associated with "being open with the patient" ($p = <.05$) and being "attentive to psychosocial aspects" of care ($p = <.05$), while negative work feelings were associated with neither variable; and (2) 189 family planning MDs in the Philippines found MDs with low levels of task satisfaction had the lowest mean value for clinic effectiveness (defined in terms of the mean number of monthly acceptors of family planning and the efficacy of the methods selected); moderate levels of task satisfaction were associated with moderate levels of clinic effectiveness; and MDs with the highest level of task satisfaction had the highest clinic effectiveness ($p = <.01$).
Fallowfield and Jenkins 2004	(R) Systematic review, 4 dB (N) Not reported (S) Pediatrics, obstetrics, trauma, and cancer (P) Assess impact that giving sad, bad, and difficult news has on doctors and patients (D) 1993–2003	(See table 2.4 for the Fallowfield and Jenkins 2004 findings related to poor or ineffective communication by MDs.) Factors related to poor communication in "breaking bad news" include disparity among MDs in opinion about truthful disclosure; stress experienced when giving bad news; inadequate guidance and help during initial formative experiences; difficulty handling their own emotions—sorrow, guilt, identification, and feeling a failure; and traditional paternalistic attitudes where MDs censor information they give to patients about outlook on the grounds that what someone does not know cannot harm them (8 studies).

TABLE 4.2—*Continued*

Reference	Review Type (R) Number of Studies (N) Study Setting (S) Study Purpose (P) Study Dates (D)	Key Findings
Harrington, Noble, et al. 2004	(R) Systematic, 3 dB (N) 20 studies/25 articles (S) Primarily outpatient (P) Examine intervention studies designed to improve patients' communication with their MDs (D) 1966–2001	Review included 7 studies (9 articles) not reviewed previously in table 4.2. All 20 studies considered in terms of target populations; design; intervention type (face-to-face, video, written, audiotape); intervention impact on patients' participation and outcomes; and influence of patient characteristics on intervention effect. Setting: outpatient clinics, $n = 18$; inpatient, $n = 1$; community, $n = 1$. Designs: 17/20 RCTs, with 11 placebo controls, 2 quasi experimental, and 1 unclear. 18/20 assessed impact of the communication process on visit; 3/30 influence of patient characteristics on intervention response; and 15/20 post-intervention measurement only. 15/20 interventions delivered immediately pre-appointment, with 5 up to 3 months pre-appointment. 9/20 did not report the duration of the interventions, with duration of others from 10 to 25 min for video to 2-hour combined face-to-face and written. Communication process effects measured by interaction analysis systems in 12/20 studies, however "nearly half" measured only 1 or 2 categories of communicative behavior; 5/20 measured 10 or more categories. Process effects: (1) patient participation, 10/16 SIG increase (5/6 SIG face-to-face, 3/3 SIG video, 2/10 SIG written); (2) question asking, 5/11 SIG increase; (3) requests for clarification, 4/6 SIG increase; (4) visit length, 5/7 no effect; (5) expressed negative affect, 2/2 SIG increase; (6) MD encourages patient participation, 2/2 SIG increase. Outcome effects: (1) satisfaction, 2/13 SIG increase (generally high level of satisfaction); (2) knowledge, no effect, 0/5; (3) accuracy of visit recall, 3/5 SIG increase; (4) perceptions of control over health and preferences for an active role in health care, 4/4 SIG increase; (5) perceived health or adjustment to illness, 1/5 SIG increase; (6) anxiety, 3/5 SIG decrease; (7) adherence to medications and behavioral treatment, 1/1 SIG increase; (8) attendance, 2/3 SIG increase; (9) disease control, 1/1 SIG improvement in HTN and DM. Influence of patient characteristics on the impact re-

TABLE 4.2—*Continued*

Reference	Review Type (R) Number of Studies (N) Study Setting (S) Study Purpose (P) Study Dates (D)	Key Findings
		ported in 3/20 studies: 1 study reported increase in question asking higher for patients from social classes I and II (professional, managerial, and technical professions); and in visit length in younger, male, and from social classes I and II. "Many" studies did not explain the process of care or health professionals providing care; report whether patients attended for more than one visit; describe patients' previous experience with the service; report intervention timing in relation to patients' previous experience with the service. Research priorities: establish which interventions are most effective and practical, for which patient groups; improved methods to include appropriate control groups, appropriate sample size, proper use of randomization and blinding, and use of valid and reliable measures.
Weiner and Cole 2004	(R) Focused review (N) Not reported (S) Oncology (P) Review literature on clinician-centered obstacles to advance care planning and propose a conceptual framework of interacting emotional, cognitive, and skill barriers (D) Not reported	Caring for the terminally ill patient often evokes powerful emotional responses in MDs (1 study) and these responses can trigger a cascade of clinician avoidance, hopelessness, and burnout, thus impairing patient care (4 studies). Barriers include (1) adverse clinician emotional responses and obstructive beliefs: personally difficult patient death (e.g., unexpected or untimely, correlated with treatment disagreements, or hastened by medical intervention when MD feels very positively or negatively toward the patient) (1 study); more intense emotional reactions by female MDs or by having a long relationship with the patient (1 study); in 2 studies with AIDS patients, a discomfort discussing death, belief that discussing death can harm the patient or undermine hope, MD is not ready for the patient to die, and lack of time. (2) Maladaptive beliefs: inadequate or maladaptive behavior role modeling in medical school and training that undermines engagement with patients (5 studies). (3) Skill deficits: lack of self-awareness in emotions, thoughts, and behaviors used to avoid advance care planning (7 studies) and emotional avoidance strategies (6 studies).

TABLE 4.2—*Continued*

Reference	Review Type (R) Number of Studies (N) Study Setting (S) Study Purpose (P) Study Dates (D)	Key Findings
Baile and Aaron 2005	(R) Selective review (N) Not reported (S) Oncology (P) Emphasize outcomes of communication studies and implications for MD training (D) Not reported	(See table 2.4 for Baile and Aaron 2005 findings related to poor or ineffective communication by MDs.) Barriers to communication include (1) time, due to bureaucratic insurance and reimbursement issues (1 study), also noting that better oncology care has come at the price of more complex information for the patient to understand and less time for the MD to spend with the patient and family (1 study); (2) MDs struggle to provide accurate information and hope in the face of grave or uncertain prognosis and they may not understand the patient's preferences or may disclose only partial information for fear of upsetting the patient (1 study), also noting that high stakes interviews such as breaking bad news are stressful and require skills with which the oncologist may not be comfortable; (3) disconnect between MDs and patients about how much information patients want, because MDs may feel it is up to the patient to bring up problems whereas patients may feel that if it is important the MD will bring it up (1 study); (4) MDs often miss opportunities to empathically respond to a patient's feelings because they either fail to identify them or lack the knowledge of how to respond to them (3 studies); and (5) cultural competence—global and geographical differences regarding "truth telling" exist that reflect prevailing religious, social, and cultural norms aimed at "protecting" the patient from the psychological impact of adverse information or determining that the family is the principal decision maker for care (4 studies).
Hack, Degner, et al. 2005	(R) Systematic review, 2 dB (N) Not reported (S) Oncology (P) Critique the empirical literature on the communication needs and goals of cancer patients (D) 1992–2004	(See table 2.4 for Hack, Degner, et al. 2005 findings related to poor or ineffective communication by MDs.) MD factors related to poor communication include (1) busy patient workload and a lack of familiarity with the patient; (2) MDs differ in level of communication skill, with those who are deficient in their skills being less effective at conveying disease information; (3) tendency to ignore symptom assessment unless clinical information is not clear and to ignore patients' symptom reports when

TABLE 4.2—*Continued*

Reference	Review Type (R) Number of Studies (N) Study Setting (S) Study Purpose (P) Study Dates (D)	Key Findings
		positive clinical information is available; (4) MDs may believe it is better to withhold, distort, or soften potentially negative and emotionally upsetting information from patients interest of fostering patient hope and well-being; (5) lack ability to assess levels of patient depression and anxiety; (6) time constraints in busy clinics and MDs' belief that they know the amount and kind of information that is best for their patients to receive may contribute to consultations that are MD directed and MD dominated.
Mystakidou, Tsilika, et al. 2005	(R) Systematic review, 5 dB (N) Not reported (S) Oncology (P) Investigate the communication context through which health care professionals and families with cancer patients interact (D) 1970–February 2004	MD ethnicity and culture are a factor in how bad news is delivered to patients and family, including truth telling, informed consent, and individuals' rights in health care decision making. While guidelines generally recommend individualized disclosure, most MDs in northern Europe and in Anglo-Saxon countries usually reveal the diagnosis both to the patient and (with the patient's permission) to the spouse. In the South and East of Europe, MDs often conceal the diagnosis from the patients (7 studies 1980–2002). 5 studies of Greek MDs found little change 1980–99 in MD attitude in truth telling to cancer patient. A 1999 survey of 1,500 Greek MDs found that 78% very rarely or never disclosed cancer diagnoses to patients and 76% informed relatives. MDs in these studies reported they had inadequate training on communication skills (61%–100%). Authors conclude that there is a tendency for Greek MDs toward increased openness, although the majority prefer to disclose the truth to patients' families. One of the major causes of MDs' attitudes regarding nondisclosure is the lack of education on communication skills.
Parker, Davison, et al. 2005	(R) Descriptive, 2 dB (N) Not reported (S) Outpatient, oncology (P) Examine empirical literature on current knowledge about information giving and skills-	Studies are "a representative sample of the empirical literature." Among studies reported, only skills-based interventions are included in this review, $n = 10$ studies. (1) Prompt sheets, 8 studies found variable results in number of questions asked by patients; no association between patient satisfaction and total number of questions asked

TABLE 4.2—*Continued*

Reference	Review Type (R) Number of Studies (N) Study Setting (S) Study Purpose (P) Study Dates (D)	Key Findings
	based interventions designed to facilitate cancer patients' communication with healthcare providers (D) Not reported	or speaking times; may increase disease/treatment specific questions; no effect when prompt sheet combined with coaching. (2) Community-based, 2 studies, a 2-hour workshop with written materials found an increase in self-reported confidence scores; a 1-day workshop for cancer patients and families found participants assessed the workshop as beneficial using a post-intervention brief survey. Methodological issues include (1) interventions are not theoretically based or based on a conceptual model of the patient-provider relationship, limiting selection of appropriate outcome measures; (2) studies may measure the same construct (e.g., satisfaction), but are often assessed with different measures, limiting across study comparisons; (3) measures lack established reliability and validity and are often developed for individual studies. With respect to study methods, authors state that interventions (1) need to be flexible enough to meet individual patients' desire for information, communication style, personal strengths, demographic characteristics, health literacy, and disease/treatment stage; (2) need to be tested in real-world clinical settings; and (3) recognize that family members are often involved in clinical visits and decision making.
Haywood, Marshall, et al. 2006	(R) Systematic, 1 dB (N) 137 controlled trials (S) Not reported (P) Describe range and effectiveness of intervention strategies designed to enhance patient participation in the visit process (D) 1996–2004	While authors review both patient and provider targeted interventions, only patient targeted CST interventions, $n = 44$ studies, are included in these key findings: checklists, 11/44; coaching, 16/44; educational materials, 14/44; group education, 3/44. Individual studies are not compared. Data are synthesized by intervention type, and their impacts (SIG $p = >.05$) reported as percent effective in 7 domains of potential effects. (1) Communication: checklists 4/9 (44%), coaching 8/9 (89%), educational materials 7/9 (78%), group education 1/1 (100%). (2) Concordance (patient participation in decision making, patient-provider concordance, and patient decisional conflict/regret): checklists 0/1 (0%), coaching 2/4 (50%), educa-

TABLE 4.2—*Continued*

Reference	Review Type (R) Number of Studies (N) Study Setting (S) Study Purpose (P) Study Dates (D)	Key Findings
		tional materials 0/2 (0%), group education 0/1 (0%); (3) self-efficacy, adherence, and behavior change: checklists 1/2 (50%), coaching 1/5 (20%), educational materials 3/5 (60%), group education 0/2 (0%). (4) Increased provider diagnosis and management: checklists 2/2 (100%). (5) Patient satisfaction: checklists 4/8 (50%), coaching 0/6 (0%), educational materials 2/9 (22%), group education 0/1 (0%). (6) Health status: checklists 1/1 (100%), coaching 3/7(43%), educational materials 2/6 (33%). (7) Resource use: checklists 0/2 (0%), coaching 1/2 (50%), educational materials 2/3 (67%), group education 0/1 (0%). While the review supports previous findings that various interventions can have a positive impact on key processes of care, there is insufficient evidence to advocate one approach to enhancing patient participation in the visit process. Authors identify study limitations as unclear intervention specification; failure to measure outcomes, especially cost and long-term effects; and no inclusion of external factors such as a patient's previous encounter with the health care system.
Irwin and Richardson 2006	(R) Focused review (N) Not reported (S) Asthma patients (P) Review evidence on patient-focused care in asthma management (D) Not reported	Barriers to care and communication include MD underestimating patients' needs for information (3 studies); pulmonary patients' need for greater continuity of care between MDs (1 study) and continuity of care with patient's MD (1 study); limited time for complex patients; and failure to elicit patient's agenda and expectations (2 studies)
Roter, Frankel, et al. 2006	(R) Focused review (N) Not reported (S) Nonspecified MD type (P) Review on the expression of emotion through nonverbal behavior in MD-patient relationships (D) Not reported	Authors argue that emotions play a part in the process of medical care because MDs and patients have and show emotions, as well as judge each other's emotions. Measurement of nonverbal sensitivity has shown that females are better at judging nonverbal cues and are more skilled in conveying emotions via nonverbal cues, but the literature is lacking about how aware MDs are of their own emotions. In 1 study, following communication skills training, female medical students were able to describe their emotional reactions to videotape clips of patients with greater awareness

TABLE 4.2—*Continued*

Reference	Review Type (R) Number of Studies (N) Study Setting (S) Study Purpose (P) Study Dates (D)	Key Findings
		of complex and ambivalent feelings than their male counterparts. Another study showed that MDs judged their patients to experience more negative emotion, and less positive emotion, than the patients themselves reported. A study where MDs and patients were asked to rate their liking of one another (feelings of warmth and friendliness, and enthusiasm for seeing someone) found a modest degree of accuracy. Research also suggests that primary care MDs generally do poorly at recognizing patients' emotional distress. The authors suggest that "nonverbally skilled MDs engage in more appropriate nonverbal behaviors, are more sensitive to patient nonverbal cues of distress or confusion, and are more effective in conveying emotional messages of caring and sincerity to their patients."
Schouten and Meeuwesen 2006	(R) Systematic review, 2 dB (N) 14 observational studies (S) Primary care (P) Gain insight into the effects of patient and MD cultural/ethnic backgrounds on the medical communication process (D) 1974–2004	Participating MDs were mostly residents in their second or third year of medical training (in the US) or general practitioners. All studies found SIG differences in MD affective and instrumental verbal behavior as well as consultation length behavior when comparing consultations with white patients and ethnic minority patients. MDs showed less affective behavior when communicating with ethnic minority patients (6 studies), but 1 study found MDs were more affective toward ethnic minorities. SIG higher ratings of positive patient affect (i.e., friendliness, interest, responsiveness and engagement) were found in race-concordant as opposed to race-discordant visits (1 study). There was SIG decreased empathy with ethnic minority patients compared to white patients (3 studies), but 1 study found MDs expressed more empathy with ethnic minority patients during pediatric consultations, and 1 study did not detect SIG differences in MDs' expressions of empathy Hispanic vs. white American patients. Compared to white patients ethnic minority patients had SIG lower scores on MD social talk and rapport building, friendliness and concern, and responsiveness to patient comments (6 studies). No relationship was found be-

TABLE 4.2—*Continued*

Reference	Review Type (R) Number of Studies (N) Study Setting (S) Study Purpose (P) Study Dates (D)	Key Findings
		tween linguistic factors and variations in communication (7 studies). Patient ethnicity is suggested to have an independent and negative effect on health outcomes, regardless of the communication process (3 studies). Authors conclude that it is difficult to reach definite conclusions about the cultural variability of doctor-patient communication; a research model is presented.
Weiner and Roth 2006	(R) Focused review (N) Not reported (S) Palliative care (P) Define common unintended clinician behaviors which impair discussion about goals of care near the end of life (D) Not reported	Based on the authors' experience and literature review 5 common counterproductive MD behaviors in palliative care are identified. The clinician (1) initiates the discussion about goals of care without assessing the readiness of patient and family to consider death and dying issues; (2) unintentionally links relief of suffering with a demand upon the patient or family to accept limited lifespan, disrupting trust; (3) misdiagnoses patients and families as being "in denial" of medical reality, when they are actually experiencing normative grief and conflict; (4) engages in a distracting and sometimes destructive debate with the patient or family over the medical reality of impending death; (5) presents value-laden medical decisions without "right or wrong" answers in a hypothetical, impersonal, and binary manner. The authors suggest that MD communication barriers may impair clinical decision making and cause unintentional suffering to the patient, family, and clinician; improved communication should diminish the occurrence of depression, anxiety, and complicated grief in the patient and survivors, potentially improving medical outcomes.
Frantsve and Kerns 2007	(R) Focused review (N) Not reported (S) General clinical (P) Identify general trends in how MDs engage in shared decision making in chronic, nonmalignant pain treatment (D) Not reported	Related to pain management, authors emphasize the interpersonal communication factors: gender bias against women in treating pain (4 studies); underestimation of patients' pain (2 studies); and chronic pain patients and their MDs having opposing attitudes, goals, treatment preferences (4 studies) and expectations of the role of the MD in treatment (2 studies)

TABLE 4.2—*Continued*

Reference	Review Type (R) Number of Studies (N) Study Setting (S) Study Purpose (P) Study Dates (D)	Key Findings
Wetzels, Harmsen, et al. 2007	(R) Cochrane review (N) 3 RCTs or quasi RTs (S) Primary care (P) Assess effects of interventions that improve the involvement of older patients (65 years) in their health care (D) 1966–2004	3 studies met inclusion criteria. No meta-analysis possible. (1) Quasi randomized trial is included in above reviews. (2) RCT ($n = 45$) using interactional analysis, pre-visit interview with researcher to help patient formulate and write questions found that intervention group asked at least one question (64%) vs. control 35% ($p = <.001$); asked different questions vs. control. Control group did not ask about purpose, proper use, monitoring of effectiveness, side effects perceived, or what to do if prescribed therapy dose was missed. (3) RCT ($n = 355$), 2-hour community setting workshop up to 3 months pre-visit, using subjective, self-reported measures, found program attendance SIG associated with greater number of self-reported active behaviors, controlling for relevant characteristics, during the MD visit ($p = <.05$); active behaviors SIG correlated with younger age and female gender; intervention patients SIG more satisfied with visit interpersonal aspects ($p = <.05$); no effect on overall satisfaction. No health related outcomes or long-term follow-up were reported in all 3 studies. Authors conclude (1) the effects of written or face-to-face preparation for visits with MDs led to more questioning behavior by older people and more self-reported active behavior; (2) there is little evidence on the effects of interventions for improving older patients' involvement in their health care.
Kinnersley, Edwards, et al. 2008	(R) Cochrane review, with meta-analysis (N) 33 RTs in 35 publications (S) 31 outpatient, 1 inpatient (P) Assess effects on patients, clinicians, and the health care system of interventions before visits to help patients or their representatives	30/33 RTs reported on patients consulting doctors, 3/33 on patients consulting MDs or nurses. Interventions: 18/33 written materials, with 8/25 adding coaching and 1/33 adding brief instructions at consultation; 5/33 coaching alone; 1/33 audiotape of previous consultation. Interventions delivered just before visit, 25/33; up to 3 months before visit, 8/33. 26/33 interventions targeted patients alone; 7/33 included clinician training. Methods: number of randomized patients ranged from 32 to 1,208. Data were pooled across studies and meta-analyses conducted for the five main

TABLE 4.2—*Continued*

Reference	Review Type (R) Number of Studies (N) Study Setting (S) Study Purpose (P) Study Dates (D)	Key Findings
	gather information in visits by question asking (D) 1966–2006	outcomes: question asking, anxiety, knowledge, satisfaction, and length of visit. Standardized mean differences used for ES. Outcomes: (1) Question asking measured in 17/33, with SIG increase 6/17. ES of 1/17 studies = .27 ($p = <.001$), small, SIG. (2) Anxiety before visits measured in 4/33, with 2/4 reduction, 1/4 increase, 1/4 no effect on anxiety. ES on 3/4 studies = 1.56 ($p = .58$), large, NS; anxiety after visit in 9/33, with 2/9 reduction, 1/9 increase, 6/9 no effect on anxiety; ES on 6/9 studies = .08 ($p = .25$), small, NS. (3) Knowledge measured in 5 studies, with 2/5 reduction, 3/5 no change in knowledge; ES 5/5 studies = .34 ($p = .26$), small, NS. (4) Patient satisfaction measured in 23/33 studies, with 5/23 increase, 14/23 no change, 2/23 increases occurred only for particular aspects of satisfaction (depth of relationship, interpersonal satisfaction), 1/23 satisfaction of child patients was increased but parental satisfaction was unchanged, 1/23 no immediate effect was found but satisfaction was increased at 3 months. ES for overall satisfaction immediately after visit on 17/23 studies = .09 ($p = .007$), small, SIG. (5) Visit length measured in 17/33, with 3/17 SIG increase, 13 no effect, 1/17 length of first of 3 linked visits was decreased whereas the third was increased. ES of 13/17 studies = .10 ($p = .19$), small, NS. Additional analyses on effect modifiers found SIG small to moderate increases in question asking for written materials (ES = .42) and coaching (ES = .36). Written materials led to a SIG small increase in visit length of consultations (ES = .13), and coaching produced a NS smaller change (ES = .07). Written materials produced a NS small increase in satisfaction (ES = .08); for coaching the effect was SIG small increase (ES = .23). Other analyses suggested that providing clinicians with training either combined with interventions directed at patients or delivered before the implementation of interventions directed at patients has no clear benefits. Authors conclude that interventions for

TABLE 4.2—*Continued*

Reference	Review Type (R) Number of Studies (N) Study Setting (S) Study Purpose (P) Study Dates (D)	Key Findings
		patients before visits produce small benefits for patients. Further research is needed to (1) identify those patients in whom interventions are likely to be most beneficial or harmful (e.g., increasing anxiety); (2) explore changing the visit culture, aimed at empowering patients, rather than delivering a one-time intervention delivered prior to the visit; (3) explore the effect on patients and MDs with MD training in parallel with interventions directed at patients. Authors state that "There appears to be no clear benefits from clinician training in addition to patient interventions, although the evidence is limited."
Mauksch, Dugdale, et al. 2008	(R) Systematic review, 3 dB (N) 9 studies (S) Primary care (P) Explore how to combine effective relationship development and communication skills with time management to maximize efficiency (D) 1973–2006	Earlier research found that although PCPs have expressed frustration about time limitations (2 studies), more time does not guarantee better communication, as evidenced by patient perception of time use (1 study) and poor communication found in 30- to 60-minute health maintenance visits (1 study); no SIG difference in visit length across the biomedical to psychosocial continuum (1 study); no difference in visit length comparing patient-centered and MD-centered styles (2 studies); and MD communication styles seem to remain constant irrespective of visit length (4 studies). Based on review of 9 studies, authors present a model for blending the quality-enhancing and time management features of selected communication and relationship skills.
Leatherman and Warrick 2008	(R) Systematic review, 5 dB (N) 15 reviews and 18 studies (S) Primary and specialty care (P) Assess the effectiveness of decision aids in screening and treatment (D) 1997–2007	Screening decision aids (DAs) primarily used for PSA, prenatal and genetic testing, and mammography, colorectal, and cervical cancer screening in primary care settings. SIG positive effects were on knowledge acquisition and on health behavior outcomes as measured by intent to have screening or uptake in screening. There was little measurement of patient experiences with decision making. Notably, how patients use DAs in communication with their provider was not explored. There was scant evidence of the effect of screening DAs on health status and health care utilization. Treatment DAs found positive effects on patient knowl-

TABLE 4.2—*Continued*

Reference	Review Type (R) Number of Studies (N) Study Setting (S) Study Purpose (P) Study Dates (D)	Key Findings
		edge about a condition and/or treatment option and on patient perceived risk estimation. There was mixed evidence of DA effects on treatment choice. Evidence from 2 studies found a decreased effect on resource utilization, and 1 study found a SIG effect on reducing adjuvant therapy in breast cancer treatment. Authors conclude that additional research is needed on the effect of DAs on patient outcomes and health care costs.
Quinn, Vadaparampil, et al. 2008	(R) Focused review (N) Not reported (S) Oncology (P) Discuss the current difficulties in communicating information about fertility preservation in the United States (D) Not reported	MD awareness/knowledge of fertility preservation options (1 study) and facilities (3 studies). MD comfort in addressing cancer fertility options (1 study) and concern about the delay in treatment necessary for fertility preservation to occur (2 studies). Financial barriers: egg harvesting or sperm banking procedures, as well as the treatments and applications for post-cancer patients to attempt pregnancy, are generally not covered by insurance carriers (1 study). Limited visit time may interfere or compete with issues related to the diagnosis, treatment, and prognosis that must be discussed in the already lengthy initial oncology visit (1 study). MDs may practice in settings/centers lacking resources to offer patients interested in pursuing fertility preservation (2 studies); 1 study found that only 14% of National Cancer Institute–designated comprehensive cancer centers had standards of care or counseling concerning fertility and/or sexual concerns.

Note: ES .2 = small, .5 = moderate, .8 or greater = large.
CST(s) = communication skills training(s)
dB = database(s)
DM = diabetes mellitus
ES = effect size: 0.2 = small, 0.5 = moderate, 0.8 or greater = large

HTN = Hypertension
MD(s) = physician(s)
n = number
NS = non-significant
RT = randomized trial
RCT(s) = randomized control trials(s)

TABLE 4.3.   Evidence from Empirical Studies Relating to Factors That Lead to Poor or Better Physician Communication ($n = 48$)

Reference	Study Design (S) Study Purpose (P) Study Setting (T) Study Date (D) Country (C)	Method	Final Sample Size	Main Measures	Key Findings
Calam, Far, et al. 2000	(S) Qualitative (P) Explore the experiences of FP residents and practicing MDs in establishing code status (T) Hospital (D) 1998–99 (C) US	Audiotaped semistructured in-depth interviews using grounded theory approach to identify ideas and themes	$n = 5$ family MDs and 5 family practice residents in a university-affiliated urban tertiary care hospital	MD perceived barriers to discussing code status	Barriers to code-status discussions included personal discomfort with confronting mortality, fear of damaging the doctor-patient relationship or harming the patient by raising the topic of death, limited time to establish trust, and difficulty in managing complex family dynamics
Curtis, Patrick, et al. 2000	(S) Descriptive (P) Determine the barriers to and facilitators of patient-clinician communication about end-of-life care (T) University and private clinics (D) 1996–97 (C) US	Structured interview	$n = 31$ MDs, 2 NPs, and 5 PAs $n = 57$ patients with AIDS	3 categories of potential interventions: education about end-of-life care, counseling to help address end-of-life concerns, and health care system changes to facilitate patient-clinician communication	Barriers that may be overcome with an education intervention: (1) s/he isn't ready to talk about the care s/he wants if s/he gets sick (25%); (2) s/he has not been very sick yet (21%); (3) s/he doesn't know what kind of care s/he wants if s/he gets sick (14%); (4) his/her ideas about the kind of care s/he wants change over time (14%); (5) discussing end-of-life care with patient takes considerable energy and preparation (14%); (6) s/he is very young to be thinking about end-of-life care

135

TABLE 4.3—*Continued*

Reference	Study Design (S) Study Purpose (P) Study Setting (T) Study Date (D) Country (C)	Method	Final Sample Size	Main Measures	Key Findings
					(12%); (7) I'm not ready to give up an aggressive approach with him/her at this time (9%). Barriers that may require a counseling intervention: (1) I worry that discussing end-of-life care will take away his/her hope (35%); (2) my role as a clinician is to make patient feel better (26%); (3) I worry that patient will think I am not being aggressive enough (21%); (4) I don't like to talk about end-of-life care (12%); (5) I feel like s/he is trying to protect me (5%). Barriers that require a change in culture or in the health care system: (1) there is too little time during our appointments to discuss everything we should (47%). Clinicians identified far more barriers to communication about end-of-life care than did patients, suggesting that clinician barriers may be more important to the occurrence of end-of-life communication than patient barriers.
van Dulmen 2000	(S) Descriptive (P) Investigate the relationship between the	Patient surveys pre- and post-visit; post-visit MD survey; video record-	n = 14 salaried and 7 fee-for-service pediatricians	(1) Length of visit; (2) verbal communication analyzed by RIAS	Salaried pediatricians: (1) visits lasted almost 3–4 minutes longer (initial visits 22 vs. 18, p = <.05; and follow-

	nature of the reimbursement system and structure and content of medical visits (T) Pediatric outpatient (D) 1996 (C) Netherlands	atricians $n = 207$ visits to salaried MDs and 95 visits to fee-for-service MDs	ings of visit	up visits 15.4 vs. 12.1; $p = <.001$), with time used to provide more information and advice; (2) engaged in more empathic behavior toward the patient, thereby facilitating a therapeutic relationship; (3) spent more time on exchanging information ($p = <.001$) with their patients and paid more attention to patient concerns and emotions ($p = .006$); and (4) gave more agreements ($p = <.001$), reflections ($p = .002$), and reassurances ($p = <.001$) than fee-for-service MDs. No differences were found in the number of diagnostic tests and investigations or in patient satisfaction.
Dosanjh, Barnes, et al. 2001	(S) Qualitative (P) Examine residents' perceptions of barriers to delivering bad news to patients and their family members (T) Hospital residents (D) Not reported (C) Canada	$n = 7$ MDs, representing four medical disciplines: family medicine, internal medicine, general surgery, and emergency	2 focus groups consisting of first- and second-year medical and surgical residents	Analysis of focus group transcripts using grounded theory approach	Most residents were aware of guidelines in the delivery of bad news, but they experienced difficulty when applying them in practice. Personal and institutional barriers as well as differing perceptions of bad news were identified as important barriers to breaking bad news. Residents' personal fears included: making mistakes, not being prepared, shame in asking for support, personal attachment to the news, awkwardness, nervous, stress, telephone delivery, confrontations, being misunderstood, and unable to follow up. Resi-

TABLE 4.3—*Continued*

Reference	Study Design (S) Study Purpose (P) Study Setting (T) Study Date (D) Country (C)	Method	Final Sample Size	Main Measures	Key Findings
					dent perceptions that affect appropriate delivery of bad news: uneasiness with death and dying; whether they are prolonging life vs. prolonging death given their orientation to cure; biases or stigmas as to what constitutes bad news may leave him/her unprepared for a patient's or family member's reaction; unusual circumstances such as telephone delivery of bad news may make it difficult to respond to family; and uncommon patient or family reactions. Institutional barriers included lack of support and time constraints. Residents reported they were often unclear on their role in delivering bad news and indicated that specific training and hospital supports were needed.
Makoul, Curry, et al. 2001	(S) Comparative (P) Assess MD-patient communication patterns with EMR (T) Internal medicine out-	Videotape analyzed with SEGUE framework, medical record review	*n* = 6 MDs (3 using EMR and 3 using paper record) *n* = 204 pa-	(1) Outline patient's agenda; (2) explore psychosocial and emotional issues; (3) discuss how the health	(1) Outline the patient's agenda (NS); (2) explore psychosocial/emotional issues (NS); (3) discuss how health problem affects the patient's life (NS); (4) check/clarify information

138

	Study details	Sample	Measures	Findings
	patient (D) 1997–98 (C) US	tients	problem affects the patient's life; (4) check and clarify information; (5) encourage patient questions; (6) ensure encounter completeness	(EMR 99% vs. control 91%, p = .009); (5) encourage the patient to ask questions (EMR 25% vs. control 8%, p = .001); (6) ensure completeness (EMR 36% vs. control 13%, p = .000). Authors caution that some of the communication behaviors of the EMR MDs may be a function of the EMR use, others probably reflect styles established prior to EMR use.
Vegni, Zannini, et al. 2001	(S) Qualitative (P) Explore GPs' perspectives on giving bad news during consultations (T) Community (D) Not reported (C) Italy	n = 168 GPs	GPs were instructed to give a written report of a doctor-patient relationship in which they were personally involved Data analyzed for linguistic content and relational style	2 relational styles emerged: (1) MD-centered style where GPs talk about signs and symptoms, diagnosis and treatment regimens; they decide for themselves whether or not to tell the truth; and (2) patient-centered style where GPs consider it to be their duty to take care of the ill persons, trying to respect each patient's right to decide. In both these relational patterns, GPs feel it is a fundamental professional duty to reassure the patient; and they feel the most difficult aspect is managing their own emotional responses.
Bylund and Makoul 2002	(S) Qualitative (P) Study gender and empathy in medical encounters (T) Internal medicine (D) Not reported (C) US	n = 20 general internists	100 videotaped interviews, coded using Empathic Communication Coding System	(1) Patient empathic opportunities and gender, number and specific emotional content, and intensity of empathic opportunities; (2) MD responses and gender (1) No SIG difference in emotion-specific content ratios across gender: both male and female patients named emotions in approximately half of their empathic opportunities; (2) female patients created more intense empathic opportunities vs.

TABLE 4.3—*Continued*

Reference	Study Design (S) Study Purpose (P) Study Setting (T) Study Date (D) Country (C)	Method	Final Sample Size	Main Measures	Key Findings
					male patients (p = .05); (3) acknowledgment was MDs' most frequent responses to the empathic opportunities created by patients (71%); (4) on a scale from 1 to 5, female MDs gave higher empathic responses vs. male MDs (mean = 3.27 vs. 2.90, p = <.01).
Collins, Clark, et al. 2002	(S) Descriptive (P) Explore patients' perceptions of their communication with MDs about cardiac testing and treatment recommendations (T) VA clinics (D) Not reported (C) US	4 focus groups stratified by race (white vs. black)	n = 13 cardiac patients who had (1) undergone stress tests or (2) undergone stress test followed by invasive cardiac procedure	Identify MD-patient communication domains	(See table 2.5 for Collins, Clark, et al. 2002 findings related to poor or ineffective communication by MD.) Black patients consistently expressed a need for building a relationship with physicians (trust) before agreeing to an invasive cardiac procedure and complained that trust was lacking. White patients tended to emphasize that they were inadequately convinced of the need for recommended procedures.
Lukoschek, Fazzari, et al. 2003	(S) Descriptive (P) Assess effectiveness of MD-patient health information exchange (T) Urban academic PCP	Post-visit survey of patients and MDs	n = 19 MDs n = 145 patients	(1) Patient perceived health information delivery by MDs; (2) MD attitude about health information delivery to	(1) MD sociodemographic factors (age, gender, ethnicity, and years of practicing medicine) not SIG associated with patient comprehension; (2) 29% of MDs disagreed with patients

practices
(D) Not reported
(C) US

patients; (3) MD self-effectiveness in health communication; (4) language barrier, satisfaction, health participation, and patients' comprehension of health information

about patient ability to comprehend health information, overestimating their patients' ability to comprehend ($p = <.001$); (3) MDs who believed health information delivery to be important had fewer patients with comprehension difficulties; (4) MDs who assessed themselves as very effective educators efficient in dealing with cultural influences on communication and diverse educational topics had SIG more patients with lack of comprehension, compared with MDs who did not feel as effective; (5) differences between these 2 MD groups were not explained by sociodemographic factors, time spent teaching patients, or attitude about health information delivery to patients; (6) MD predictors of low patient comprehension included MDs who perceived that patients had difficulties comprehending health information (OR = 3.7, $p = .005$), who did not feel it is important to deliver health information (OR = .3, $p = <.001$), and who rated themselves as effective health educators (OR = 2.7, $p = <.001$).
In multiple linear regression analyses, patient older age (beta = .08, $p = .001$) and Hispanic ethnicity (beta =

Maly, Leake, et al. 2003
(S) Descriptive
(P) Assess MD provision of health information

Interview (unclear if by telephone or in person) within 6 months of

$n = 117$ surgeons
$n = 222$ newly

Receipt of information and perceived helpfulness

141

TABLE 4.3—*Continued*

Reference	Study Design (S) Study Purpose (P) Study Setting (T) Study Date (D) Country (C)	Method	Final Sample Size	Main Measures	Key Findings
	and assess differences by age and ethnicity (T) Oncology outpatient clinic (D) Not reported (C) US	breast cancer diagnosis and/or within 1 month post-treatment	diagnosed breast cancer patients of Anglo (64%), African American (12%), and Hispanic (12%) ethnicities		1.21, $p = .003$) had a negative association with MD provision of interactive informational support, controlling for patient and MD sociodemographic characteristics, practice characteristics, breast carcinoma stage, comorbidity, number of MDs seen, visit length, social support, and patient self-efficacy in interacting with MDs. Authors suggest possible explanations for the results are ageism and bias toward ethnic minority women by MDs. Notably, language barriers (65% of Hispanic patients reported speaking Spanish better than English) cannot be discerned from this study.
McIntosh and Shaw 2003	(S) Qualitative (P) Ascertain patient and MD experiences and expectations of information regarding low back pain (T) Community (D) Not reported	Semistructured GP interviews and focus groups comprising patients with low back pain	$n = 15$ GPs $n = 37$ patients with low back pain	Analysis of focus group transcripts	There were differences in opinions among MDs as to their role and responsibility as information providers, and uncertainty among MDs in terms of the value, availability, prioritization, and funding of information materials. Some GPs supported use of informational materials

Author	Study descriptors	Method	Sample	Variables	Findings
	(C) UK				and others believe that they may promote the "medicalization" of low back pain. MD diagnostic uncertainty about back pain led to poor communication with patients and patients' lack of understanding of their problems.
Shapiro, Hollingshead, et al. 2003	(S) Descriptive (P) Identify resident perceptions of competent cross-cultural doctor-patient communication (T) General practice (D) Not reported (C) US	Questionnaire	$n = 57$ MDs (20 family medicine residents and 37 internal medicine residents)	MD perceived (1) relevance of sociocultural factors in practice; (2) competence in sociocultural issues; (3) use and helpfulness of cross-cultural communication techniques; and (4) problematic patient cross-cultural characteristics	5-point Likert-type rating scale. MDs rated sociocultural issues as relevant to clinical practice (mean = 4.01); (2) rated themselves as competent in cross-cultural communication skills (mean = 3.45); (3) used cross-cultural communication techniques frequently (mean = 4.01), and found them helpful (mean = 4.26); (4) over half rated patient characteristics as a moderate to serious problem interfering with effective culturally competent communication; (5) insufficient time (92%). Authors comment that resident attitude of perceiving patient deficiencies and shortcomings to explain cross-cultural communication difficulties suggests a lack of true cross-cultural sensitivity and a tendency to hold patients, rather than MDs, responsible for "crossing cultures."
Verhoeven, Bovijn, et al. 2003	(S) Descriptive (P) Identify and quantify the barriers MDs en-	Postal survey with 69 items	$n = 122$ PCPs	Barriers in (1) sexual counseling practices; (2) circumstances and	MD barriers include (1) insufficient training (69%); (2) not familiar with sexual practices (e.g., gay patients)

TABLE 4.3—*Continued*

Reference	Study Design (S) Study Purpose (P) Study Setting (T) Study Date (D) Country (C)	Method	Final Sample Size	Main Measures	Key Findings
	counter in discussing STIs with their patients (T) Community (D) Not reported (C) Belgium			patient characteristics; (3) perception of the counseling atmosphere; (4) competence	(43%); (3) lack of time (61%); (4) general discomfort in taking a sexual history (18%); (5) presence of the patient's partner (89%) or mother (94%); (6) first contact with a patient (61%); (7) fear of embarrassing the patient (31%); (8) patient without genital complaints (71%); (9) patient characteristics, e.g., language and comprehension problems (74%), ethnic differences (68%), and age (31%) or opposite gender from patient (18%–64% depending on risk); and (10) female MDs feel more uncomfortable vs. male MDs with male HIV testing (54% vs. 23%, $p = <.05$). "About half" of MDs fail to counsel an asymptomatic patient with obvious STI risk.
Arber, McKinlay, et al. 2004	(S) Descriptive (P) Investigate whether patient age, gender, class, and race influence MD questioning style and advice giving	Video simulation of a patient consulting with CHD symptoms, designed to systematically alter patient age, sex, class, and race	$n = 256$ MDs (128 UK GPs and 128 US PCPs)	After viewing 1 of 16 video-simulated consultations, MD interviewed about their management of the patient, e.g., "Would you	Patient characteristics have little influence on the likelihood of asking about indicators of pathology, medical and risk factor history, or symptoms of pain and discomfort. Gender and age SIG influence MD question-

Author/year	Study design	Sample	Purpose/analysis	Results
	(T) Primary care (D) 2001–2 (C) UK, US	ask the patient any additional questions before you decide what's going on? Anything else?"		ing of CHD patients. Male patients are asked more questions ($p = <.01$), particularly about smoking ($p = <.001$), drinking ($p = .005$), and stress and psychological state ($p = .007$). Middle-aged patients vs. older patients are asked more about smoking ($p = .001$) and alcohol consumption ($p = <.001$). Advice about smoking is given to more men than women ($p = .01$), and to more mid-life vs. older patients ($p = .006$). Women doctors question patients about their lifestyle more often (smoking, $p = .003$; alcohol, $p = .025$), and give more advice to patients about their diet ($p = .004$).
Chibnall, Bennett, et al. 2004	(S) Qualitative (P) Identify MD barriers to the psychosocial spiritual (PSS) care of end-of-life patients (T) University-based health sciences center (D) Not reported (C) US	Group discussion, 2 groups for twenty 75-minute discussion sessions over the course of one year using transcribed audiotapes	$n = 17$ MDs representing 10 areas of medical specialty	Qualitative analysis to identify emerging PSS domains and themes that are psychosocial spiritual care of dying patients
				3 primary domains, cultural (48% of text units), organizational (33%), and clinical (19%), and 7 themes emerged. Cultural domain themes: medical training (21%), selection (12%), medical practice environment (8%), and debt/delay (7%). MDs believed that medical school selection and training combine to marginalize PSS. Practice environment does not encourage PSS care, and debt/delay kills idealism. Organizational domain themes: dissatisfaction with medicine (19%) and time/busyness (15%). Dissatisfaction with reim-

TABLE 4.3—*Continued*

Reference	Study Design (S) Study Purpose (P) Study Setting (T) Study Date (D) Country (C)	Method	Final Sample Size	Main Measures	Key Findings
					bursement and time pressures contribute to the tendency to avoid patient PSS issues and discussion. Clinical domain consisted of the theme of communication (19%), with the tendency to avoid nonmedical issues because of emotional investment and risks. Authors conclude that "the culture that selects and trains technically competent MDs does not value PSS needs and creates a work environment hostile to PSS concerns; and that these forces may act directly, by marginalizing PSS aspects of terminal care, and indirectly, through their effects on the emotional, relational, and spiritual lives of the MDs themselves."
Deveugele, Derese, et al. 2004	(S) Descriptive (P) Describe the features of GPs' short, moderate, and long consultation (T) Community GPs (D) Not reported	Questionnaire administered to GPs at beginning of study and a short questionnaire after each consultation Patient questionnaires at the beginning of the	$n = 183$ GPs from 6 European countries $n = 2,801$ patients with videotaped	(1) Visit time; (2) 16 RIAS categories of communicative behavior	There was little variability in the content (task oriented behavior [59%] and socioemotional behavior [37%]) among short (5 min), moderate (5–15 min), and long (>15 min) visits, suggesting that GPs develop a "standard operating procedure." On

(C) Europe, 6 countries	audiotaped consultation, analyzed using RIAS	consultations		average communication was 8% social behavior, 15% agreement, 4% rapport building, 10% partnership building, 11% giving directions, 28% giving information, 14% asking questions, and 7% counseling. Proportion of "giving information" and "psychosocial talk" increased SIG when visit duration increased; proportion of "partnership building," "giving directions," and "counseling" decreased SIG with increased visit time ($p = <.01$). Authors conclude that MDs adopt a general communicative style that only shows to some degree a relationship with visit length.
Farber, Urban, et al. 2004	(S) Descriptive (P) Identify MD perceived skills in palliative care (T) Palliative care (D) 2000 (C) US	National survey of internal medicine and family practice MDs Questionnaire on 4-point scale	$n = 462$ MDs	Frequency and skill in palliative care: (1) cultural aspects; (2) advance directives; (3) giving bad news; (4) pain management; (5) physical symptoms; (6) psychological and cognitive symptoms; (7) social support; (8) economic demands and the caregiver needs; (9) patient expectations/hope; (10) spiritual needs	(See table 2.5 for Farber, Urban et al. 2004 for evidence of poor communication in palliative care.) Interest in palliative care was associated with an increased frequency in performing palliative care items ($p = .036$), as having training in palliative care was associated with better perceived performance ($p = .05$).

TABLE 4.3—*Continued*

Reference	Study Design (S) Study Purpose (P) Study Setting (T) Study Date (D) Country (C)	Method	Final Sample Size	Main Measures	Key Findings
Gott, Galena, et al. 2004	(S) Descriptive (P) Identify barriers perceived by GPs and practice nurses to inhibit discussion of sexual health issues (T) Primary care (D) 2001–2 (C) UK	Semistructured interviews	$n = 22$ MDs $n = 35$ PNs	Clinician and patient barriers to discussing sex; patient barriers to discussing sex and the influence of external factors on sexual health management within primary care	(1) GP attitudes: GPs expressed concerns about whether sexual health was actually a "medical" issue or not, concerns as to whether patients would perceive sexual issues as legitimate topics for discussion within a medical consultation, and fear that it would jeopardize the MD-patient relationship; (2) primary care priority had to be diagnosing health conditions and prescribing medication with limited time available to discuss the impact of the condition upon the patient's life or sex life; (3) discomfort, stereotyped ideas, and/or prejudice in discussing sexual health with patients of the opposite gender, patients from black and ethnic minority groups, middle-aged and older patients, and nonheterosexual patients; and (4) limited training in managing sexual health in past education and currently available, and training competed for time and resource demands

| Frankel, Altschuler, et al. 2005 | (S) Qualitative
(P) Evaluate the impact of exam-room computers on communication between clinicians and patients
(T) Primary care office
(D) Not reported
(C) US | Longitudinal design using videotapes of regularly scheduled visits from 3 points in time: 1 month before, 1 month and 7 months after introduction of computers into the exam room | $n = 9$ clinicians (6 MDs, 2 PAs, 1 NP)
$n = 54$ patients | Using basic communication concepts from the Four Habits Communication Model as a base, an iterative consensus-building process was used to identify additional themes | Exam room computers changed the verbal, visual, and postural relationships between providers and patients. Results found 4 broad factors that influenced the impact of computers on communication. For (1) visit organization (managing the cognitive, physical, and socioemotional tasks that constitute the medical encounter); and (2) verbal and nonverbal behavioral factors, "facilitators and barriers that were present before the introduction of computers were carried forward and amplified when exam-room computers were used." In contrast, (3) computer navigation and mastery skills; and (4) spatial organization of the exam room "were unique to the introduction of the computer. The effects of all of the factors on communication could be either positive or negative." |
| Li and Lundgren 2005 | (S) Controlled trial
(P) Assess effect of short patient training session on various ways of requesting physicians to clarify a piece of previously elicited information during medical visit
(T) Clinic | Post-visit survey/usual care vs. 10–15 minute training, based on Conversational Grounding theory
Brochure noting 5 questions to clarify a previously elicited piece of information provided by MD during visit, and | $n = 114$ adult volunteers from clinic
$n = 57$ females
$n = 57$ males | 13 item questionnaire measuring patient (1) overall satisfaction; (2) relationship satisfaction; (3) communication satisfaction; (4) expertise satisfaction | (1) Intervention vs. control SIG increased overall satisfaction ($p = <.0001$); relationship satisfaction ($p = <.0001$); communication satisfaction ($p = <.0001$); expertise satisfaction ($p = <.0001$). (2) Females vs. males had more relationship satisfaction ($p = <.05$). (3) SIG correlates of satisfaction in the intervention group: greater age with relationship, |

TABLE 4.3—*Continued*

Reference	Study Design (S) Study Purpose (P) Study Setting (T) Study Date (D) Country (C)	Method	Final Sample Size	Main Measures	Key Findings
	(D) Not reported (C) Canada	rehearsal with re- searcher			communication and compliance sat- isfaction; increased educational level with expertise satisfaction; in- creased compliance with communi- cation satisfaction. (4) SIG correlates of satisfaction in the control group: both greater age and poorer health with communication satisfaction.
Knauft, Nielsen, et al. 2005	(S) Descriptive (P) Identify patient and MD barriers and facili- tators to end-of-life communication (T) University, county, VA clinics, and oxygen de- livery company (D) Not reported (C) US	In-person patient inter- views and mail survey of MDs. MDs completed a separate question- naire for each patient.	n = 56 MDs n = 115 pa- tients with oxygen-de- pendent COPD	15 barriers and 11 facili- tators of communica- tion	MD endorsed barriers: (1) there is too little time during our appointments to discuss everything we should (64%); (2) I worry that discussing end-of-life care will take away her/his hope (23%); (3) patient is not ready to talk about the care she/he wants if she/he gets sick (21%); (4) patient has not been very sick yet (20%); (5) patient doesn't know what kind of care she/he wants if she/he gets sick (15%); (6) patient's ideas about the kind of care she/he wants change over time (11%); and (7) my role as a doctor is to make him/her feel better (10%). Female MDs were more likely to en-

	(S)/(P)/(T)/(D)/(C)	Methods	Sample	Measures	Findings
					dorse "I work in a system that expects me to have end-of-life discussions with my patients" (p = .001). Non-white MDs were more likely to endorse (1) patient doesn't know what kind of care he wants if he gets sick (p = .04); (2) patient is not ready to talk about the care he wants if he gets sick (p = .02); (3) patient's ideas about the kind of care he wants change over time (p = .01); and (4) I worry that discussing end-of-life care will take away his hope (p = .03).
McCauley, Jenckes, et al. 2005	(S) Descriptive (P) Measure MD beliefs and identify barriers to integrating spirituality into patient care (T) Primary care (D) Not reported (C) US	30-item survey distributed at the annual, mandatory, off-campus, staff meeting	n = 78 MDs from a statewide staff model, managed care group	(1) Spiritual Barriers scale; (2) Spirituality in Patient Care scale	MDs believed that a patient's spirituality affects health (95%); addressing spirituality concerns is part of the MD's role (68%); spirituality should be a part of a routine patient history (agree 47%, uncertain 32%). Barriers included lack of time (95%); lack of training (69%); low priority compared to medical issues (64%); personal discomfort (57%); fear of offending patients (51%); fear of projecting personal beliefs (37%); fear of colleague opinion (21%); and fear of administrative response (21%).
Park, Betancourt, et al. 2005	(S) Qualitative (P) Explore residents' training and capabili-	Transcribed videotapes of 7 focus groups and audiotapes of 10 individ-	n = 68 resident MDs (residents in in-	MD perceptions of (1) preparedness to deliver care to diverse pa-	(1) Most MDs noted the importance of cross-cultural care yet reported little formal training; (2) MDs wanted

TABLE 4.3—*Continued*

Reference	Study Design (S) Study Purpose (P) Study Setting (T) Study Date (D) Country (C)	Method	Final Sample Size	Main Measures	Key Findings
	ties to provide quality care to diverse populations (T) Community (D) 2003 (C) US	ual in-depth interviews	ternal medicine, family practice, pediatrics, ob/gyn, psychiatry, emergency medicine, and general surgery were represented)	tients; (2) educational climate; (3) training experiences	more formal training yet expressed concern that culture-specific training could lead to stereotyping; (3) most had developed ad hoc, informal skills to care for diverse patients; (4) indicated they lacked the support (e.g., cultural aspects not included in case reviews, not evaluated on cultural competence, and lack of translators) needed to enable them to provide the best-quality care, and thus interpreted effective cross-cultural care as a lower priority; (5) most believed their institutions did not provide the needed time and resources to assist them with optimally treating diverse patients
Street, Gordon, et al. 2005	(S) Descriptive (P) Examine the influence of patient characteristics, MD communication style, and clinical setting on patient participation in medical interactions	Post hoc analysis of data from 3 empirical studies on physician-patient communication with coded audiotapes	n = 279 patients n = 135 primary care n = 79 SLE n = 65 lung cancer	(1) Active patient participation; (2) MD partnership building; (3) prompted vs. self-initiated patient participation	(1) 84% active participation behaviors were patient-initiated vs. prompted by MD partnership building or supportive talk; (2) predictors of active participation: MD partnership building (p = <.001); MD supportive talk (p = .001); higher patient education (p = .02); clinical setting, lung cancer

	(T) Primary and specialty care (D) Not reported (C) US			patients more active vs. SLE and primary care patients ($p = .001$); (3) predictors of patient-initiated and MD-prompted patient participation: white greater than nonwhite ($p = .01$); clinical setting, lung cancer patients vs. SLE and primary care patients ($p = .001$); no SIG significant predictors of MD-prompted active participation; (4) predictors of physician partnership building and supportive talk: female MDs used more supportive talk ($p = <.01$); MDs used more supportive talk with white vs. nonwhite patients ($p = <.01$); MDs used more partnership building and supportive talk with lung cancer patients vs. SLE and primary care patients ($p = .01$). Authors conclude: MDs can have a powerful influence on patient involvement but underuse behaviors that can optimize patient participation in medical encounters, and more research is needed to examine how specific clinical practice features may influence MD and patient communication.
Travado, Grassi, et al. 2005	(S) Descriptive (P) Examine MD communication skills and related psychosocial orientation, and burnout	$n = 125$ MDs	Researcher administered survey	Self-Confidence in Communication Skills (SCCS), Expected Outcome of Communication (EOC), MD belief	(1) MDs (86%) reported minimal training in communication, although they tended to describe themselves as quite skilled in their relationships with cancer patients; (2) MDs were

TABLE 4.3—*Continued*

Reference	Study Design (S) Study Purpose (P) Study Setting (T) Study Date (D) Country (C)	Method	Final Sample Size	Main Measures	Key Findings
	variables (T) 2 general and 1 cancer hospital (D) Not reported (C) Italy, Portugal, and Spain			(PBS), Maslach Burnout Inventory (MBI)	not convinced about the importance of the psychosocial aspects in health care or they were still attached to traditional biomedical values; they were uncertain about their patients' psychosocial needs and about their own reactions to the patients if they discussed psychosocial issues, wondering if patients would approve of their questioning; (3) low MD psychosocial orientation and burnout symptoms were SIG ($p = <.01$) associated with lower confidence in communication skills, higher expectations of a negative outcome following MD-patient communication ($p = <.01$), and lower expectations of obtaining positive outcomes ($p = <.01$); (4) high MD psychosocial orientation was associated with less negative expectations of the outcome of communication with patients and less burnout ($p = <.01$); (5) MDs with a greater sense of personal accomplishment (vs. burnout) corre-

					lated with higher self-confidence in their ability to communicate effectively, more positive expectancies, and fewer negative expectancies (p = ‹.01). Authors conclude that low psychosocial orientation and burnout of MDs negatively influence their communication skills with patients.
Wetzels, Wensing, et al. 2005	(S) Cluster randomized trial (P) Evaluate effects of program to enhance the involvement of older patients in their general practice consultations (T) 25 general practices (D) 2002 (C) Netherlands	Pre-post test randomization of 25 GPs from 20 practices who selected patients with recent consultation. Patients mailed leaflet to help prepare for the visit; GPs received a 30-minute outreach visit to encourage their patients' involvement during visit and to instruct them in the use of the patient leaflet.	n = 263 patients aged ›70 years n = 121 intervention group n = 142 control group, usual care	Questionnaires measuring (1) involvement (satisfaction with information given, opportunities to ask questions, give their opinion, and take part in decisions); (2) enablement (patients enabled to deal with their health problem after consultation); (3) satisfaction with care	(1) No effect of leaflet on involvement, enablement, or satisfaction. (2) 47/121 patients used the leaflet appropriately; their outcome scores did not differ SIG between intervention or control groups. (3) Intervention group reported more psychological symptoms to their GP vs. control (p = .034). Patients were not stimulated to discuss any other health problems.
Burd, Nevadunsky, et al. 2006	(S) Descriptive (P) Examine the impact of MD gender on sexual history taking (T) Specialist and primary care (D) Not reported (C) US	Questionnaire	n = 69 OB/GYNs, family practitioners, internists, pediatricians, and surgeons (40 male and 29 female)	Identification by MD of self-comfort during sexual health interviews and perceived comfort of patients	(1) No SIG difference found between male and female MDs in frequency of obtaining sexual histories or in rate of identification of sexual dysfunction. (2) MDs reported factors causing discomfort as patient's age ‹18 and ›65, patient's academic achievement below college level, and patient's divorced or single marital sta-

TABLE 4.3—*Continued*

Reference	Study Design (S) Study Purpose (P) Study Setting (T) Study Date (D) Country (C)	Method	Final Sample Size	Main Measures	Key Findings
					tus. (3) Both MD and patient gender influence comfort level of the MD and MD perceived comfort level of male patients: SIG difference (p = <.05) between male and female MDs reporting their discomfort when interviewing male patients (19% and 50%, respectively) and female patients (35% and 12%, respectively). SIG difference in MD perception of female patient discomfort 53% male MD vs. 24% female MD (p = <.05). Authors suggest that MDs perceive their own comfort level and that of their patients are best during same-gender interviews.
Farmer and Higginson 2006	(S) Qualitative (P) Describe MD perceptions of decision making for ACS and ways in which patient characteristics influence diagnosis (T) Emergency department	Semistructured interviews, analyzed using a grounded theory approach	n = 18 MDs serving ethnically diverse and lower-income patients	Identification of emerging categories and themes in diagnosing and treating coronary heart disease	In making a diagnosis, MDs emphasized the medical history and interpreted patient complaints by comparing their clinical impressions to a "classic" or "textbook" norm. MDs' perceptions of patients' articulateness about their symptoms, culture, language barriers, cognitive impairment, age, gender, and health issue

Author, year	Study characteristics	Method	Sample	Focus	Findings
	(D) 1995–96 (C) UK				influenced the data gathered, the interpretation of the data, and the reference against which those data were compared. MD perceptions stemmed from their training, experiences, "gut feelings," beliefs, and cultural values, and these were highly variable among individual MDs. MDs held stereotyped impressions about 1 or more patient groups, "and in some cases MD perceptions appeared to reflect some degree of condescension and may be a source of bias."
Farmer, Roter, et al. 2006	(S) Observational (P) Describe patient-provider interactions for patients in an emergency department with ACS (T) Emergency department (D) 1995–96 (C) UK	Hand recorded observations, evaluated using domain analysis, taxonomic analysis, and theme interpretation methods	$n = 74$ patients (68% white, 18% Afro-Caribbean, and 15% South East Asian)	Identification of barriers to the quality of historical data obtained during the medical interviews	Barriers to effective communication were (1) use of leading questions to define chest pain based on MD's preconceived ideas about the basis of the patient's chest pain; (2) patient-MD conflict as a result of, and contributor to, poor communication (e.g., where providers believed patients presented "inappropriately" to the emergency or patients nonadherent to prescribed treatment); and (3) frank miscommunication due to language barriers and translational difficulties. Miscommunication occurred frequently, and MDs rarely clarified or further explored inconsistencies in patient histories. Authors conclude that data quality obtained in the

TABLE 4.3—*Continued*

Reference	Study Design (S) Study Purpose (P) Study Setting (T) Study Date (D) Country (C)	Method	Final Sample Size	Main Measures	Key Findings
					medical interview is a critical part of diagnosing ACS. Authors conclude that when diagnostic shortcuts are taken to overcome educational, cultural, or language barriers in the medical interview, they may contribute to health care disparities.
Frich, Malterud, et al. 2006	(S) Qualitative (P) Explore barriers to diagnosis and treatment experienced by women at increased risk of CHD (T) Outpatient lipid clinic (D) 2000–2002 (C) Norway	Semistructured interviews	*n* = 20 women diagnosed with heterozygous familial hypercholesterolemia	Analysis based on a coding scheme developed for the data	Results found gender differences in how women at risk of coronary heart disease are treated. Barriers to diagnosis and treatment: (1) women experienced MD resistance when they asked for a cholesterol test; (2) women's symptoms of CHD were misinterpreted and downplayed when they consulted doctors for evaluation and treatment; (3) they experienced delays in treatment.
Park, Betancourt, et al. 2006	(S) Qualitative (P) Assess internal medicine residents' perceptions of cross-cultural care, barriers to care, training experiences, and recommendation	Transcribed semistructured interviews with thematic content analysis	*n* = 26 MDs (third-year internal medicine residents)	(1) Perceptions of cross-cultural care; (2) barriers to care; (3) training experiences; and (4) recommendations	(1) Most residents expressed interest in learning cross-cultural skills and acknowledged the salience of cultural factors on medical care. Some residents did not endorse the usefulness of cross-cultural training. (2) Barriers to cross-cultural care in-

Study	Design/Purpose/Setting	Sample	Methods	Analysis	Findings
	(T) Outpatient (D) Not reported (C) US				cluded patient gender, age, sexual orientation, limited English proficiency, and low socioeconomic status; different patient belief system or perspectives about the importance of following a medical regimen; MD's background, e.g., religion or minority status; and language and interpreter limitations. (3) Most residents had very little cross-cultural training during residency. (4) Residents recommended increasing community-based opportunities, involving patients in the teaching process, training staff and attendings, and integrating cross-cultural care into their existing training (e.g., journal clubs, case presentations).
Rosenberg, Richard, et al. 2006	(S) Qualitative (P) Describe the challenges for immigrant patients and their MDs and MD skills in inter-cultural communication (T) Primary care (D) Not reported (C) Canada	$n = 12$ MDs $n = 24$ psychologically distressed, ethnically diverse patients	Videotaped consultation with MD and patient, each separately, viewing videotape of their clinical encounter and commenting on important moments	6 predetermined analysis categories address MD-patient relationship	Individual MDs (1) lacked knowledge of the effects of culture on the MD-patient relationship, expressions of distress, and the effects of immigrant-specific stress on health, and were not motivated to elicit cultural information; (2) used an ethnic stereotype to guide care; (3) did not consider that the patient might have a different view and did not look for other causes of the patient's difficulties; (4) were motivated to have an interpersonal, rather than an intercultural, encounter. Authors con-

TABLE 4.3—*Continued*

Reference	Study Design (S) Study Purpose (P) Study Setting (T) Study Date (D) Country (C)	Method	Final Sample Size	Main Measures	Key Findings
					clude that lack of formal training partly explains why most MDs demonstrated an elementary level of cultural competency.
Siminoff, Graham, et al. 2006	(S) Qualitative (P) Examine if patient characteristics are associated with communication patterns between oncologists and breast cancer patients (T) Oncology (D) Not reported (C) US	Audiotaped interviews with analysis using RIAS system	$n = 58$ oncologists $n = 405$ newly diagnosed breast cancer patients	12 mutually exclusive communication variables; 6 MD and 6 patient variables	(1) MDs provided more biomedical information to younger vs. older patients ($p = <.01$), white vs. nonwhite patients ($p = <.01$), patients with higher educational achievement ($p = <.01$), and higher income patients ($p = <.01$); (2) MDs provided little psychosocial counseling and education overall, but more to white vs. nonwhite patients ($p = <.01$) and to high and medium income patients ($p = <.05$); (3) MD emotional expressions also varied by patient's demographic variables, with white, younger, and more educated patients receiving more emotional utterances ($p = <.05$); (4) MDs engaged in more relationship building with white vs. nonwhite patients ($p = <.01$), more educated patients ($p = <.05$), and more affluent patients ($p = <.05$). Authors

Author	Study characteristics	Method	Sample	Measures	Results
Wachtler, Brorsson, et al. 2006	(S) Qualitative (P) Examine how consultations with immigrant patients are understood and managed by GPs (T) Community outpatient primary care (D) 2003 (C) Sweden	Semistructured interviews, with transcribed audiotapes with thematic analysis	$n = 20$ GPs	(1) GP understanding of consultation; (2) GP management of consultation	Results found GPs did not acknowledge culture, conduct their consultations with immigrant patients in the same way that they conduct all their consultations, and tend to avoid even pronounced cultural differences. GPs focus on the individual and use a western humanist attitude. However, when GPs described their worst consultations, where they believed that they barely communicated with their patients, cultural difference played a central role.
Barnhart, Lewis, et al. 2007	(S) Descriptive (P) Identify barriers affecting the provision of recommended coronary risk factor therapies in women (T) Community (D) 2002–3 (C) US	MD survey conducted prior to Grand Rounds educational programs	$n = 529$ internists; $n = 529$ internists and OB/GYNs	(1) Screen women <40 for CHD risk factors; (2) for smoking patients: ask for a quit date, provide nicotine replacement; (3) for smoking and overweight patients: counseling and services	Communication barriers: MDs (1) had limited knowledge of practice guidelines for optimal lipid levels, underestimated the impact of tobacco use as a risk factor for CHD in young women, and needed to improve their counseling and referral services for tobacco cessation and obesity; (2) identified lack of time (OR = 1.5–1.7) and training (OR = .070–.72) as barriers to primary prevention among women patients
Cegala, Street, et al. 2007	(S) Descriptive (P) Assess impact of pa-	Post hoc analyses of data from 3 empirical stud-	$n = 210$ patients with	(1) Amount of information MD provides; (2)	(1) MDs provided SIG greater amount of information to high participants vs.

The top of the first row (continuation): conclude that differences may mean a less adequate decision-making process for patients who are members of racial or ethnic minorities and for patients who are less affluent, older, and have less education.

TABLE 4.3—*Continued*

Reference	Study Design (S) Study Purpose (P) Study Setting (T) Study Date (D) Country (C)	Method	Final Sample Size	Main Measures	Key Findings
	tient participation on MD information provision during a medical interview (T) Primary care (D) 2000, 2001 (C) US	ies on effects of patient PACE CST. (Study adapted the original PACE system into PACE for Parents and PACE for Physicians, companion booklets designed to enhance physician-parent communication about the diagnosis and treatment of childhood illness. Coding system included.) Patients classified as high or low participants in interview. PACE coding system used to analyze MD and patient discourse during medical interview.	CST $n = 38$ MDs	amount of question-elicited information MD provides; (3) amount of volunteered information MD provides	low ($p = <.001$); (2) MDs provided SIG greater amount of question-elicited information to high participants vs. low ($p = <.001$); (3) MDs provided SIG greater amount of volunteer information to high participants vs. low ($p = <.001$) about treatment and tests or procedures; (4) post hoc analysis found high vs. low-participation patients engaged in SIG more expression of affect, e.g., worries, anxieties ($p = <.001$), and when MDs communicated with high vs. low participation patients, they used SIG more supportive utterances ($p = <.001$). The authors conclude that communicatively active patients set direction for MD communication.
Cox, Smith, et al. 2007	(S) Qualitative (P) Examine effect of child, MD, and parent genders, visit length on communication	Sociodemographic survey of MD and parents, transcribed videotapes	$n = 7$ family MDs and $n = 8$ pediatricians $n = 100$ pa-	RIAS analysis for (1) information giving; (2) information gathering; (3) relationship building	Girls did twice as much relationship building as boys (IRR = 2.33), and their MDs did 34% more information gathering (IRR = 1.34, 1.16–1.55). Female MDs did 29% less informa-

Author/Year	Study details	Methods	Sample	Measures	Findings
	(T) MD office (D) Not reported (C) US		tients		tion giving (IRR = .71). Having the father accompany the child reduced child relationship building 76% (IRR = .24) and reduced MD information giving 14% (IRR = .86), compared to having mother accompany. After adjusting for participants' genders, longer visits were associated with more participation for all participants.
Harrington, Norling, et al. 2007	(S) Descriptive (P) Report development and evaluation of an MD and parent CST programs designed to improve communication regarding antibiotic prescribing for children (T) Pediatric clinic (D) Not reported (C) US	Interactional analysis of "sick child" office visits audiotapes using PACE coding system. Data on comparison group collected before MD training. Pre-visit, waiting room training on PACE for parents. 45-min MD training on PACE for pediatricians.	$n = 81$ parents $n = 42$ control $n = 39$ treatment $n = 4$ pediatricians	Parents: (1) information giving; (2) information seeking; (3) information verifying; (4) express more concerns Pediatricians: (1) address positive treatment options; (2) address parents' feelings, concerns, and expectations; (3) create partnership with parents; (4) encourage questions. Visit length	(See table 5.2 for MD effects.) Parent effects: CST parent vs. control SIG more likely to verify information ($p = .04$) and SIG more likely to express concerns ($p = .04$).
Kelly and Haidet 2007	(S) Descriptive (P) Investigate possible MD overestimation of patient literacy level (T) Primary care, VA hospital (D) 2004	Patient testing and MD estimation of patient literacy	$n = 12$ PCPs $n = 100$ patients	Post-visit: (1) Rapid Estimate of Adult Literacy in Medicine by patients; (2) MD categorical rating on a scale 1–4 of patient literacy level	Patient literacy level was not SIG associated with patient race/ethnicity or gender. MDs overestimated the literacy level for 54% of African American, 11% of white non-Hispanic, and 36% of other race/ethnicity patients ($p = <.01$). Authors conclude MD

TABLE 4.3—*Continued*

Reference	Study Design (S) Study Purpose (P) Study Setting (T) Study Date (D) Country (C)	Method	Final Sample Size	Main Measures	Key Findings
	(C) US				overestimation of patient literacy level may be an important barrier to high quality communication during the medical encounter.
Liu, Sawada, et al. 2007	(S) Descriptive (P) Compare MD-patient communication in telemedicine vs. face-to-face clinical consultations (T) University medical center (D) Not reported (C) Japan	Patient had both a face-to-face and telemedicine consultation with a different doctor on the same day, videotaped	n = 5 MDs	(1) Transcribed video-taped consultation characteristics and MD verbal behavior; (2) visit time; (3) MD and patient satisfaction questionnaire	(1) Telemedicine consultation was SIG longer than face-to-face consultation (p = .01); (2) no SIG differences found in the number of MD closed- or open-ended questions between consultation types; (3) empathy utterances (p = .01), praise utterances (p = .05), and facilitation utterances (p = .05) SIG less in the telemedicine consultations than in the face-to-face consultations; (4) MDs rated good communication with patients 40% in the telemedicine consultation vs. 90% face-to-face (p = .01), and understood what was on the patient's mind 45% telemedicine vs. 85% face-to-face (p = .05); (5) no SIG differences in patient satisfaction between consultation type
Rosen and Kwoh 2007	(S) Descriptive (P) Assess use of a patient-MD e-mail service	Patient survey 2 years post enrollment in patient-MD e-mail pro-	n = not reported pediatric rheuma-	(1) Urgency of message; (2) subject matter; (3) message volume; (4)	(1) Answering patient questions by e-mail was 57% faster vs. telephone for the MD (p = <.0001); (2) SIG more

Study	Characteristics	Sample	Measures	Results
	(T) Pediatrics (D) 2004–6 (C) US	gram; comparison e-mail vs. telephone messaging	tologists $n = 121$ families who used service	time of day of messaging; (5) time to generate response; (6) patient satisfaction	requests for test results and more patient updates ($p = <.001$) via e-mail vs. telephone messages; (3) MD received 1.2 e-mails per day from patients; (4) agreed patient-MD e-mail increased access to the MD and improved the quality of care; (5) families did not believe patient-MD e-mail distanced them from MD
Rouf, Whittle, et al. 2007	(S) Descriptive (P) Determine if MD experience modifies the impact of exam room computers on the MD-patient interaction (T) Primary care, VA hospital clinic (D) 2003 (C) US	MD questionnaire, post-visit patient and MD questionnaire	$n = 11$ faculty internists and 12 residents $n = 155$ patients	(1) To what extent (a) use of computer decreased the time MDs spent talking to, looking at, and examining the patients; (b) computer interfered with the MD-patient relationship; and (c) MD use of the computer made the visit feel less personal; (2) patient satisfaction with visit and quality of care	(1) Residents' patients vs. faculty patients were SIG (a) more likely to agree that the computer adversely affected the amount of time the MD spent talking to (34% vs. 15%, $p = .01$), looking at (45% vs. 24%, $p = .02$), and examining them (32% vs. 13%, $p = .009$), (b) less likely to strongly agree they were satisfied with their overall relationship with the MD (50% vs. 71%, $p = .02$); (c) less likely to rate the quality of the index visit as excellent (38% vs. 62%, $p = .005$); (2) patients were more likely to agree that the computer made the visit feel less personal (20% vs. 5%, $p = .017$); (3) few patients thought the computer interfered with their relationship with their MDs (8% vs. 8%). Authors suggest differences in MD-patient interaction between residents and faculty may be due to MD experience.

TABLE 4.3—*Continued*

Reference	Study Design (S) Study Purpose (P) Study Setting (T) Study Date (D) Country (C)	Method	Final Sample Size	Main Measures	Key Findings
Schmid Mast, Hall, et al. 2007	(S) Descriptive (P) Investigate the effect of MD sex and communication style on patient satisfaction (T) Experimental, laboratory (D) Not reported (C) Switzerland	Students engaged in an interaction with a virtual MD, male or female; MD communication style was varied along the dominance and the caring dimension, with satisfaction measured on a 5-point scale	n = 167 college students randomly assigned to one of 8 experimental conditions: male vs. female, and high and low dominance and caring 80 male and 87 female students, mean age 26.5 years	36-item patient satisfaction questionnaire	Results showed a SIG main effect of MD caring (p = .009) with participants being more satisfied with the high caring (mean = 3.39) as compared to the low caring (mean = 3.06) MD. There were no main effects of physician or patient gender, and physician dominance. Male MD caring and dominance communication style did not affect satisfaction of male or female participants, but there was a SIG interaction effect (p = .005) indicating that female participants were less satisfied with a male physician who adopted a noncaring and dominant communication style. Female participants were SIG (p = .0001) more satisfied with a caring female vs. a noncaring female MD. For a female MD interacting with a male participant, there was no effect of physician communication style on satisfaction.
Deep, Griffith, et al. 2008	(S) Descriptive (P) Explore how patients, their family members,	Semistructured interviews with transcribed audiotapes	n = 26 MD-patient dyads of residents and	(1) Perceptions of prognosis; (2) patient/surrogate understanding of	Results found discrepant interpretations of patients' preferences for life-sustaining treatment. In 6 dyads

	and MDs interpret the discussion of the patient's preferences for CPR (T) Medical center inpatient medical units (D) 2006 (C) US	seriously ill patients/surrogates		resuscitation; (3) MD beliefs about appropriateness of attempting resuscitation; (4) agreement between patient or surrogate and MD	(21%), the participants reported differing results of the discussion: 2 patients had orders to limit their care based on the MD's interpretation of their discussion; 2 patients who did not want resuscitation lacked a DNR order; 2 patients did not recall having the conversation. Authors conclude that discrepancies could be attributed to the MD misconstruing the patient's wishes, interference of a family member, and fluctuating preferences. "Complicating discussions are the numerous colloquialisms used by patients, family members and MDs such as 'CPR,' 'life support,' or being 'on a machine' which assumed different meanings for the various participants. These meanings are rarely explicated when discussing a patient's wishes" and "MDs focus solely on dichotomizing the patient's preferences to 'Full Code' or 'DNR.'"
Harding, Selman, et al. 2008	(S) Qualitative (P) Identify barriers to communication with congestive heart failure patients (T) Cardiology (D) Not reported (C) UK	n = 7 MDs, 5 cardiologists, and 2 palliative care MDs	Transcribed, taped semi-structured interview with patients, caregivers, MDs, and staff	Caregiver perceived communication barriers	(See evidence of poor communication from this study, table 2.5.) Results include (1) MD curative focus; (2) MD lack of confidence and skills in discussing end of life; (3) MD fear of taking away hope; (4) MD confusion and misapprehension regarding palliative care; (5) lack of knowledge of

TABLE 4.3—*Continued*

Reference	Study Design (S) Study Purpose (P) Study Setting (T) Study Date (D) Country (C)	Method	Final Sample Size	Main Measures	Key Findings
					when to refer to palliative care; (6) MD lack of time and resources to communicate complex issues; (7) role confusion among specialists.
Haskard, Williams, et al. 2008	(S) RCT (P) Assess the effects of a communication skills training program for physicians and patients (T) Primary care (D) Not reported (C) US	Patient post-visit survey, measured at 3 months. MDs randomized into 4 groups: control, MD trained, patient trained, MD and patient trained. Patients: at 3 months, one 20-minute pre-visit, waiting room intervention of audiotape and patient guidebook. MDs: three 6-hour interactive workshops and coaching.	n = 2,196 patients n = 156 MDs	Patient perception of (1) choice; (2) decision making, information; (3) lifestyle counseling; (4) overall satisfaction	(See table 5.2 for MD effects.) Patient effects: (1) No effects of patient training on patient satisfaction or on MD stress and life satisfaction scores; (2) patient training SIG increased MD satisfaction with the data collection process (p = .002).
Johnson, Serwint, et al. 2008	(S) Comparative (P) Investigate impact of a computer-based documentation tool on parent–health care provider communication	Pre-post study design with control group visits chosen randomly from earlier data set evaluating a training intervention. Audiotaped or videotaped visits.	n = 59 pediatric residents	(1) Audiotapes and videotapes scored using RIAS coded categories; (2) patient centeredness scores	No SIG difference in the provider/parent talk ratio between cohorts after controlling for visit length. Computer group had (1) improved use of open-ended questions (p = .002), (2) more dialogue about anticipatory guidance (p = .001); (3) greater amounts

(T) Pediatric teaching clinic (D) Not reported (C) US				of social development counseling (p = .001); (4) greater use of partnership strategies (p = .001) and patient centeredness (p = .001); (5) increased parent dialogue (p = .007). Visit length was 5 minutes greater for the computer group, even after >6 months of use.
Kaduszkiewicz, Bachmann, et al. 2008	(S) Descriptive (P) Investigate differences between GPs and specialists about disclosing the diagnosis of dementia (T) Community (D) Not reported (C) Germany	Postal survey and 30 semistructured interviews with GPs. Qualitative analysis of interview data formed basis of survey instrument.	n = 211 GPs and 96 specialists (neurologists and psychiatrists)	9 questions related to ways of disclosing diagnosis and prognosis and beliefs about disclosure and communication	GPs identified communication barriers in interviews: (1) fear of inflicting damage on the patient (12 interviewees); (2) opinion that disclosure carries no benefit for the patient (6); (3) fear of ruining the doctor-patient relationship (6); (4) feeling that the patient would not understand the diagnosis anyway (6); (5) uncertainty about the course of the disease (5). Survey results found only minor differences between GPs and specialists, both groups being equally in favor of a timely disclosure: (1) GPs (70%) and specialists (77%) strongly agreed that "patients with dementia should be informed early because of the possibility to plan their lives"; (2) only SIG difference was that specialists reported to use the terms "dementia" and "Alzheimer" more often in the communication with the patient. GPs (50%) expressed a SIG greater interest in communication

TABLE 4.3—Continued

Reference	Study Design (S) Study Purpose (P) Study Setting (T) Study Date (D) Country (C)	Method	Final Sample Size	Main Measures	Key Findings
					training vs. specialists (30%) (p = <.001). Authors contrast their results of MDs' basic positive attitude toward disclosure to previous studies showing greater reluctance for both GPs (6 studies, 1995–2004) and specialists (6 studies, 1995–2002).

ACS = acute coronary syndrome
CHD = coronary heart disease
CST(s) = communication skills training(s)
CPR = cardiopulmonary resuscitation
DNR = do not resuscitate
ED = emergency department
EMR = electronic medical record
FP = family practice
GP(s) = general practitioner(s)
IRR(s) = adjusted incidence rate ratios
MD(s) = physician(s)
n = number

NP(s) = nurse practitioner(s)
OR = odds ratio
PA(s) = physician assistant(s)
PACE = Patient education system (Prsesenting, Asking, Checking, Expressing). Study adapted the original PACE system into *PACE for Parents* and *PACE for Physicians*, companion booklets designed to enhance physician-parent communication about the diagnosis and treatment of childhood illness. Coding system included.
PN(s) = practice nurse(s)
PSS = psychosocial spiritual

RCT(s) = randomized control trial(s)
RIAS = Roter Interaction Analysis System, method of coding doctor-patient interaction using frequency counts of communication "utterances"
SEGUE = Set the stage, Elicit information, Give information, Understand the patient's perspective, End the encounter
SIG = significant(ly)
SLE = Systemic Lupus Erythematosus
STI = sexually transmitted infection
UK = United Kingdom
VA = Veterans Administration

5 | How Effective Are Strategies to Improve Physician Communication?

In chapter 4, we discussed the factors that seem to be associated with the quality of physician communication. Some physician characteristics, such as age and gender, clearly are not subject to change through educational programs or skill-building efforts. Other physician characteristics associated with physician communication, such as physician knowledge and communication skills, can be altered, at least in theory, by programmatic interventions (Maguire and Pitceathly 2002).

In this chapter, we discuss research findings regarding efforts to improve physician communication through education and training (see the left part of fig. 1.1, logic model). Studies that evaluate the effectiveness of educational programs vary widely in their scope and sophistication, as do the programs themselves. A good portion of the literature consists of studies that use a simple test of physician knowledge before and after a course. Relatively few studies measured the impact of skill-building or other educational programs on physician communications with actual patients. Studies of the impact of instructional programs on patient outcomes focused on patient-reported satisfaction with physician visits or patient adherence to treatment recommendations. We found no studies documenting a relationship between skill-building programs on physician communication and patient biologic markers of health status, self-reported health status, utilization, or costs of care.

Identifying Relevant Literature

We sought to identify published evaluations, in English, of programs intended to improve physician communication through knowledge and skills. We searched Medline, JSTOR, and the Cochrane Library database for review articles. We also include in this chapter individual evaluations published between 2002 and 2008 but not included in review articles. We used a combination of such keywords as "physician-patient relations," "communication," "patient-centered care," "education, medical, undergraduate," "education, medical, graduate," "education, medical, continuing," and "evaluation." Our initial search yielded over 600 unduplicated references. After eliminating articles not directly related to developing physician communication through knowledge and skills, we examined over 400 articles and abstracts. We identified a small number of additional relevant articles through examination of references at the end of the reviews and individual studies.

Our search process yielded 14 review articles (which reviewed 138 studies) and 42 individual studies (in 46 articles). The studies covered in the review articles were directed at programs for medical students (80), residents (24), and practicing physicians (38), with some studies addressing programs targeting more than one category of student. Six of the 14 review articles focused on programs for medical students (undergraduate or graduate), 5 included only educational programs for experienced physicians, and 3 summarized findings from programs for both experienced physicians and students. Five of the 14 review articles addressed only educational programs for physicians treating cancer patients. Nine reviews encompassed programs seeking to upgrade the general communication skills of physicians. The other reviews addressed programs with more limited objectives with respect to improving communication skills: empathy (2), competence in the delivery of bad news (1), cultural competence (1), and emotion management (1).

The Impact of Programs Directed at Improving Physician Communication

In table 5.1, we summarize the evidence from review studies regarding the effectiveness of programs that are designed to improve physician communication. We discuss the evidence from reviews in two categories: 1) reviews that address evaluations of communication knowledge and skill-building programs for physicians working with all types of patients and 2) reviews that focus only on evaluations of communication programs for physicians treating cancer patients. Table 5.2 presents findings from individual evaluations of programs. The findings in this table are quite consistent overall with findings from the review articles, so we discuss only a small number of evaluations that are noteworthy because they are illustrative of the larger body of research or because of their methodological approach or the significance of the communication program that they evaluate.

Evidence from Reviews—General Programs. For the most part, the authors of the nine general reviews (addressing programs not directed specifically at improving physician communication skills in treating cancer patients) reached similar conclusions. They found some evidence of improvements in knowledge and skills for programs enrolling undergraduate or postgraduate medical students, with little evidence relating to the effectiveness of programs for more experienced physicians. Evaluations of programs for practicing physicians were few. Cheraghi-Sohi and Bower (2008) reviewed the impacts of four programs, where the measure of effectiveness was patient satisfaction, and found positive effects for one. A common thread in programs directed at practicing physicians was the use of very time-limited interventions, presumably to accommodate physician work schedules. Hulsman, Ros, et al. (1999) also found limited impacts for programs directed at practicing physicians; where effects were significant, they were related to physicians' own assessments of improvements in their knowledge, attitudes, and skills.

The reviews contained more evidence of significant impacts associated with programs for medical students. Rosenbaum, Ferguson, et al. (2004), in their review of programs designed to help physicians communicate bad news, found that participants reported greater self-confidence after the programs and felt better prepared to communicate bad news to patients. The most effective interventions were those that described basic steps for delivering bad news and provided opportunities for students to discuss their concerns and to receive feedback on their skills. In their review of programs designed to improve cultural competence in physician communications with patients, Beach, Price, et al. (2005) found significant effects on participant knowledge, attitudes, and skills in about half of the programs, concluding that the programs showed promise. Smith, Hanson, et al. (2007) reviewed 15 randomized clinical trials using meta-analysis techniques. Six of the programs used structured feedback based on recorded student-patient interviews, 6 used lectures and small-group discussions, and the rest used other instructional techniques. Students' abilities to establish rapport improved in most of the programs, as did data-gathering abilities. Based on these and other results, the authors concluded that medical students could be taught communication skills, with the most effective methods being structured feedback using a recorded interview and small-group discussion.

There was considerable consensus on the part of the authors that the individual studies included in their reviews had significant limitations including small sample sizes (Stepien and Baernstein 2006), lack of control groups in many instances (Stepian and Baernstein 2006), limited follow-up periods (Hulsman, Ros, et al. 1999), lack of detail regarding methodology (Lewin, Skea, et al. 2001), lack of a theoretical framework to guide the intervention (Cegala and Lenzmeier Broz 2002), incongruity between the stated objectives of the intervention and the instrument chosen by the evaluators to measure change (Cegala and Lenzmeier Broz 2002), and lack of evidence of effects on patients (Beach, Price, et al. 2005). Their comments reflect the extreme variation in both the complexity of the educational interventions and the sophistication of the evaluation designs. However, as far as we could determine, the review articles did not include any large-scale, rigorous evaluations of well-defined, theory-based educational programs to improve physician communication.

Evidence from Reviews—Oncology Programs. Five different review articles assessed the effectiveness of educational programs to improve the knowledge and skills of physicians in the treatment of cancer patients. The review that included the largest number of studies was conducted by Butler, Degner, et al. (2005); 47 randomized clinical trials and before-and-after studies with control groups. The studies included educational efforts directed at physicians and at other health professionals as well. While the evaluations reported positive results, the review authors cited several limitations similar to those previously listed. They also noted that it was not clear if the initiatives described in the studies could be adopted on a widespread basis, based on the information provided. Kennedy (2005) reported significant impacts on different components of physician communication but called for more use of control groups and standardized measures of outcomes. Merckaert, Libert, et al. (2005a) reported improved physician attitudes toward skill development after the completion of training courses and, in a smaller number of studies, behavioral improvements as well. Gysels, Richardson, et al. (2004) also reported generally positive findings related to programs intended to improve physician (and other health professional) communication with cancer patients, but they suggested that more effort should be devoted to tracking outcomes over a longer time period.

Evidence from Individual Studies. We selected several individual studies to describe in detail. These studies were chosen, as a group, to illustrate the breadth of the types of intervention described in this literature, as well as the variation in sophistication of the methods used by the evaluators.

Cooper and Hassell (2002) described a half-day skills workshop in the United Kingdom that was designed to expose 14 specialists in rheumatology to skills training in physician communication. The workshop consisted of 1) small-group discussions about physician knowledge of and experience with communication skills and problems, 2) discussion of videotapes of actual consultations, and 3) role playing involving a "patient," a physician, and an "observer," using different scenarios relevant to a rheumatologist's practice. At the end of the half-day, physicians completed a questionnaire in which they evaluated the workshop along several dimensions. Their responses indicated that the workshop had been valuable, that they believed communication skills could be taught, and that they thought their own skills had improved. The specialists agreed that good communication was important for specialists as well as primary care physicians. This study illustrates one type of evaluation found relatively frequently in the literature, as well as relatively common study limitations. The intervention was very modest in scope and objectives; the sample size was small; the outcomes measured were extremely limited, with no real comparison group; and data were collected only from physician participants, with no follow-up data collection. In particular, there was no attempt to assess whether the workshop improved actual communication with patients or patient outcomes. The study was somewhat unusual in that it focused only on practicing specialists.

Rodriguez, Anastario, et al. (2008) also designed an intervention targeted at practicing physicians, in this case with the objective of teaching them "agenda setting." As with Cooper and Hassell (2002), the number of physicians participating in the intervention was small—10 physicians from a large multispecialty group practice in California who were identified through patient surveys as relatively poor performers. Again, the intervention was relatively modest, consisting of a single three-hour workshop followed by 45-minute follow-up teleconference calls conducted at three and seven weeks after the intervention. In this study, however, the authors used a more sophisticated evaluation design. The physicians receiving the intervention were compared to 11 "matched" physicians. All physicians received feedback on patient evaluations of their performance prior to the intervention. They also were evaluated after the intervention using surveys of random samples of 100 commercially insured patients associated with each physician. The authors used relatively sophisticated "multilevel" regression models in their analysis, to control for the clustering of patients with physicians. The study found significant post-workshop improvements (relative to control physicians) in physician ability to explain things clearly, and it found "marginally significant" improvements in the overall quality of physician-patient interactions. The authors concluded that a "simple and modest intervention . . . can have a positive impact on the quality of physician-patient interactions." While the authors noted that the improvements were relatively small in magnitude, they pointed out that improvements of that magnitude could significantly increase a medical group's scores on public reports of group performance with respect to "patient experience." Thus, they suggested that there was a very tangible organizational benefit to sponsoring skill-building interventions on physician communication for practicing physicians.

Gulbrandsen, Krupat, et al. (2008) explored whether a well-known model for improving physician communication—the Kaiser Four Habits Model—could be successfully implemented in a different cultural setting. While the Kaiser model and its several variations has been used since the mid-1990s by Kaiser Permanente Medical Group in the United States as well as other organizations, there is relatively little peer-reviewed evidence of its effectiveness (Stein, Frankel, et al. 2005; Krupat, Frankel, et al. 2006). Gulbransen, Krupat, et al. (2008) sought to pilot test whether the model could be effectively employed in Norway. As they describe the model, " 'Four Habits' refer to what should happen in a clinical consultation; that it has a friendly and well-planned beginning, a search for the patient's perspective, empathetic response, and thorough information giving, shared decision-making and adherence to advice towards the end" (388). Sixteen hospital-based physicians were trained in the model in a three-day course. A sample of 210 patients received a questionnaire relating to their experience in visits before and after the training course. There was evidence of improvement, but, consistent with the pilot nature of the study, many limitations were noted by the authors, including the small number of physician participants and the fact that all the physicians in the study were enthusiastic prior to participation. Data on patient response rates were not collected in a systematic manner. These concerns led the authors to suggest that extrapolation of the results to other groups of physicians probably would not be valid. Based on their experience, the authors questioned whether patient questionnaires were useful tools to evaluate specific physician behaviors, and they suggested that coding of videotapes of actual physician-patient encounters would be a preferable approach.

Shilling, Jenkins, et al. (2003) also based their analysis of a physician communication intervention in the United Kingdom on responses of patients to questionnaires, but they measured physician satisfaction as well. They compared patient satisfaction scores for 160 physicians in 34 outpatient cancer treatment centers, half of whom were randomized into an intervention group. Patient satisfaction data were collected prior to the intervention for both groups of physicians, after the intervention for the group receiving training, and after three months for the control group of physicians. The questions were adapted from well-known, previously validated instruments used to measure patient satisfaction with physician visits. The training course lasted three days and involved analysis of videotapes of physician encounters with patients. The authors found no significant increase in patient satisfaction as a result of the training, despite measurable changes in physician behavior. However, they did note that patient satisfaction scores increased for the physicians who attended the training but not for physicians in the control group. Given the relatively rigorous design of this study and the sophisticated statistical methodology used, the lack of significant results related to patient satisfaction raises concerns. The authors speculated that a "ceiling effect" may have been present; that is, the scores were high at baseline for patients of all physicians in the study. They also observed that patients may be reluctant to criticize their physicians, which could skew patient satisfaction data, making these data less useful in measuring the impact of training programs in communication.

Hobma, Ram, et al. (2006) took a different approach to measuring the impact of an intervention on physician communication skills; instead of relying on findings from patient surveys, they evaluated videotapes of physician consultations before and after training. One hundred general practitioners in the Netherlands participated in their study. While the physicians participated in the study as individuals, randomization of physicians took place at the practice level. This avoided possible "contamination" of physicians in the control group who might be in the same practice as physicians receiving the training. Although physicians were randomized, the authors selected the first 100 responding physicians as study participants. Thus, all physicians in both the treatment group and the control group were volunteers who were particularly interested in the topic. The educational program was unusual in that it was individualized, focusing on improving aspects of communication where improvement was judged to be the most likely to be beneficial, based on initial assessment of videotaped interviews. The group receiving the educational intervention demonstrated a significant improvement relative to the physicians in the control group, with the greatest improvement occurring for those physicians who were the most involved in the training program (i.e., who received the largest "dose" of training). Interestingly, the scores of the control group at baseline were similar to the scores of physicians in the intervention group after the training program, and the scores in the control group deteriorated over the study period. The authors were not able to explain this pattern in the control group scores, and they also noted that the design of the study did not permit them to assess whether improvements in behaviors of the physicians in the intervention group persisted past the six-month follow-up period.

Roter, Larson, et al. (2004) implemented a sophisticated physician communications program for 28 physician residents in a pediatric training program in the United States. Simulated patient interviews, combined with tailored feedback, were used in the training program, which took place over a four-week period. Standard coding procedures from the Roter Interaction Analysis System (RIAS) were employed to analyze content of the visits with simulated patients, but these procedures were embedded in a new software program that facilitated individualized feedback. Paired *t*-tests were used to analyze the data. The authors reported significant improvement in the communication skills of residents in all four areas of communication that they investigated: "listening more/talking less, more open-ended data gathering techniques, more sensitive response to patient's emotions, and building an active patient partnership related to problem solving" (Roter, Larson, et al. 2004, 154). The average length of time taken for the simulated interviews increased by two minutes, and, interestingly, this increased time reflected almost entirely an increase in patient talk. The authors acknowledged limitations in their study. Specifically, it was not a randomized trial (raising issues relating to the impact of "selection effects" on their results), and there were no follow-up data that could be used to assess the impact of the training over time and with actual patients. These limitations reflect the fact that the study was designed largely to test the feasibility of using the new software to facilitate individualized feedback on communication skills.

Carter, Lewis, et al. (2006) studied the impact of participation by 196 third-year US medical students in small-group workshops that involved didactic presentations and vignettes portraying ineffective and effective physician communication. In many ways, this approach is representative of large numbers of programs that educate medical students on issues of physician communication as part of their overall training. In their study, rather than measuring patient satisfaction or actual physician performance, the authors measured student attitudes and knowledge of communication techniques before and after participation in the workshops. There was a special focus on improving cultural awareness among students. The students agreed that the workshop was effective, and there was evidence that participation in the workshop increased cultural awareness relating to communications with patients. Recognizing the limitations of the study, the authors encouraged future research that would assess whether increased cultural awareness transferred into better communication in practice. While this would be desirable, most evaluations of training programs for medical students have similar limitations. Students are essentially a "captive audience" for communications training, but the training programs are limited in their content, and it is difficult for evaluators to move beyond assessments of participant opinions or knowledge when evaluating program impacts.

Conclusions

Drawing clear conclusions from the literature summarized in this chapter is challenging, for three main reasons. First, the methodological quality of the evaluations varies considerably. A large portion of the literature consists of before-and-after comparisons with relatively few participating physicians. While there are studies based on randomized designs, the number of participants in these studies is also quite small, and participants generally consist of volunteers who presumably think that improving communication with patients is an important goal. Together, these factors make it difficult to generalize study findings.

Second, the studies use a wide range of measures for assessing what constitutes a "successful" intervention. In studies of interventions aimed at medical students, improvement of knowledge relating to communication skills and techniques is a typical measure of success. In some cases, role playing is used to assess whether skills have improved in practice as a result of training programs for both students and practicing physicians. Patient perceptions of physician communication before and after skills training are used to measure success in a large number of studies, but this seems problematic for a number of reasons. The most rigorous attempts to measure program impacts involve coding physician communications using audio or video recordings made before and after training and then comparing changes to a control group. For logistical reasons, these studies frequently involve limited numbers of physicians and patients.

Third, the studies reviewed in this chapter assess quite different interventions, for the most part. Where the interventions consist of multiple components, it is difficult to determine the incremental impact of any single component. This is not unique to studies of physician communication. For example, attempts to learn from evaluations of organizational efforts at quality improvement and of physician pay-for-performance programs typically face the same obstacle.

Perhaps the clearest and most important lessons to be drawn from this chapter's review of the existing literature on the effectiveness of communication skill-building programs are that 1) little is known about the degree to which any initial positive results persist over time and 2) the impact of these programs on any patient outcomes, beyond post-visit measures of patient satisfaction, has been largely unexplored. Therefore, decision makers who want to invest in programs to improve physician communication will likely need to base their decisions on simulations that combine information from program evaluations with results from studies that have explored associations between physician communication and specific patient outcomes of interest (see chapter 3). Our conclusions should be tempered by the fact that we took a conservative approach to defining physician communication training, requiring that improvement of physician communication skills be the sole focus for the intervention. Using this approach, we did not identify a consistent and positive effect that skills training in physician communication had on patient adherence to treatment. A recent review (Zolnierek and Dimatteo 2009), however, reaches more positive conclusions. Using a broad search of training programs in communication skills—including articles on shared decision making, health literacy, brief training for smoking cessation, cultural competency, and building trust—an analysis of 21 studies (1976–2007) found support for a positive impact of physician training on patient adherence to treatment.

TABLE 5.1. Evidence from Review Studies Relating to Success of Interventions Aimed at Improving Physician Communication ($n = 14$)

Reference	Review Type (R) Number of Studies (N) Study Setting (S) Study Purpose (P) Study Dates (D)	Summary of Findings
Hulsman, Ros, et al. 1999	(R) Systematic, 2 dB (N) 14 studies (S) General practice and internal medicine (P) Overview of evaluation studies of communication skills training programs for clinically experienced MDs (D) From 1985	8 of 14 studies included trainee/resident MDs and 6/14 practicing MDs. Although the training objectives were not always clearly described, programs focused on enhancing communication skills. Training objectives were classified into 3 categories: receptive behaviors, information behaviors, and interpersonal and affective behaviors. 5 types of educational methods were identified: instruction, modeling, skill practice, feedback, and discussions on communication skills. Evaluation designs included pre- post-test randomized (3) and non-randomized (2) control group design; pre- post-test (5); post-test control group (3); and test during training (1). Evaluation of MD behavior was by video recording ($n = 8$) or audio recording (4) supplemented with analytic instruments (11). In 2/12 studies which include behavioral observations, no conclusion can be drawn about training effects on communication behavior. 9/12 studies report some training effects. Only a short (4.5 h) intervention Levinson did not result in detectable changes in communication behavior. The behavioral observations show that overall training effects were found on less than 50% of the observed behaviors. The average percent of SIG improvement is interpersonal and affective behavior (56%); receptive behaviors are (46%); and information behaviors (40%). 1 study using both simulated and real patients to evaluate the course effects on MD behavior found more effects in the simulated interactions Smith 1998. 6 studies measuring MD recognition of patient psychosocial problems reported improved recognition. 1 of 6 studies reported at 15 months follow-up that residents' improved attitudes toward psychosocial medicine had remained consistent, while self-assessment of psychosocial skills had declined. The authors conclude that clinically experienced MDs can be trained in communication skills; however evidence of behavioral changes is limited and most training effects are based on MDs' subjective

TABLE 5.1—*Continued*

Reference	Review Type (R) Number of Studies (N) Study Setting (S) Study Purpose (P) Study Dates (D)	Summary of Findings
		evaluation of their knowledge, attitudes, and skills. Follow-up evaluation of training effects needs to be extended beyond post-course assessment.
Lewin, Skea, et al. 2001	(R) Cochrane Review, 5 dB (N) 17 studies (S) Primarily PCPs (P) Assess the effects of interventions for health care providers that aim to promote patient-centered approaches in clinical consultations (D) 1966–99	All of the studies used training for health care providers (MDs, residents, and nurses) as an element of the intervention; 10 studies evaluated training for providers only; 7 utilized multifaceted interventions where training for providers was one of several components. 13/17 focused on the consultation process. 8 of 13 consultation studies have been described in other tabled reviews. Outcomes assessed included MD humanistic and empathic behaviors, a range of MD and patient verbal behaviors, and MD detection and/or management of emotional distress. No study mentioned whether consumers were consulted regarding the most important or relevant outcomes for consumers in terms of assessing the effects of the proposed interventions. Reporting of key methodological features often was not sufficiently detailed or complete to determine whether studies had adhered to good practice, e.g., failure to adjust for potential unit of analysis error; small sample size. Multifaceted interventions made it difficult to ascertain which components, or combination of components, were responsible for the measured effect. No study measured intervention effects on organizational changes (e.g., visit time or follow-up procedures) as part of the evaluation. There was variability across the studies in the intensity of the interventions (teaching/training approaches and patient centeredness) and in patient age and conditions. The authors conclude that there is fairly strong evidence to suggest that some interventions to promote patient-centered care in the clinical consultation may lead to significant increases in the patient centeredness of consultation processes, as indicated by a range of measures relating to clarifying patients' concerns and beliefs; communicating about treatment options; and levels of empathy.

182

TABLE 5.1—*Continued*

Reference	Review Type (R) Number of Studies (N) Study Setting (S) Study Purpose (P) Study Dates (D)	Summary of Findings
Cegala and Lenzmeier Broz 2002	(R) Systematic, 1 dB (N) 26 studies (S) Practicing MDs, residents, or other postgraduate providers (P) Examine MD communication skills training with respect to the communication objectives and behaviors that are addressed (D) 1990–present	Review focuses on issues relating to the studies' communication objectives and skills and not on research designs, methods, or results. The authors observed that (1) there was little consistency across the studies in what is considered to be a communication skill; (2) little effort made to provide an overarching framework for organizing provider communication skills; (3) little information reported about specifically what communication skills were taught; often when skills are reported there is incongruity between the stated objectives of the intervention and the instrument used to assess communication effects; (4) generally studies offer a focus, but it is not explicit enough to convey specifically which communication skills were taught; (5) unclear in the majority of studies which specific communication skills were addressed by the intervention, and lack of confidence that assessment items reflect the communication skills actually taught; (6) little specificity of communication skills even among the studies that report skills and do not have apparent problems of misalignment. The authors offer 3 recommendations, to (1) enhance clarity and interpretability of results, need to use and report assessment instruments that are closely matched with the communication skills taught; (2) drive decisions about which communication skills to address, provide a theoretical framework for the communication skills addressed in interventions; (3) provide an additional structure for skills along the lines of interview stages and communicative functions and explicate how the communication process is viewed, and ultimately reflected, in interventions, including when, during the interview, skills might be most effectively used.
Gysels, Richardson, et al. 2004	(R) Systematic, 6 dB (N) 13 studies, 16 articles (S) Oncology (P) Assess the effectiveness of different com-	4 of 13 studies focused on nurses; 2/13 addressed in other tabled review articles. Of the remaining 7 studies: (1) 1 RCT focused on improving attitudes of senior oncologists showed an increase in effective communication skills in the areas of the ex-

TABLE 5.1—*Continued*

Reference	Review Type (R) Number of Studies (N) Study Setting (S) Study Purpose (P) Study Dates (D)	Summary of Findings
	munication skills training courses for health professionals (D) 1966–2003	pression of empathy (p = .2), use of open questions (p = 001), appropriate responses to cues (p = .005), and psychological probing (p = .041). (2) 2 descriptive studies (1 with medical students and 1 with oncologists) with the objective of enhancing skills in giving bad news had positive outcomes. 1 study compared a post-evaluation questionnaire on solutions to problems provided by the medical students prior to training and found that 38% had a change of opinion toward the responsibility for giving distressing information. 1 study found oncologist confidence improved in 18 of 21 communication outcome items and on 11 of the 45 communication outcome issues for managing difficult patient situations. (3) 2 descriptive studies focused on improving interviewing skills of health professionals, including MDs, showed increased confidence in assessment and counseling skills in pre-post in 1 study with n = 20 MDs and nurses and, in the second study (n = 212 various health professionals), SIG increases in the use of open, directive questions, questions with a psychological focus, and clarification of psychological aspects. Improvement in questions and clarification was maintained 6 months after the intervention. A SIG reduction was found in questions with a physical focus, clarification of physical aspects and premature advice was found; no reduction in the giving of advice or the use of leading questions. At 6 months, these inhibitory behaviors were still used. The more effective the course attendees became in eliciting feelings, the more worried they became about exploring patients' feelings further. (4) 1 RCT with medical students and a 2-year follow-up, Klein and 1 pre-post comparison targeting senior oncologists and using videotape with simulated patients, addressed improvement in attitudes, knowledge, and general skills. The RCT found that students in the experimental group (being trained with cancer patients vs. patients with other diagnoses) had higher self-report rat-

TABLE 5.1—*Continued*

Reference	Review Type (R) Number of Studies (N) Study Setting (S) Study Purpose (P) Study Dates (D)	Summary of Findings
		ings on an attitudes questionnaire toward the ability to listen to patients and trust in doctor-MD relationship as essential. At 2 years experimental students believed the ability to communicate with patients and that clinical decisions should reflect patients' wishes more important vs. control group. At 2 years the experimental group, when rated by instructors, were SIG more likely to introduce themselves to the patient, respond empathically, show regard and concern for the patient, and assess the impact of the symptoms on the patient's life. The comparative study found confidence ratings for key communication areas SIG improved and at 3 months SIG positive shifts in attitude toward patients' psychosocial needs and more patient centered in practice. The authors conclude that health professionals can be trained to communicate more effectively with cancer patients but caution that maintenance of program effectiveness over time is an important understudied issue.
Rosenbaum, Ferguson, et al. 2004	(R) Focused review, 1 dB (N) 26 studies (S) Medical students and residents (P) Describe effective models of teaching the delivery of bad news to medical students and residents to serve as a guide to medical educators (D) Not reported	Strategies to teach delivery of bad news include (1) lecture (1 study); (2) small group discussion (5); (3) small group peer role play (4); (4) small group standardized patient role-play (8); (5) one-to-one standardized patient encounters (7); and (6) teachable moments in clinical settings (1). 13/26 studies reported learner satisfaction as the measured outcome. 2/5 small group discussion studies measured pre-post outcomes with 1 finding SIG improvement in knowledge and attitude and 1 finding no SIG difference in self-assessed self-confidence. 1/4 small group peer role play studies measured standardized patient ratings of knowledge and humanistic skills and faculty rated humanistic skills and found intervention group did SIG better on skills, no difference on knowledge. 4/8 small group, standardized, patient role play studies evaluated outcomes using a pre-post questionnaire. Learners experienced (1) SIG increase in comfort; (2) SIG increase in having a plan for delivering bad news; (3) SIG increase in

TABLE 5.1—*Continued*

Reference	Review Type (R) Number of Studies (N) Study Setting (S) Study Purpose (P) Study Dates (D)	Summary of Findings
		self-confidence in delivering bad news; and (4) SIG increase in more comprehensive listing of steps to be followed when delivering bad news. 4/7 studies using one-on-one-learning with standardized patient encounters, 3 studies found standardized patient ratings SIG improved; 1 study used pre-post questionnaire and found SIG less self-assessed learner confidence after one encounter. Authors conclude that all interventions were rated highly by learners and improved learner self-confidence and, in some cases, learner knowledge and behaviors. Based on adult learning principles and findings, the most effective interventions present basic steps to effectively deliver bad news, and provide learner opportunities to discuss concerns, practice, and receive feedback on their skills.
Beach, Price, et al. 2005	(R) Systematic, 6 dB (N) 14 studies (S) Medical students and residents (P) Evaluate interventions designed to improve cultural competence (D) 1980–2003	14 studies on MDs, 1988–2003, in a broader review on health professionals. 12/14 focused on medical students, 1/14 on medical students and residents, 1/14 on residents and fellows. 6/14 studies measured 7 knowledge outcomes: 6/10 had SIG beneficial effect, 1/7 had non SIG beneficial effect. 12/14 studies measured 22 attitude outcomes: 8/22 had SIG beneficial effect, 7/22 had non SIG beneficial effect, and 7 /22 had no or unclear effect. 7/14 studies measured 10 skills outcomes: 8/10 had SIG beneficial effect, 1/10 had non SIG beneficial effect, and 1 /10 had no or unclear effect. 1/14 studies measured patient satisfaction and found 4 outcomes measured all had SIG beneficial effect. Authors conclude that cultural competence training shows promise as a strategy for improving the knowledge, attitudes, and skills of health professionals. However, evidence that it improves patient adherence to therapy, health outcomes, and equity of services across racial and ethnic groups is lacking.
Butler, Degner, et al. 2005	(R) Systematic (N) 47 RCTs or controlled before and after studies	Studies are those excluded in the Fellowes, et al. 2004 Cochrane review for not meeting inclusion criteria. 16/47 studies involved graduate MDs and

TABLE 5.1—*Continued*

Reference	Review Type (R) Number of Studies (N) Study Setting (S) Study Purpose (P) Study Dates (D)	Summary of Findings
	of communication skills training in cancer health professionals, measuring changes in behavior/skills using objective and validated scales (S) Oncology (P) Show how communication competency has been studied, from the perspectives of the health care provider and the knowledge gaps which exist (D) to 2003	4/47 medical students; however, these studies were not discussed as separate groups. Review results are discussed for all health professionals, including nurses, nursing students, social workers, chaplains, and home care workers. Although all 47 studies claimed that effective communication skills can be learned through a variety of experiences and result in positive interactions with patients and families, the authors identify several limitations. (1) Definition of communication and skills was rarely found. (2) Indicators used to measure successful communication skills outcomes were most often survey type, self-report questionnaires measuring such factors as change in knowledge, skills, and attitudes (3 studies), needs assessment (1 study), discussing death and dying (1 study), and sustainability of skills over time (3 studies). Patients were interviewed solely as a method of applying information taught within a communications program to improve learner communication skills, and patients were excluded from evaluating outcomes. (3) There was wide variability in training program time and timing of outcome measures. (4) Outcomes for most of the studies supported the need for further training in order to achieve and enhance quality patient care. (5) Some studies identified lack of emotional support from colleagues and employers to assist the transfer of communication skills learned in the training sessions into the workplace. (6) Few studies showed any resemblance to consensus recommendations for communication program structures and core skills that should comprise communication training programs. The authors conclude that desired core competencies need to be articulated. It is also unclear how feasible the application to practice of successful interventions might be in terms of efficiency (cost), human resource development (intensive preparation of trainees), and long-term effectiveness.

TABLE 5.1—*Continued*

Reference	Review Type (R) Number of Studies (N) Study Setting (S) Study Purpose (P) Study Dates (D)	Summary of Findings
Kennedy 2005	(R) Systematic, 4 dB (N) 21 studies (S) Oncology (P) Evaluate the literature regarding the efficacy and outcomes of communication skills training programs for health care providers (D) 1982–2004	10 of 21 studies focused on MD communication skills training and 7 of these have been addressed in other tabled reviews (Merckaert, Libert, et al. 2005a; Gysels, Richardson, et al. 2004). Of the remaining 3 studies: (1) 1 study that focused on skills to promote patient disclosure using audio-taped interviews with simulated patients before and after training ($n = 169$ MDs) found increased use of open directive questions (e.g., focusing on and clarifying psychological aspects, empathic statements, and summarizing) vs. inhibiting behaviors. (2) 1 study ($n = 63$ MDs) found SIG increased use of facilitative behaviors and acknowledgments ($p = .01$), as well as empathetic statements ($p = .02$) and a decrease in premature reassurance with a 2.5-day communication skills training followed by six 3 hour, consolidation workshops. (3) 1 RCT conducted two 4-hour sessions ($n = 15$ MDs, 9 trained and 6 not trained) focusing on open-ended questions and facilitative behaviors using pre-post questionnaires. It found increased provider confidence and a non SIG trend toward more use of open-ended questions and increased facilitative behaviors. Author identifies need for additional controlled studies and standardized observational instruments.
Merckaert, Libert, et al. 2005a	(R) Systematic, 8 dB (N) 13 studies, 22 articles (S) Oncology (P) Review recent studies on effectiveness of communication skills training programs for health care professionals (D) 2002–5	9 studies addressed graduate (6), resident-trainee (1), or medical students (2) communication skills training; 2 studies were RCTs. One RCT compared cancer specialists with basic training ($n = 33$) and basic training plus a consolidation workshop providing further practice of skills learned during basic training ($n = 29$). Utterance-by-utterance analysis of audio recorded (1) simulated patient interview and (1) actual patient interview found improvements in both cases with the workshop group: increased use of open, open directive, and screening questions and eliciting and clarifying psychological concerns directed toward pa-

TABLE 5.1—*Continued*

Reference	Review Type (R) Number of Studies (N) Study Setting (S) Study Purpose (P) Study Dates (D)	Summary of Findings
		tients; decrease in premature information directed toward relatives; increase in the use of supportive skills (empathy, educated guesses, alerting to reality, confronting, and negotiating and summarizing) directed toward both patient and relative. A second RCT with 12-month follow-up had 4 groups: written feedback on videotaped consultations plus 3-day course ($n = 39$), course alone ($n = 41$), feedback alone ($n = 41$), and control ($n = 39$). Counts of communication behaviors of 2 consultations at 3 months found course attendance SIG improved key outcomes. Most changes observed were maintained 12 months after the course, and some new changes were observed. Gysels, Richardson, et al. (2004) report that at post-test, participants used SIG more focused questions (RR = 1.34), more focused and open questions (RR = 1.27), more expressions of empathy (RR = 1.69), and more appropriate responses to patients' cues (RR = 1.38) and fewer leading questions (RR = .76) compared with individuals randomly selected to receive no course. A case-control study of 21 oncologists found no effect of four 1-hour, computer-assisted modules on MD behavior, as analyzed by video recordings of consultations. Of 6 nonrandomized studies including 3 studies of practicing MDs and 1 each of MDs recruiting for clinical trials, teaching medical students end-of-life skills, (and participating in mandatory family medicine residents training) 5/6 reported improved MD attitudes toward skills development following the interventions; 2/6 reported behavioral improvements. 1/6 measured attitudes at 6 months follow-up and found retention of improvement. Authors conclude that effective training should include learner-centered, skills-focused, and practice-oriented techniques, be organized in small groups, and be at least 3 days long.

TABLE 5.1—*Continued*

Reference	Review Type (R) Number of Studies (N) Study Setting (S) Study Purpose (P) Study Dates (D)	Summary of Findings
Gaffan, Dacre, et al. 2006	(R) Systematic, 7 dB (N) 12 studies on commu- nication (S) Oncology (P) Review literature re- garding teaching oncol- ogy to undergraduate medical students (D) 1993–2004	2 of 12 studies were covered in other tabled review articles. For the other 10 studies, study designs included control (1); descriptive (7); cohort (2). The number of students ranged from 15 to 369. 3 studies, using pre-post ratings of interviews with simulated patients or student feedback or summative assessment, found the use of role play improved oncology-specific communication skills. Of 6 studies using role play to teach how to give bad news, 1 controlled study found that the ability to give bad news was transferable from cancer scenarios to other scenarios. Trained in-tervention students performed SIG better vs. un-trained students. The training scenarios with standardized patients involved either cancer or a miscarriage, but all students were evaluated us-ing the miscarriage scenario. Within the interven-tion group, the cancer-trained students per-formed as well as the miscarriage-trained students. 5/6 studies using pre-post designs found increase in the number of students who had a plan for giving bad news; SIG increase in student self-reported comfort in delivering bad news; SIG better score on objective structured clinical examination; increase in knowledge and competence; and the use of real patients sensi-tized students to the need for empathy. 1 cohort study offered a short course in "truth telling" and found reduction in paternalistic attitudes using a pre-post questionnaire on attitudes toward truth telling. Authors conclude that students who learn communication skills from patients with cancer have better skills and attitudes than students learning from non–cancer patients.
Stepien and Baernstein 2006	(R) Systematic, 1 dB (N) 13 studies (S) Medical school (P) Identify effective strategies to enhance empathy in undergradu-	7 of 13 studies were studies covered in other tabled review articles. Of the remaining 6 stud-ies, designs included use of control group (2), RCT (1) cross-sectional (2), and case study (2 studies, 9 students and 69 students). The con-trolled studies included (1) a workshop given in

TABLE 5.1—*Continued*

Reference	Review Type (R) Number of Studies (N) Study Setting (S) Study Purpose (P) Study Dates (D)	Summary of Findings
	ate medical students (D) "No time limit"	12 hours over 1 semester to 43 preclinical students, with SIG changes pre- and post-intervention using a nonvalidated empathy scale; (2) an audiotape-led communication skill workshop given in 16 hours to 112 preclinical students with ES 9.1 vs. control group 6.1 observing students and rating them on a validated empathy scale pre- and post-intervention; (3) a lecture-workshop over 11 hours to 55 clinical year 1 students, with students evaluated using a written self-evaluation of empathy and videotape interviews rated with 2 observational measurement tools (history taking and empathy scales). Of these 3 measurement instruments, only the 5 items which address empathy on a history taking rating scale detected SIG improvement in empathy following training. The cross-sectional study found a decline in empathy as individuals advance through medical training. The survey of 1,181 premedical students, medical students, residents, clinical faculty, and alumni found that empathy was highest in premedical and first-year medical students, decreased in second- and fourth-year students, and was lowest in residents. Medical alumni (unknown graduate year) scored lower than first year medical students but higher than medical residents. Authors conclude that current studies are challenged by varying definitions of empathy, small sample sizes, lack of adequate control groups, and inadequacy of existing empathy measurement instruments.
Satterfield and Hughes 2007	(R) Systematic, 4 dB (N) 26 studies (S) Medical school (P) Identify various emotion skills training methods and outcomes in medical student curricula studies	Emotion skills were defined as being (1) "other-directed" cognitive and behavioral strategies intended to improve the awareness, understanding, and/or management of emotional states in others, e.g., making empathic statements or eliciting patient emotions; and (2) "self-directed" that enhance awareness, understanding, and/or management of emotions in the self, e.g., impulse control

TABLE 5.1—*Continued*

Reference	Review Type (R) Number of Studies (N) Study Setting (S) Study Purpose (P) Study Dates (D)	Summary of Findings
	(D) 1980–2006	or awareness of one's own emotions. Undergraduate emotion skills courses varied by total number of contact hours (2–64 hours), session frequency (from 1 session per day to 1 session every 6 months), duration (2 weeks to 2 years), pedagogy, patient populations targeted (e.g., HIV, oncology, end-of-life), and educational outcomes (e.g., empathy, performance on objective structured clinical examinations). Outcome measures included none (3 studies), anecdotal reports or informal impressions of improvement, student reports of recommendations, and student and teacher satisfaction surveys; 15 of 26 studies used objective emotion skills measures. No 2 studies used the same measure of emotion skills. 6/26 studies included a control or comparison condition and 5/26 used a RCT design. All 5 RCTs demonstrated a modest positive effect on empathy and other-directed emotion skills for as long as 3 years postintervention. In these 5 studies, contact time comprised a minimum of 8 hours and teaching methods included small group discussions, role plays, videos, case discussions, and practice interviews. The year of medical school training did not predict emotion skills outcomes. Authors conclude that there is little agreement among educators about the relative importance of emotion skills and the amount of educational resources that might justifiably be used to provide the support or infrastructure needed to make an emotion skills program effective. They suggest that emotion skills, much like physical examination skills, can be viewed as a properly defined, teachable, and measurable skill set.
Smith, Hanson, et al. 2007 Cheraghi-Sohi and Bower 2008	(R) Systematic, 3 dB (N) 15 RCTs (S) Medical school (P) Evaluate the effects of teaching on medical students' patient communication skills using	Studies were classified according to teaching method: (1) structured feedback about student performance during a recorded student-patient interview (6 of 15 studies); (2) lecture and small group discussion (6/15); and (3) other method (3/15). Communication skills were grouped into three categories: establishing rapport, data gath-

TABLE 5.1—*Continued*

Reference	Review Type (R) Number of Studies (N) Study Setting (S) Study Purpose (P) Study Dates (D)	Summary of Findings
	meta-analysis (D) 1966–April 2005	ering, and patient education. (1) Establishing rapport: Students' ability to establish rapport SIG improved in most studies after teaching vs. preclinical students, and students who were taught a specific curriculum had large improvement in skills vs. usual or clerkship experiences. Skills improved in 5 of 6 studies using structured feedback as the educational intervention (ES = .88, *p* = <.00001). 1 study reported SIG differences in student performance after receiving feedback, but ES was not SIG. Using small groups was effective in 5 of 5 studies (ES = .88, *p* = <.0001). Using other methods (3 studies) did not improve student skills. (2) Data gathering abilities: Instruction improved students' abilities in 4 of 5 studies (ES = .79, *p* = <.0001). Interviewing patients followed by specific feedback on the videotaped interview SIG improved skills in 3 studies (ES = .73). Small group teaching also SIG improved skills in 1 study. (3) Patient education: 1 study examined the effects of teaching on students' ability to educate patients by comparing students' abilities to counsel patients about HIV/AIDS after a 3-hr workshop using a small group format and found SIG differences in abilities in trained vs. not trained students at 3 months. No effects were found at 12-month follow-up. Authors conclude that communication skills can be effectively taught to medical students; the best studied and most effective methods were giving structured feedback about student performance during a recorded student-patient interview and small group discussion.
	(R) Systematic, 3 dB (N) 9 RCTs (S) Primarily primary care and pediatric practicing MDs (P) Review efficacy of feedback and brief training	4 of 9 studies addressed communication skills training. The outcome reported in this review was patient satisfaction. 1 study (1987) reported a SIG positive effect. The intervention consisted of two 3-hour seminars using both written and oral methods. 3 studies reported no SIG positive effect on patient satisfaction. Training interventions included (1) 1 hour including 15 minutes of video-

TABLE 5.1—*Continued*

Reference	Review Type (R) Number of Studies (N) Study Setting (S) Study Purpose (P) Study Dates (D)	Summary of Findings
	on improving interpersonal care (D) Not clear	tape presenting research on communication and vignettes on rapport building, 3 booster sessions with content not specified; (2) workplace program of three 90-minute sessions at 2-week intervals consisting of readings, lecture, discussion videotape review, and role playing; (3) two 4-hour workshops using oral and written methods and role play.

dB = database(s)
ES = effect size
GP(s) = general practitioners
MD(s) = physician(s)
n = number

PCP = primary care physician
RCT = randomized control trial
SDM = shared decision making

TABLE 5.2. Evidence from Empirical Studies Relating to Success of Interventions Aimed at Improving Physician Communication ($n = 42$ studies/ $n = 46$ articles)

Reference	Study Design (S) Study Purpose (P) Study Setting (T) Study Date (D) Country (C)	Methods/Interventions	Final Sample Size	Main Measures	Key Findings
Undergraduate, Medical School and Residency Training					
Greco, Brownlea, et al. 2001	(S) RCT (P) Assess effect of systematic patient feedback on sustaining interpersonal skills (T) GP training (D) 1994–97 (C) UK	18-month longitudinal study of GP trainees. Varying intensities of patient feedback to trainees on interpersonal skills.	$n = 196$ trainees $n = 62$ control patient feedback at 3 and 18 months $n = 69$ serial (6, 12, and 15 month) patient feedback $n = 65$ serial feedback plus preceptor discussion	Patient completed score on the Doctors' Interpersonal Skills Questionnaire which measures interpersonal skills on a 5-point scale using a patient-completed questionnaire	Overall interpersonal skills index showed that the control group did not SIG improve ($p = <.05$) in patient ratings pre-post test. The serial feedback and serial feedback plus discussion groups SIG improved their scores, especially in the earlier stages of training. 5 variables were "more resistant to change": (1) explanation skills; (2) consideration of patient context; (3) concern for patient as a person; (4) warmth of greeting; and (5) respect shown to patient.
Oh, Segal, et al. 2001	(S) Comparative (P) Evaluate the acquisition and long-term use of patient-centered interviewing skills (T) Internal medicine residents	Observed interviews pre-post CST and at 2 years. Cross-sectional survey on self-reported use of skills. CST consisted of 20 core sessions incorporating	$n = 42$ residents $n = 14$ residents receiving CST during internship,	(1) Flow of the initial interview (opening and exploration of problems); (2) interpersonal skills (facilitation and relationship skills)	The study had two components: (1) a prospective study of the retention of CST skills two years after the intensive training and (2) a cross-sectional survey comparing the use of CST skills between residents who received CST and those who had not.

195

TABLE 5.2—*Continued*

Reference	Study Design (S) Study Purpose (P) Study Setting (T) Study Date (D) Country (C)	Methods/Interventions	Final Sample Size	Main Measures	Key Findings
	(D) 1996–98 (C) US	seminars, role plays, and supervised interactions with patients.	evaluated before, immediately after, and 2 years after their CST *n* = 14 interns prior to CST *n* = 14 residents no CST		(1) Skills acquisition and retention: Scores on both the immediate post CST and at 2 years showed SIG improvement in all areas vs. pre CST. No SIG loss of skills on 2-year vs. immediately post CST, with the exception of respect in relationship skills. (2) Comparison groups results: Self-reported use of skills found CST group scored better than did the two comparison groups on all 5 scales the survey evaluated. However, SIG differences were found only for the use of reflection of patients' emotions.
von Gunten 2003	(S) Comparative (P) Evaluate end-of-life care skills (T) Hospice (D) 1998–99 (C) US	Pre-post program survey. Residents participate in the care of patients in the inpatient care setting and make joint home visits with physicians and other team members, plus lectures and conferences.	*n* = 65 internal medicine and family practice residents from 5 different training programs	27-item self-assessment evaluation tool developed for the study	Comparison of the combined pre-post mean ratings of self-perceived competence (e.g., comfort with communication, caring for a dying patient, and taking a pain history and writing orders for pain medications) showed a SIG difference (*p* = <.0001). Post assessment included items that asked for the residents' assessment of the instruction and the curriculum:

Author, Year	Study characteristics	Methods	Sample	Outcomes measured	Results
Mukohara, Kitamura, et al. 2004	(S) RCT (P) Examine impact of short intensive seminar on communication (T) Medical students (D) 2001–2 (C) Japan	Post CST, 1 week–5 months, with control group using videotape with standardized patient rated by checklist. 2-day, small group seminar on the medical interview and communication skills based on western principles; first Japanese medical school program on communication skills building.	$n = 97$ students doing a clerkship in internal medicine. $n = 50$ CST students. $n = 47$ students, control with no CST	16 core communication skills	(1) effective clinical faculty (93%); (2) interdisciplinary interactions valuable (87%); (3) rotation covered about the right amount of content (81%) and right duration (78%). Results found SIG difference between groups on asking how the illness or problems affected the patient's life (53% vs. 30%, $p = .02$). No SIG differences in 15/16 core communication skills.
Rosen, Spatz, et al. 2004	(S) Comparative (P) Assess effect of workshop on cross-cultural awareness (T) Medical students (D) Not reported (C) US and Israel	Pre-post using survey of medical students before workshop and 6 weeks following the workshop. 1 and ½-day workshop using instruction, small group discussion, and case study with simulated patients.	$n = 32$ medical students	(1) Student-perceived improved attitudes and skills; (2) 36-item self-evaluation survey on 7 domains measuring elements of attitude, knowledge, and perceived skill	(1) Post workshop students: "strongly agreed" or "agreed" that they improved in the following areas: understanding a patient's perception of illness (92%); eliciting patients' expectation of treatment (96%); asking about cultural issues that affect treatment (83%); and understanding of their own cultural bias (71%). (2) Pre-post self-evaluation students showed SIG improvement in health-belief assessment, sexual history taking, and biopsychosocial inter-

TABLE 5.2—*Continued*

Reference	Study Design (S) Study Purpose (P) Study Setting (T) Study Date (D) Country (C)	Methods/Interventions	Final Sample Size	Main Measures	Key Findings
					viewing skills ($p = <.05$), and breaking bad news and approach to treatment ($p = <.001$); no SIG change in communication with patients' family members and working with an interpreter.
Roter, Larson, et al. 2004	(S) Comparative (P) Evaluate a brief CST using new video feedback interactive Pediatrics (T) Pediatrics (D) Not reported (C) US	Pre-post CST videotaped interviews with simulated patients, coded by RIAS. 4-hour CST using instruction, role play, and feedback using RIAS interactive software.	$n = 28$ first year pediatric residents	17 items in 4 communication categories: (1) data gathering; (2) building a relationship; (3) activating and partnering; (4) problem solving/negotiation	SIG improvements in resident performance with simulated patients pre and post CST: (1) reduced verbal dominance with ratio of the MD to patient dialogue decreasing from 2.1:1 to 1.7:1; (2) overall increased use of open-ended questions ($p = <.001$); (3) increased use of empathy ($p = .05$); (4) increased partnership building on 3/4 items ($p = .05$ to $p = <.001$); and (5) increased problem solving skills on all 3 items ($p = .05$ to $p = <.001$). Female residents demonstrated greater communication change than males.
Han, Keranen, et al. 2005	(S) Comparative (P) Test feasibility of observational CST to improve skills in delivering bad news and	Attitudes measured before and 1 week after CST and end of the intern year. Faculty precounseled, observed,	$n = 44$ residents	(1) Faculty checklist of 18 observed items in resident discussions with patients; (2) resident survey, 4-point scale on	(1) Faculty ratings of observed behaviors ranged from 59% to 95%; 7 criteria fell below satisfactory (70%); attempted to elicit patient's goals; suggested a follow-up plan; con-

Author/Year	Study	Method	Sample	Outcome Measure	Results
	discussing code status (T) Hospital, internal medicine residents (D) 2002–3 (C) US	evaluated, and gave feedback to house staff on a discussion with patients and families.		attitudes toward CST and on self-reported competence and confidence	cluded with review and plan; gave "warning shot" prior to giving bad news; used appropriate level of directiveness; discussed particular treatment options; included discussion of prognosis. (2) Resident self-ratings of communication competence and self-confidence showed SIG ($p = .02$) improvement 1 week after the CST for delivering bad news; no difference for code status (the limitation of life-sustaining medical interventions).
Alexander, Keitz, et al. 2006	(S) Controlled trial (P) Evaluate effect of a short course CST in delivering bad news and eliciting patients' preferences for end-of-life care (T) Internal medicine residents at VA hospital clinic (D) 1999–2001 (C) US	Pre-post CST using coded audio recorded standardized patient encounters. 16-hour CST using small group teaching with lecture, discussion, and role play.	$n = 56$ residents $n = 37$ CST residents $n = 19$ control residents	Scores based on the "standards of practice" for palliative care, derived from the literature, for communication skills relating to delivering bad news and eliciting patients' preferences for end-of-life treatment	(1) CST group summary scores were SIG higher than the control group (9.6 vs. 8.4, range 0–17, $p = .04$). (2) Pre-post CST group scores found SIG ($p = .001$) increases in their overall skill ratings, with improvement in the specific areas of delivering bad news ($p = <.0001$) and responding to emotional cues ($p = .003$). (3) Cumulative scores for eliciting patient preferences for life-sustaining care did not differ between CST and control groups or between pre and post CST overall scores. There was a SIG increase in eliciting patient preferences in the pre-post CST group (1.1 vs. 1.8, $p = <.0001$, range 0–5). Control group scores not reported. Pre-post analysis found SIG changes in
Carter, Lewis, et al	(S) Comparative	Pre-post using self-as-	$n = 196$ third	(1) 11-item scale de-	

TABLE 5.2—*Continued*

Reference	Study Design (S) Study Purpose (P) Study Setting (T) Study Date (D) Country (C)	Methods/Interventions	Final Sample Size	Main Measures	Key Findings
al. 2006	(P) Develop and evaluate effectiveness of an interactive workshop to improve medical student attitudes, beliefs, and cross-cultural communication skills (T) Medical students (D) Not reported (C) US	sessment of cultural attitudes and beliefs. 6-week small group workshop using instruction, interactive self-assessment exercises, tools for interacting with culturally diverse patient groups, and role play.	year medical students	signed for study to assess student cultural attitudes and beliefs on a 5-point scale; (2) student rating of program on 5-point scale	7/11 items (all *p* values *p* = <.05), with 3/11 items indicating "a strong trend" (all *p* values *p* = <.056) in the desired direction. No change was found in 1/11 item ("I am likely to behave in a culturally competent manner when seeing patients"). The majority of students agreed or strongly agreed that the program was valuable (55%), appropriate (70%), and effective (67%).
Claramita and Majoor 2006	(S) Comparative (P) Compare communication skills of resident MDs with and without CST (T) Hospital outpatient clinics (D) Not reported (C) Indonesia	Post CST resident and patient survey. Compare residents with and without CST in post-graduate practice in Indonesia.	*n* = 48 GP and specialist residents *n* = 18 residents with CST *n* = 30 residents without CST	Questionnaire developed for the study consisted of 39 items scored on a 5-point scale after a consultation; 4.0 on the Likert scale was defined as "satisfactory"	No effect was found for CST and item ratings were not satisfactory (below 4 on the Likert scale); patients did not observe any difference in communication behavior among intervention and control groups. There was no difference in self-evaluation ratings by intervention and control MDs. A SIG difference was found between MD communication behavior skills as observed and desired by their patients (*p* = <.001).
Furman, Head, et al. 2006	(S) Comparative (P) Evaluate an educa-	Chart audit 10 days pre- and 5 days post CST. 1-	*n* = 8 residents *n* = 79 patient	Documentation of DNR discussion between	Before the CST, 32% of the patients had a documented advance directive

Study	Description	Method	Sample	Measures	Results
	tional CST on teaching residents skills for discussing advance directives. (T) VA medical center (D) 2000 (C) US	time instruction and role play exercise.	records	patient and resident or intern	discussion vs. 34% of the patients had a discussion after the CST, demonstrating minimal improvement. Authors conclude that MDs need more interactive, experiential learning opportunities and related supervision.
Hart, Drotar, et al. 2006	(S) Comparative (P) Evaluate effectiveness of a brief CST to enhance interpersonal communication skills (T) Pediatric hospital outpatient clinic (D) Not reported (C) US	Pre-post CST using RIAS coded audiotapes (1 pre and 2 post pediatric visits) and parent rating of communication. One 1½- hour instruction and role play.	n = 28 pediatric residents	(1) RIAS categories of 34 utterance types; (2) 23-item validated parent-report measure of parents' perceptions of the consultation; (3) 27-item measure of parent satisfaction with the consultation	(1) The total amount of interpersonal communication utterances (i.e., positive affect, empathy/reassurance, and partnership combined) increased over time ($p = <.03$, ES = .17); (2) parents perceived residents as communicating well and their perceptions of residents' communication skills did not change over time (mean = 15.1, range 0–16); (3) parents were SIG more satisfied with care post CST ($p = <.01$), with SIG change in the distress relief subscale of the measure ($p = <.01$).
Rosen, Kountz, et al. 2006	(S) Comparative (P) Evaluate short-term workshop on sexual communication skills and management of sexual problems (T) Residents (D) Not reported (C) US	Pre and post workshop participant surveys and 6-month follow-up. ½-day workshop using faculty presentations and patient-MD panels.	n = 34 family practice and specialty residents	(1) Questions on self-perceived comfort and ability in sexual interviewing; (2) post workshop program evaluation	(1) Pre workshop, 46% stated they rarely or never discussed sexual issues with their patients; 90% agreed that sexual problems can have a major impact on the overall quality of life; 48% were moderately or very uncomfortable in managing patient sexual problems but 75% believed it was moderately important or very important to know about a patient's sexual health. (2) Post workshop,

TABLE 5.2—*Continued*

Reference	Study Design (S) Study Purpose (P) Study Setting (T) Study Date (D) Country (C)	Methods/Interventions	Final Sample Size	Main Measures	Key Findings
					67% had attained a greater awareness of sexual problems; 52% were more comfortable in sexual history taking; and 74% understood the role of specialist evaluation in sexual problem management. (3) 9 residents responded to a 6-month follow-up: 8/9 rated their comfort level in sexual interviewing as moderately improved; 5/9 used referral services for sexual medicine; 6/9 participated more actively in the management of these patients. No tests of SIG performed.
Brinkman, Geraghty, et al. 2007	(S) RCT (P) Evaluate effect of multisource feedback on communication skills and professionalism (T) Pediatrics, inpatient children's hospital (D) 2005 (C) US	Baseline and 5-month evaluation. Standard feedback plus end-of-rotation reports summarized evaluations and comparison to peers, plus 30-minute coaching sessions vs. standard, 1-monthly written evaluation by supervisory MD.	$n = 36$ first year pediatric residents $n = 18$ CST residents $n = 18$ control residents	Parent and nurse ratings of, e.g., friendliness, using plain language, being respectful, being truthful, showing interest, communicating effectively during the physical examination, sharing decisions, explaining problems, encouraging questions,	Both groups had comparable baseline characteristics, and parent and nurse ratings. Parent ratings increased for both groups. While parent ratings increased more for the CST group, differences between groups were not SIG. Nurse ratings increased for the CST group and decreased for the control group. The difference in change between groups was SIG for communicating effectively with the

Author/Year	Study Description	Method	Sample	Measures	Results
Dow, Leong, et al. 2007	(S) Controlled trial (P) Assess if residents can learn empathy techniques from theater professors (T) Ambulatory clinic at urban university and health system (D) 2004 (C) US	Pre-post CST observations members of the Theater Department of a primary care patient visit. Four 90-minute classroom and workshops with professors of theater.	$n = 20$ internal medicine residents $n = 14$ CST group $n = 6$ control group	Measures of 33 parameters within 6 subscores: (1) empathic communication; (2) relating to the listener; (3) verbal communication; (4) nonverbal communication; (5) respect for dignity; and (6) overall impression and listening carefully	Results showed SIG improvement ($p < .011$) in CST group across all subscores pre vs. post measurement. After adjusting for pre-CST scores, the post-CST subscores in the CST group were SIG better ($p = <.01$) vs. control group for empathy ($p = .004$, ES $= 1.7$), relating to the listener ($p = .01$, ES $= 1.8$), nonverbal communication ($p = .01$, ES $= 1.4$), respect for dignity ($p = .002$, ES $= 1.9$), and overall impression ($p = .007$, ES $= 1.5$). Verbal communication improved CST group vs. the control group, but not SIG ($p = .058$, ES $= 1.0$). patient and family.
Fischer and Arnold 2007	(S) Comparative (P) Assess effectiveness of workshop on teaching delivering bad news and discussing end-of-life goals of care (T) University-based interns (D) Not reported (C) US	Pre-post survey. 3-hour workshop using group discussions, brief lecture, videotape review, and role play.	$n = 43$ interns taking pre-test $n = 29$ interns taking post-tests No difference between those who completed both the pre-test and post-test and drop-outs on gender, race, workshop rat-	Measures of knowledge, attitudes, and self-reported confidence in delivering bad news and discussing advance care plans	Pre-post mean knowledge score, bad news subscore, and advance care planning subscore all increased SIG ($p = <.001$). Interns reported increased confidence in their ability to discuss advance care plans with clinic patients ($p = .001$), discuss limitation of treatment with hospitalized patients ($p = .002$), handle emotional responses that may arise in the discussion of advance care planning ($p = .036$), deliver bad news to patients ($p = .002$), and handle emotional responses that may arise while delivering bad news ($p = .001$). No change in intern attitudes.

TABLE 5.2—Continued

Reference	Study Design (S) Study Purpose (P) Study Setting (T) Study Date (D) Country (C)	Methods/Interventions	Final Sample Size	Main Measures	Key Findings
			ings, baseline knowledge, attitudes, or confidence		
Klaristenfeld, Harrington, et al. 2007	(S) Comparative (P) Evaluate program to teach surgical residents about palliative care and end-of-life issues (T) Hospital (D) Not reported (C) US	Pre-post, and 3-month follow-up surveys. Three 1-hour sessions on palliative care using lecture, discussion, and role play, including strategies for improving MD-patient interactions and methods for breaking bad news.	$n = 47$ surgical residents at university medical center	15 items on a 5-point scale measuring understanding, importance of, and ease with palliative and end-of-life care	2 items showed a SIG ($p = <.01$) change: (1) 57% of residents felt "comfortable speaking to patients and patients' families about end-of-life issues," vs. post-test (81%) and 3 months (84%). (2) 9% of residents at pre-test thought that they had "received adequate training in palliation during residency," vs. post-test (86%) and at 3 months (84%). 92% percent of residents at 3-month follow-up "had been able to use the information learned in clinical practice."
Lown, Sasson, et al. 2008	(S) Comparative (P) Evaluate effect of CST on radiologists' communication skills (T) Diagnostic mammography	2-case, 2-station OBSE: (1) making diagnosis; (2) communicating bad news to patient-teachers. Three 1-hour workshops facilitated by fac-	$n = 9$ resident radiologists	(1) Baseline self-assessment scores on communication skills and confidence and stress in communicating abnormal findings; (2) 7	(1) Baseline results on a 4-point scale: self-assessed communication skills (2.3), confidence (1.6), and stress (2.6) in communicating abnormal findings. (2) Post-CST ratings for 2 OBSE cases (5-point scale) found

	(D) Not reported (C) US	...ulty patient-teacher, using discussion and videotape.	post CST skills scores and debriefing themes	mean scores for both cases were lowest for the skill "understands the patient's perspective" (acknowledging the patient's personal or family history of breast disease and eliciting the patient's thoughts and emotions or concerns about findings and recommendations) (3.2) and highest for "manages the flow" (efficient time management without rushing or interrupting the patient) (3.9). (3) Residents identified 9 themes involving verbal and nonverbal suggestions for improving communication skills. No tests of SIG performed.

Graduate, Practicing Physicians and fellows

Guadagnoli, Soumerai, et al. (2000)	(S) RCT (P) Evaluate effect of using medical opinion leaders and performance feedback to reduce the proportion of women who reported that surgeons did not discuss options prior to surgery for early stage breast cancer (T) Hospital (D) 1993–95 (C) US	Pre-post survey of patients having Stage I or II breast cancer. Opinion leader strategies included slide presentations at meetings, one on one discussions and data review, and dissemination of graphic as decision aids.	$n = 28$ hospitals $n = 18$ opinion leader group (experimental) $n = 10$ performance feedback group (control) pre-$n = 763$ women in opinion leader group and $n = 287$ in perfor-	(1) Proportion of women who said their surgeons did not discuss surgical treatment alternatives; and (2) proportion of women who underwent breast conserving surgery	Hospital level change: (1) proportion of women who said their surgeons did not discuss surgical treatment alternatives: NS change 33%–17% opinion leader hospitals vs. 31%–13% for performance feedback hospitals; proportion declined SIG over time for both hospital groups ($p = <.001$). (2) NS change between hospital groups in proportion of patients who underwent breast-conserving surgery (34%–43% for opinion leader hospitals vs. 41%–46% for performance feedback hospitals); rate of breast-conserving surgery increased SIG over time for both hospital groups (p

TABLE 5.2—*Continued*

Reference	Study Design (S) Study Purpose (P) Study Setting (T) Study Date (D) Country (C)	Methods/Interventions	Final Sample Size	Main Measures	Key Findings
			mance feedback group post-*n* = 920 women in opinion leader group and *n* = 344 in performance feedback group		= <.05).
Moral, Alamo, et al. 2001	(S) RCT (P) Evaluate effect of CST for MDs caring for fibromyalgic patients (T) Primary care (D) 1997 (C) Spain	Post CST videotaped encounter with a fibromyalgic simulated patient, and 1 to 2-month follow-up telephone query to the patient. 18-hour CST using instruction, role play, and videos.	*n* = 20 FP MDs *n* = 10 CST MDs *n* = 20 control MDs	(1) 13-item checklist for videotape; (2) 3 patient questions on how fully patient was able to present problem, MD discussing cause of pain, and listening	Mean post-CST videotape scores were 11.3 (range 10–12) for CST group vs. 9 (range 4–12) for control group (p = <.01). Results of patient questionnaire found CST group scores SIG higher for patient ability to present problem (p = .03), MD clear explanation (p = .001), and MD listening (p = .004).
van Dulmen and van Weert 2001	(S) Comparative (P) Evaluate CST for gynecologists (T) Gynecology, outpatient (D) Not reported (C) Netherlands	Pre-post CST videotaped consultations analyzed using RIAS. 3-day CST using instruction, role play, and pre CST videotapes of MDs.	*n* = 18 gynecologists *n* = 272 pre CST videotapes *n* = 256 post CST video-	Scoring of 16 RIAS categories, e.g., social talk, agreements, concerns, medical questions, psychosocial questions	Post-CST MDs. SIG differences were found in 4 of 16 RIAS categories: (1) increased sensitivity to psychosocial aspects of communication (p = .01); (2) gave more signs of agreement; (3) asked fewer medical questions (p

				tapes	= .01) and were less directive (p = .05). No difference was found in the duration of the outpatient visits. MDs believed that (1) GP and specialist consultations have comparable communication skills; (2) communication skills can be taught and learned; (3) the workshop had improved their skills; (4) MDs should spend more time discussing what to tell patients and how to do it; and (5) use of a videotape of their consultations was threatening. No tests of significance performed.
Cooper and Hassell 2002	(S) Descriptive (P) Design, implement, and evaluate CST for rheumatologists (T) Rheumatology outpatient (D) Not reported (C) UK	Post-workshop attitudinal questionnaire. 1/2-day workshop using small group discussion, videotapes, role play.	n = 14 MD senior specialist trainee rheumatologists	6 items measuring attitudes toward communication	
Sliwa, Makoul, et al. 2002	(S) Comparative (P) Evaluate the effectiveness of a rehabilitation-specific CST program for MDs (T) Rehabilitation hospital (D) 1992–93 (C) US	Pre-post CST. 3 groups of patients or family members were interviewed by telephone 3 months after discharge, 1 group before and 2 groups post CST. Six 1-hour semimonthly seminars using discussion and videotapes.	n = unspecified number of attending and resident MDS n = 245 patients n = 73 pre CST n = 172 post CST, 2 groups were combined for analysis	Patients' perceptions of the extent to which MDs accomplished 18 communication tasks using a 4-point scale	SIG results found on 14 of 18 items, with the greatest differences (all p = .005) associated with "provides you with choices when treatment is required"; "involves you in deciding on a treatment plan"; "discusses how you felt your disability affects your life"; "gives you a chance to talk about your concerns"; "encourages you to ask questions"; "asks for your views about your progress"; and "fully explains recommendations for the rehabilitation program."
Back, Arnold, et al. 2003 Back, Arnold, et al. 2007	(S) Comparative (P) 3-year evaluation of CST for senior fellows (T) Oncology (D) 2002–4	Pre-post retreat CST audiotaped encounter with simulated patients using each MD as his or her own control. 4-day	n = 115 medical oncology fellows participating in training ses-	Measures of 14 skills using audiotapes coded, observable behaviors in (1) giving bad news and (2) discussing tran-	(1) MDs acquired a mean of 5.4 giving bad news skills (p = <.001) and a mean of 4.4 discussing transitions skills (p = <.001). E.g., percentage of MDs learning bad news skills: use

TABLE 5.2—Continued

Reference	Study Design (S) Study Purpose (P) Study Setting (T) Study Date (D) Country (C)	Methods/Interventions	Final Sample Size	Main Measures	Key Findings
	(C) US	retreat using instruction, role play, and self-awareness exercises on relationship building, giving bad news, transitions to palliative care, and DNR.	sions 2002–4	sitions to palliative care	word cancer (50%), remaining silent for 10 seconds after giving news (65%), making empathic statement after news (75%); transition skills learned: elicits patient values (60%), respond to "how much time" (58%), and assesses patient understanding (42%). (2) SIG changes were found in 10 of 12 communication categories pre-post assessment for both bad news and transitions skills, e.g., names an emotion that the patient seems to be experiencing but has not explicitly articulated at any point ($p = .001$) and expresses respect or praise about how the patient is handling the situation ($p = .001$).
Shilling, Jenkins, et al. 2003	(S) RCT (P) Identify factors that influence patient and MD satisfaction with consultation and if satisfaction can be improved with CST (T) Oncology	Pre-post CST patient satisfaction. 3-day CST using structured feedback, videotape review, role play with simulated patients, interactive group demonstrations, and discussion.	$n = 160$ MDs $n = 80$ MDs CST $n = 80$ MDs control $n = 1,816$ patients	(1) 51-item validated patient satisfaction questionnaire; (2) 5-item questionnaire that included one question asking, "how satisfied were you with the interview?"	Satisfaction data are part of the Fallowfield, Jenkins, et al. (2002 and 2003) RCT on CST evaluation (addressed in review articles, table 5.1). Results on satisfaction were related to patient's age ($p = <.0001$), psychological morbidity ($p = .02$), and length of wait in clinic ($p = <.0001$). MD satisfaction

Author/year	Study characteristics	Design/Intervention	n	Measures	Results
	(D) 34 cancer centers (C) UK				was SIG greater for males (p = <.025), surgeon specialty vs. medical or clinical (p = <.0001), site of cancer (p = <.0001), and type of treatment discussed, with the least satisfaction with palliative care. No SIG relationship to patient age or gender. CST had no SIG effect on patient satisfaction or consultation time.
Theunissen, de Ridder, et al. 2003 de Ridder, Theunissen, et al. 2007	(S) Comparative (P) Evaluate CST on MD-patient communication on hypertension control aimed at increasing patient adherence to treatment (T) General practice (D) Not reported (C) Netherlands	Quasi-experimental design, usual care compared to 2 items: discussion of patient beliefs or of action plans. Two 3-hour CSTs on presenting a semi-structured protocol for hypertension management on items 1 or 2.	n = 10 GPs n = 5 GPs protocol for item 1, patient beliefs n = 5 GPs protocol for item 2, action plans	(1) Adherence to experimental protocol; (2) scores on 16 communication categories using RIAS	Visit time SIG longer than usual care by 17 and 18 minutes. In both experimental items the proportion of affective GP utterances was higher while patients contributed more to the conversation (p = <.001). When GPs changed their communication style, patients did accordingly. The authors conclude that the study provided GPs with a tool to discuss illness representations and action plans of patients with hypertension.
Harms, Young, et al. 2004	(S) Comparative (P) Evaluate CST effect on patient outcomes of satisfaction and anxiety (T) University anesthesia department (D) Not reported (C) Switzerland	Pre-post CST patient survey. 20-hour program using videotape reviews of actual preoperative visits and role play.	n = 59 resident and faculty anesthesiologists n = 1,228 patients	86 questionnaire items yielding 6 summary variables related to patient satisfaction and patient preoperative anxiety	Overall satisfaction with the pre-operative visit was high with (79%) and without CST (78%); anesthesia anxiety low with and without CST (2.0, range 0–10), and surgery anxiety with and without CST (2.3 and 2.4, respectively). After adjusting for baseline patient and MD variables, CST had no SIG effect on patient satisfaction or overall anxiety. Estimates of CST effect on each of 10 specific

TABLE 5.2—*Continued*

Reference	Study Design (S) Study Purpose (P) Study Setting (T) Study Date (D) Country (C)	Methods/Interventions	Final Sample Size	Main Measures	Key Findings
					aspects of pre-operative anxiety found SIG effects on harm from anesthesia (ES = .05, p = .04), not waking up (ES = .04, p = .05), and results of surgery (ES = .06, p = .04).
Vegni and Moja 2004	(S) Comparative (P) Evaluate effects of CST (T) Ophthalmology (D) Not reported (C) Italy	Pre-post CST videotape of simulated patient using RIAS scoring system and researcher-completed Patient Centered Score Sheet. 16-hour CST using instruction, videotape review, role play, and exercises.	n = 11 ophthalmologists	(1) Patient-centered score (range 0–1); (2) 7 categories of the RIAS scores	Results found (1) SIG increase in the mean patient centeredness score (.24 to .43, p = <.01); (2) SIG improvement in 3 categories: using open ended questions (p = <.02), process (e.g., orientation statement) (p = <.05), and social communication (e.g., personal statement) (p = <.01); (3) SIG decrease in medical and therapeutics information offered categories (p = <.01); (4) no SIG differences in categories of closed questions, emotional, and lifestyle and psychosocial information.
Welschen, Kuyvenhoven, et al. 2004	(S) RCT (P) Assess effectiveness of a multiple intervention aimed at reducing antibiotic prescription rates for respiratory	Pre-post test with usual care as control group education. GP meeting with consensus guidelines on antibiotic use, combined with commu-	n = 89 GPs n = 42 intervention n = 49 control	(1) Antibiotic prescription rates for acute respiratory tract symptoms (from claims data); (2) patient satisfaction	(1) SIG effect on antibiotic prescribing rate for respiratory tract symptoms: baseline rate did not differ SIG between intervention (27%) and control group (29%) vs. intervention (23%) and control (37%) at 9

Study	Design / Purpose	Intervention	Sample	Measures	Results
	tract symptoms (T) Primary care (D) 2000–2001 (C) Netherlands	nication skills training; monitoring and feedback on prescribing behavior; group education for assistants of general practitioners and pharmacists; and education material for patients.			months (mean difference in change $= 12\%$, 95% CI 18.9% to 4.0%). (2) Multilevel analysis confirmed the results of the unadjusted analysis (intervention effect 1.7%, 2.3% to 1.0%). (3) No effect on patient satisfaction.
Merckaert, Libert, et al. 2005b	(S) RCT (P) Assess CST impact on improving MDs' ability to detect distress in cancer patients (T) Oncology (D) Not reported (C) Belgium	Transcribed audiotapes, patient and MD assessment of patient distress. 19-hour basic CST (focused on knowledge and skills acquisition) using lecture, role play, and case discussion, plus six 3-hour consolidation workshops (for improving supportive skills).	$n = 58$ MDs $n = 30$ MDs receiving basic CST and consolidation workshop $n = 28$ MDs control, receiving basic CST only	(1) 14-item, self-report instrument to assess patient anxiety and depression on a 4-point scale; (2) MD rating of patient distress on a 10-point visual analog scale immediately after interview	(1) No change was observed in basic CST or in basic CST plus workshop in MDs' ability to detect distress in cancer. (2) Pre-CST, MDs did not adjust the use of their assessment or supportive skills to the level of distress they perceived in their patients and to the level of patient self-perceived distress. Post-CST, basic CST MDs used SIG ($r = .56$, $p = <.001$) more psychological assessment skills when MDs perceived their patients as more distressed; use of supportive skills became SIG correlated with use of assessment skills ($r = .43$, $p = <.01$). Only for basic CST plus workshop were MDs' assessment skills correlated with patients' self-assessed level of distress ($r = .64$, $p = <.001$), and MD use of assessment and supportive skills was highly SIG correlated ($r = .64$, $p = <.001$). (3) Mixed-effects modeling found MD

TABLE 5.2—Continued

Reference	Study Design (S) Study Purpose (P) Study Setting (T) Study Date (D) Country (C)	Methods/Interventions	Final Sample Size	Main Measures	Key Findings
					detection of patients' distress was associated SIG positively with MDs breaking bad news (p = .02) and with MDs using assessment skills (p = .015) and supportive skills (p = .045).
Stein, Frankel, et al. 2005	(S) Descriptive (P) Present case study of organizational efforts to optimize clinician clinical communication skills (T) Health maintenance organization (D) 1998–2003 (C) US	6 months pre and 6 months post CST clinician-specific patient satisfaction scores. Four Habits model.	n = over 400 clinicians, 6 cohorts over 6 years 1998–2003	Aggregate out- member patient satisfaction scores (MPS) on 5 items: (1) skills and abilities; (2) confidence in care; (3) listened and explained; (4) involvement in decisions about care; (5) familiar with medical history	MPS results for 6 years: (1) 65.6% vs. 68.4%; (2) 64.4% vs. 68.0%; (3) 68.7% vs. 7.6%; (4) 67.8% vs. 72.4%; (5) 66.2% vs. 7.5%; (6) 7.4% vs. 73.5%. "Aggregated MPS scores of course participants show statistically significant improvement."
Verhoeven, Avonts, et al. 2005	(S) RCT (P) Evaluate impact of CST on increasing screening for chlamydial infections (T) General practice (D) 2003 (C) Belgium	Pre-post CST observation of clinical practice CST of screening algorithm consisting of 7 questions (4 on signs and symptoms, 3 on sexual history) plus video and 1-page text on communication	n = 36 MDs n = 18 MDs with CST n = 18 MDs control, no CST n = 317 patients	(1) Number of patients who had risk assessment and test, as a measure of the ease by which GPs managed to raise the issue; (2) proportion of appropriately tested patients, as a measure of the quality	CST GPs did not include more patients (10 CST patients vs. 7.6 control patients), but the quality of the screening process was SIG better (81.6% vs. 56.2% appropriate tests, p = .02). CST GPs selected eligible candidates for screening more accurately and decreased the risk of over-screening.

Study	Design / Purpose	Intervention	Sample	Outcome measures	Results
Amiel, Ungar, et al. 2006	(S) Controlled clinical trial (P) Evaluate effectiveness of CST in breaking bad news (T) Primary care (D) Not reported (C) Israel	skills for taking a sexual history vs. control with algorithm alone Pre-post CST, using OBSE. Fourteen 90-min small group sessions using theory, attitude clarification, communication skills, practice with simulated patients.	$n = 34$ GPs $n = 17$ GPs with CST $n = 17$ control group discussions about patients and situations in their clinic that triggered emotional reactions	of the communication regarding the risk assessment Mean scores on 10–11 items using a 5-point rating scale in each of 8 OBSE	CST GPs SIG increased their mean grade pre- (58.5) vs. post-test (68.5) ($p = <.01$, ES = .94). Improvement in the control group was minimal (pre-test 57 vs. 58.1, ES = .23). The post-CST scores between the groups were SIG (68.5 vs. 58.1, $p = <.01$).
Hobma, Ram, et al. 2006	(S) RCT (P) Evaluate effect of CST focused on assessed MD needs (T) General practice (D) 2002–3 (C) Netherlands	Pre-post CST videotaped consultations. Assessment of GP skills via videotape followed by three to four 2-hour structured activities in small group meetings, aimed at remedying the identified shortcomings.	$n = 76$ GPs $n = 38$ CST GPs $n = 38$ control GPs	Communication skills rated using a validated instrument (MAAS-Global) assessing 12 MD-patient communication items and producing a summary score, on a 6-point scale	(1) Participants reported 8 items as personal improvement goals, and SIG improvement was found on 5 (ES = .66): introduction, naming patient request for help, evaluation of the consultation, exploring patient reason for consultation, and summarization of consultation; (2) mean number of meetings attended was 2.75, and regression analysis found a SIG effect of participation (beta = 1.30).
Muthny, Wiedebusch, et al. 2006	(S) Descriptive (P) Evaluate 75 CST workshops on breaking bad news of death (T) Hospital	Post CST survey. 1-day workshop using lecture, video case vignettes, self-experience, lecture role play	$n = 760$ MDs and nurses from intensive care units and sur-	1 part of a 3-part survey on self-perceived learning effects on communication with relatives, and requesting organ	Survey results indicate CST improves skills in dealing with bereaved relatives (78%); improves communication skills (66%); makes it easier to approach the relatives (56%); makes

TABLE 5.2—*Continued*

Reference	Study Design (S) Study Purpose (P) Study Setting (T) Study Date (D) Country (C)	Methods/Interventions	Final Sample Size	Main Measures	Key Findings
	(D) Not reported (C) Germany	and exercises.	gical wards	donation	it easier to decide when to ask for donation (66%); makes it easier to ask for organ donation (47%); helps to feel better after the contact with the relatives (65%); makes better long-term coping with this situation (65%); helps the relatives to cope with their loss (44%); achieves higher agreement and lower refusal rates (31%).
Stratos, Katz, et al. 2006	(S) Comparative (P) Evaluate 12 standardized CSTs on end-of-life care, including communication (T) Palliative care (D) 2000–2001 (C) US	Pre-post training evaluation. 16-hour seminar series on end-of-life issues, e.g., death and dying, psychiatric and spirituality issues, pain management, communication.	$n = 62$ MDs consisting of 33 faculty MDs and 29 residents	(1) Knowledge test; (2) attitude and confidence regarding clinical and teaching skills in palliative care on a 5-point scale	(1) Pre-post test knowledge gain: faculty: (68% vs. 82%); residents (32% vs. 75%); (2) SIG improvement in self-reported confidence in performing 12 end-of-life skills, both faculty and residents ($p = <.001$); confidence in teaching 12 end-of-life skills, both faculty and residents ($p = <.001$); attitude toward end-of-life both faculty and residents ($p = <.001$).
Cals, Scheppers, et al. 2007	(S) Comparative (P) Evaluate CST for managing acute bronchitis (T) General practice (D) Not reported	Pre-post test CST using audiotape consultations with simulated patients in routine practice before, 2	$n = 20$ GPs All 20 GPs were visited by 3 standardized patients,	11-item scale including 5 general communication items and 6 items specific to lower respiratory tract infections	Compared to baseline, GPs used SIG more communication skills, general as well as those specific to low respiratory tract infection (e.g., elicits pa-

Author, Year	Study Design/Purpose	Method	n	Measures	Results
	(C) UK	weeks, and 6 months post CST. Two 3-hour seminars using discussion, feedback of CST audiotape transcripts, video, and lecture.	generating 60 complete transcripts for analysis	communication on a 4-point scale	tient's concerns about cough problem, elicits patient's expectations about management, summarizes the consultation, checks patient's understanding of the given information, mentions both pros and cons of antibiotic treatment to the patient) in both the short term ($p = <.001$) and the longer term ($p = <.001$). Overall communication score (range 0–30) declined slightly from short- to longer-term follow-up (median score 22.00 vs. 2.00, $p = .002$). There was no SIG change in consultation time. (See table 4.3 for parent effects.) No effect on MD communication behavior. No effect on visit length.
Harrington, Norling, et al. 2007	(S) Descriptive (P) Report development and evaluation of an MD and parent CST program designed to improve communication regarding antibiotic prescribing for children (T) Pediatric clinic (D) Not reported (C) US	Interactional analysis of "sick child" office visits audiotapes using PACE coding system. Data on comparison group collected before MD training. Pre-visit, waiting room training on PACE for Parents. 45-min MD training on PACE for Pediatricians.	$n = 81$ parents $n = 42$ control $n = 39$ treatment $n = 4$ pediatricians	Parents: (1) information giving; (2) information seeking; (3) information verifying; (4) express more concerns Pediatricians: (1) address positive treatment options; (2) address parents' feelings, concerns, and expectations; (3) create partnership with parents; (4) encourage questions Visit length Patient assessment of quality of information	
Hietanen, Aro, et al. 2007	(S) RCT (P) Evaluate effect of CST	Patient survey 3½ months after entering	$n = 7$ MDs $n = 3$ CST MDs		Compared to the control group, patients in CST group were (1) more

TABLE 5.2—Continued

Reference / Study Design (S) Study Purpose (P) Study Setting (T) Study Date (D) Country (C)	Methods/Interventions	Final Sample Size	Main Measures	Key Findings
on quality of clinical trial informed consent (T) Oncology (D) 2001–3 (C) Finland	trial. 6-hour CST to MDs at 2 of 3 hospitals, using instruction and role play.	$n = 4$ MDs control group $n = 149$ patients at CST hospitals $n = 139$ patients at control hospital	given about the trial and the communication skills of MDs who had introduced the trial	satisfied with the information received (73% vs. 56%, $p = .003$); (2) more likely to consider the time given for making their decision more sufficient (98% vs. 90%, $p = .004$); recalled more often that the MD had also offered other therapeutic options than the trial treatment (91% vs. 97%, $p = .032$); and understood the main aim of the study better (89% vs. 78%, $p = .030$). The majority of patients in both groups believed they understood all aspects of the clinical trial (95% and 92%, NS); however questions on the quality of informed consent revealed misconceptions, e.g., two-thirds of both groups agreed that "treatment being researched in my clinical trial has been proven to be the best treatment for my type of cancer."
Gulbrandsen, Krupat, et al. 2008 (S) Descriptive (P) Explore effect of Four Habits model on Norwegian MDs	2-month pre and 1-month post CST patient satisfaction questionnaire and MD evaluation fo-	$n = 16$ MDs internal medicine (5), neurology (4), gy-	(1) Summary patient satisfaction; (2) MD course evaluation	Results found mean patient satisfaction 8.7 (range 0–10). Female patients SIG satisfied vs. male patients SIG satisfied vs. male patients ($p = .02$); patients 46 or older SIG

Study	Methods	n	Outcomes	Results
(T) Primary and specialty care MDs (D) 2006 (C) Norway	cus group 3 months post CST. 3-day workshop, using role play with US and Norwegian facilitators.	necology (3), pediatrics(1), psychiatry (1), surgery (1), and family medicine (1) $n = 206$ patient satisfaction questionnaires		more satisfied vs. younger patients ($p = .004$). Habits 1 and 4 were more easily recognized as important and useful than habits 2 and 3. Most of the MDs had dedicated themselves to train on habit 1 or habit 4, and these were also the habits that they believed made greatest impact on their practice. Almost all participants, across specialties, said that focusing on habit 4 had improved their consultations greatly.
Haskard, Williams, et al. 2008 (S) RCT (P) Assess effects of a communication skills training program for physicians and patients (T) Primary care (D) Not reported (C) US	MD attitude questionnaire with measures at 0, 3, 6 months. MDs randomized into 4 groups: control, MD trained, patient trained, MD and patient trained. MDs: three 6-hour interactive workshops and coaching. Patients: at 3 months, one 20-minute pre-visit, waiting room intervention of audiotape and patient guide book.	$n = 2,196$ patients $n = 156$ MDs	MD-related: (1) patient satisfaction; (2) visit satisfaction; (3) patient counseling; (4) stress and life satisfaction; (5) MD global ratings of the communication process	(See table 4.3 for patient effects.) Trained MD effects vs. nontrained MDs: (1) patient satisfaction: SIG improvement in MD information giving ($p = .03$) and overall care ($p = .04$); SIG increase in willingness to recommend MD ($p = .04$); (2) MD visit satisfaction: SIG increase in MD satisfaction with physical exam detail ($p = .004$); no effect on: visit very satisfying, felt adequately trained and confident, had enough time to care for the patient, understood what the patient wanted to say, wanted aspects of the physician-patient relationship to change; (3) patient reported counseling: SIG increase in MD counseling about weight loss ($p = .02$); exercise ($p = .02$); and quitting smoking ($p = .001$) and alcohol

TABLE 5.2—Continued

Reference	Study Design (S) Study Purpose (P) Study Setting (T) Study Date (D) Country (C) Methods/Interventions	Final Sample Size	Main Measures	Key Findings
				(p = .003); no effect on counseling with life stress; (4) stress and life satisfaction: SIG decrease in MD satisfaction with interpersonal aspects of professional life (p = .007); no effect on "rated morale" or overall work-related quality of life; (5) global ratings: SIG increase in MD sensitive communication (p = .05); no effect on MD informative and participatory, patient took initiative, or MD-patient collaboration.
Lienard, Merckaert, et al. 2008	(S) RCT (P) Assess CST impact on changes in patients' and relatives' anxiety following a three-person medical consultation (T) Oncology (D) Not reported (C) Belgium	(See Merckaert, Libert, et al. 2005b above; Merckaert, Libert, et al. 2008 below.) This is the third publication of data from the RCT and focuses on cancer patient and relative anxiety.	n = 56 MDs n = 29 MDs receiving CST and consolidation workshop n = 27 MDs receiving CST only	(1) 14-item, self-report instrument to assess patient anxiety and depression on a 4-point scale; (2) 20-item questionnaire State Trait Anxiety Inventory-State on a 4-point scale giving scores 20 to 8	Following a 3-person consultation, no SIG effect was found (1) group-by-time on changes in patients' and relatives' anxiety levels; (2) no correlation between changes in patients' or in relatives' anxiety and MD assessment skills, information skills, or supportive skills; (3) mixed-effects modeling showed (a) when MDs gave bad news patient anxiety following consultation increased (p = .03) and when information was on treatment, patient anxiety in 3-per-

| Merckaert, Libert, et al. 2008 | (S) RCT (P) Assess CST impact on MDs' detection of patients' and relatives' distress (T) Oncology (D) Not reported (C) Belgium | (See Merckaert, Libert, et al., 2005b above.) This study uses previously unreported trial data on MD ability to detect patients' and relatives' distress. | $n = 56$ MDs $n = 29$ MDs receiving CST and consolidation workshop $n = 27$ MDs receiving CST only | (1) 14-item, self-report instrument to assess patient anxiety and depression on a 4-point scale; (2) MD rating of patient and his or her relative's distress on a 10-point visual analog scale immediately after interview | son consultation decreased ($p = .009$) and when patient self-reported stress was high, the more it decreased after consultation ($p = .03$); (b) the more the relatives' self-reported distress was high, the more the relative anxiety following the 3-person consultation decreased ($p = .005$); when MDs gave bad news, relatives' anxiety following consultation was increased ($p = .001$). Authors conclude that, as expected, breaking bad news leads to an increase in patient and relative anxiety and that consultations focusing on treatment information decrease patient anxiety, not relative anxiety, suggesting this type of information restores hope.

In a 3-person interview, mixed-effects modeling of MD detection of patients' distress showed (1) a positive group-by-time effect in favor of MDs in the workshop group ($p = .02$). MD detection of patients' distress was associated negatively with patients' self-reported distress ($p = <.000$); positively with MD concurrent use of psychological assessment and supportive skills ($p = .004$); and negatively with general assessment skills ($p = <.000$). (2) Detection of relatives' |

TABLE 5.2—*Continued*

Reference	Study Design (S) Study Purpose (P) Study Setting (T) Study Date (D) Country (C)	Methods/Interventions	Final Sample Size	Main Measures	Key Findings
					distress was associated negatively (p = <.000) with relatives' self-reported distress and with general assessment skills (p = <.017). Authors conclude that on average there is an ongoing tendency of MDs to underestimate distress levels, a "breakdown in empathy." In contrast to the findings in the Merckaert, Libert, et al. 2005b study, above, this study found basic CST plus workshop (including knowledge, attitudes, and supportive skills) MDs showed an improvement in their detection of patients' distress vs. CST only group (focused on knowledge and attitudes), which showed a reduction in this ability, suggesting an added value of a 3-person interview.
Rodriguez, Anastario, et al. 2008	(S) Controlled clinical trial (P) Evaluate effect of CST on "agenda-setting" on patients' experiences with care (T) Group practice, pri-	Pre-post CST patient survey. 3-hour CST focusing on agenda setting, adapted from Four Habits model, using lecture, video, group	n = 21 MDS n = 10 MDs at or below the statewide 25th percentile of per-	Summary (range 0–100 points) measures, from Ambulatory Care Survey, of patients' experiences including the quality of MD-patient	In adjusted analyses, there was no SIG change (2.9 points) in the overall quality of physician-patient interaction scale scores of CST MDs or in control MDs (3 points). There was SIG improvement in CST MDs' ability

mary and specialty care (D) 2005 (C) US

discussion, and role play, followed by group teleconference discussion at 3 and 7 weeks post CST.

formance on patient surveys from 3 practice sites of a multispecialty MD organization $n = 11$ MDs matched controls based on survey scores, geography, specialty, and practice size $n = 2,081$ patients from 21 MDs

interaction and willingness to recommend MD

to "explain things in a way that was easy to understand" vs. control group ($p = .02$). There was no SIG change in willingness to recommend MD.

Despite the modest magnitude of changes, authors note 3-point gain in CST group scores has considerable practical significant for practices in the context of public reporting and pay-for-performance, e.g., a change of this magnitude would raise an organization's standings by about 40 points in percentile rank from the 40th to 80th percentile or 50th to 90th percentile.

CST = communication skills
DNR = do not resuscitate
FP = family practice
GP(s) = general practitioners
MD(s) = physician(s)
n = number
Four Habits Model = (1) invest in the beginning, (2) elicit the patient's perspective, (3) demonstrate empathy, (4) invest in the end

OBSE = Objected Structured Clinical Examination, an evaluation method used which uses simulated MD–patient encounters in a standardized setting
PACE = Patient education system (Presenting, Asking, Checking, Expressing). Study adapted the oiringal PACE system into PACE for Parents and PACE for Physicians, companion booklets designed to enhance physician–parent communica-

tion about the diagnosis and treatment of childhood illness. Coding system included.
RCT = randomized control trial
RIAS = Roter Interaction Analysis System, method of coding doctor–patient interaction using frequency counts of communication "utterances"
SIG = statistically significant, SIG may be stated as present or actual values provided.
SMD = shared decision making

6 | Improving Physician Communication: Insights from Skills Training Programs

In earlier chapters, we reviewed published studies relating to physician communication. We found considerable evidence of deficiencies in physician communication (chapter 2) and also evidence that poor communication is associated with lower levels of patient satisfaction, poorer adherence to treatment recommendations, and less favorable longer-term patient outcomes in some cases (chapter 3). However, the evidence regarding how physician communication affects longer-term patient outcomes such as health status or measures of resource utilization is very limited. In the previous chapter, we reviewed the evidence that programs designed to improve physician communication skills are effective, finding that there are significant limitations with respect to the conclusions that can be drawn from this literature.

In this chapter, we move away from assessing the published literature on physician communication and instead describe selected real-world programs designed to improve physician communication. We did not choose these programs to be representative of all such efforts, as we are aware of no database that catalogs the universe of physician skill-building programs that exist in practice. Instead, our intent is to use brief descriptions of a small number of programs to illustrate the issues confronted by their sponsoring organizations, as well as potential sources of organizational support for efforts to improve physician communication. In particular, these descriptions illustrate the motivations of organizations that commit resources to support improvement of physician communication. A fundamental question is, in the present environment, are there logical "organizational owners" of interventions to improve physician communication skills, and if so, what can one reasonably expect these "owners" to invest in skill-building efforts.

In chapter 1, we presented a "logic model" that linked physician characteristics to the quality of physician communication and, subsequently, to
immediate, intermediate, and longer-term patient outcomes (see fig. 1.1),
while also identifying mediating factors in the relationship between physician characteristics and the quality of physician communication. The
model was based on the assumption that the primary motivation for improving physician communication is its potential to improve patient
health outcomes. In this chapter, we modify this logic model to include a
role for sponsors of programs designed to improve physician communication skills. Instead of treating these organizations as essentially exoge-
nous to the logic model, we hypothesize that they have organizational objectives that motivate their investments in these programs and that these
objectives may shape the way in which programs are designed and carried
out in practice and therefore their potential impact on patients. We hypothesize that program goals may include improvement in patient health
status but also will encompass other organizational objectives, such as
compliance with regulatory or other standards, enhancing organizational
revenues, improving efficiency, or reducing costs. Figure 6.1 depicts this
expanded logic model.

The organizational outcomes combine two distinct organizations that
currently sponsor programs for improving physician communication
skills: medical schools/residency programs and integrated delivery systems (IDSs). We use the term *integrated delivery system* to refer to an organization that combines physicians, inpatient facilities (frequently), and
a health plan (less frequently) under a single organizational structure.

As with patient outcomes, we categorize organizational outcomes as
immediate, intermediate, and longer-term. Both IDSs and medical
schools are hypothesized to have immediate organizational outcomes
that they hope to achieve in sponsoring programs for improving physician communication skills. For medical schools, meeting curriculum
and competency requirements related to the teaching of communication skills is likely to be a highly valued immediate outcome. In addition,
as the need to improve physician communication skills becomes more
widely accepted in the medical care field, the offering of these programs
may respond to desires on the part of faculty and students to comply
with accepted norms in medical education. The development of programs perceived to be excellent at doing this could improve both student
and faculty satisfaction. Beyond these immediate outcomes, medical
schools that achieve special recognition for their work in this area could

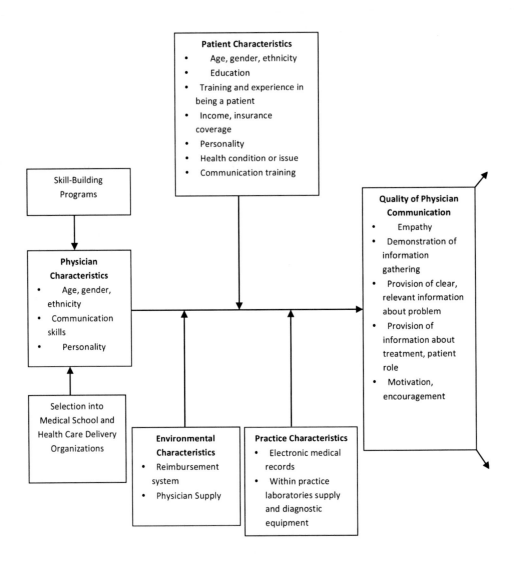

Fig. 6.1. The role of physician communication: an expanded logic model

increase their prestige among peers, which we categorize as an intermediate outcome in the logic model.

IDSs are likely to have different organizational objectives associated with sponsorship of programs on physician communication skills. We hypothesize that their immediate objectives include improvement in patient satisfaction scores and in physician work satisfaction. Patient satisfaction scores are becoming increasingly important to IDSs because health plans

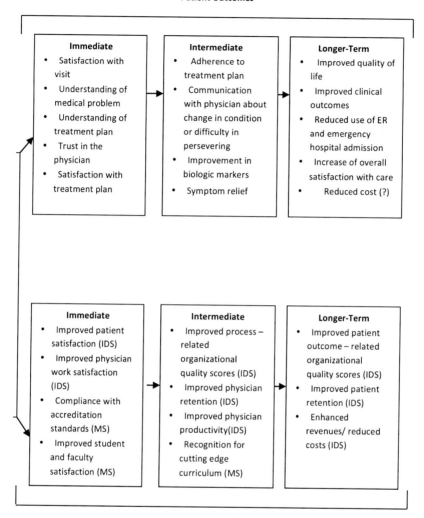

Immediate	Intermediate	Longer-Term
• Satisfaction with visit • Understanding of medical problem • Understanding of treatment plan • Trust in the physician • Satisfaction with treatment plan	• Adherence to treatment plan • Communication with physician about change in condition or difficulty in persevering • Improvement in biologic markers • Symptom relief	• Improved quality of life • Improved clinical outcomes • Reduced use of ER and emergency hospital admission • Increase of overall satisfaction with care • Reduced cost (?)

Immediate	Intermediate	Longer-Term
• Improved patient satisfaction (IDS) • Improved physician work satisfaction (IDS) • Compliance with accreditation standards (MS) • Improved student and faculty satisfaction (MS)	• Improved process – related organizational quality scores (IDS) • Improved physician retention (IDS) • Improved physician productivity(IDS) • Recognition for cutting edge curriculum (MS)	• Improved patient outcome – related organizational quality scores (IDS) • Improved patient retention (IDS) • Enhanced revenues/ reduced costs (IDS)

Organizational Outcomes

and purchasers of care value performance in this domain. It is becoming more common for information on patient satisfaction to be publicly reported, allowing potential patients to compare different medical groups and physician practices. Possible intermediate outcomes valued by IDSs include improved process-related quality scores (assuming that better physician communication improves patient adherence to treatment plans) and improved physician retention. Currently, measures of adherence to guidelines in the care process are more common in publicly available performance reports than are measures of patient satisfaction. Organizations also may believe that programs to improve communication skills of deficient physicians are more cost effective than replacing those physicians with new hires, given the costs associated with recruiting and training new physicians. A third intermediate outcome valued by IDSs could be improved physician practice productivity. In practices where physicians communicate more effectively with patients, it is possible that office visits are carried out more efficiently and that less time from nurses or office staff is required for post-visit follow-up.

We hypothesize that IDSs may be motivated by longer-term outcomes as well, but measuring the impact of better physician communication on longer-term outcomes can be problematic. For example, IDSs may expect that training in communication skills will improve biologic measures of patient health and patient loyalty. If improved scores attract new patients or retain existing ones, providing skills training for physicians might enhance revenues. For IDSs that receive global or capitated payments to care for patients, better patient adherence to treatment protocols, especially in the treatment of chronic illnesses, could reduce costs and therefore increase profits or retained earnings. Clearly, the possible relationship between improved physician communication skills and these longer-term organizational outcomes is likely to be much more tenuous, as perceived by IDSs, than the relationship to immediate and intermediate outcomes. Nevertheless, the possibility of favorable longer-term outcomes could contribute to the overall support of IDSs for skills training programs for physicians.

For clarity of presentation, the augmented logic model in figure 6.1 omits one potentially important set of relationships: the connection between valued organizational outcomes and the existence and content of programs that build physician communication skills. The orientation and content of skill-building programs supported by IDSs are likely to be influenced by the types of outcome that IDSs value most highly. For example, if improving patient satisfaction scores is the most highly valued outcome, emphasis is likely to be placed on enhancing those communication skills that map most directly onto higher patient satisfaction. However, these same skills may not be particularly effective in improving patient adherence to treatment plans or in improving long-term patient health status.

Data Collection

To explore the issues identified in the preceding section, we conducted a set of structured interviews in two communities—Seattle and Minneapolis–St. Paul—with representatives from a medical school and an IDS in each community. In addition, we interviewed respondents from an independent body that conducts courses and supplies supporting materials related to building physician communication skills. We also reviewed materials available on the website of a second independent body that conducts classes in physician communication skills and provides supporting materials. Our interview protocols were approved through an institutional review board process. Different protocols were developed to address the different responsibilities, characteristics, and activities of individuals in the organizations we selected. We used findings from these interviews, combined with material supplied by the organizations or available on their websites, to construct our organizational profiles. As noted previously, these five organizations should not be viewed as representative, in a statistical sense, of the skill-building programs in physician communication that are offered by different organizational types, as achieving this type of representativeness is not possible given the data available and the small number of organizations included. Rather, the interview results are intended to be suggestive of how these types of organization might view physician skill-building training and of the issues that can be encountered in implementing programs in different organizational settings.

Medical Schools/Residency Programs

We interviewed representatives affiliated with the University of Washington Medical School and the University of Minnesota Medical School. We chose the University of Washington because faculty members have published articles on their program in the peer-reviewed literature, suggesting the presence of a relatively aggressive physician skills-building program. We chose the University of Minnesota because our initial inquiries suggested that its approach would be fairly typical of state-funded medical schools.

Programs that train physicians to be better communicators with their patients have been offered in at least some medical schools for almost 40 years. These programs can vary widely in their approach, consisting of "various combinations of lectures, workshops, supervised encounters with real and simulated patients, and viewing and discussing videotaped doctor-patient encounters" (Baumal and Benbassat 2008). Only recently, however, have they become commonplace. In 1995, the Liaison Committee on Medical Education and the Committee on the Accreditation of Canadian Medical Schools declared that medical schools had a responsibility to teach communication skills to students. Makoul (2003) notes, however, that "the standard requires only the presence of instruction and evaluation; it says nothing about the timing, quality, or quantity" (80). Teaching interpersonal and communication skills is now a "core competency" identified by the Accreditation Council for Graduate Medical Education and the American Board of Medical Specialties, ensuring its place in postgraduate medical education as well (Makoul 2003). In the United Kingdom, the General Medical Council "encourages the acquisition of communication skills from the outset of undergraduate learning and produces guidance for general clinical training . . . and general professional training . . . , both of which stipulate the need for sound communication skills" (British Medical Association 2004, 10). It also advocates that physicians continue to upgrade their communication skills throughout their careers (British Medical Association 2004). The British Medical Association (2004) has observed, "Since 2002, the ability to communicate competently with patients has been a precondition of qualification for all healthcare professionals if they are to deliver patient care in the NHS [National Health Service]" (17).

University of Washington Medical School

The University of Washington Medical School (UW) provides undergraduate medical training to students from five states. Students complete their basic science courses at a university in their home states and complete their second-year courses at the UW campus in Seattle. They then disperse to clerkships for their third and fourth years. This presents challenges for conducting physician communication training. In the first year, students watch videotaped lectures on communication and interview patients under the supervision of preceptors. In the second year, on campus at UW, they accompany faculty on hospital visits on a weekly basis, during which they interview patients and conduct general physical examinations. These activities are carried out individually, with the faculty mentor providing immediate feedback. The student then carries out an oral case presentation at bedside to a small group. The set of competencies the students must achieve in their second year are clearly delineated. The Communications Working Group offers the faculty in the first- and second-year programs guidance on the communications skills that need to be taught to students. In the third year, all students are required to complete a "patient-centered care" curriculum online, which includes training in using the Patient Centered Observation Form (PCOF) to rate videos of physician-patient interactions. They rate the interactions, receive feedback, and then rate them again. The curriculum emphasizes relationship, communication, and efficiency. The students also observe themselves, and faculty observe them, using the PCOF. Respondents believed that, over time, faculty have become better at convincing students that training in communication skills is important, and this is due partly to continuity in the faculty involved in the program.

The UW has a well-developed training program in communication skills for residents in family medicine as well. It motivates resident participation by emphasizing the importance of communication skills for physician time management, a point that has been successful in "selling" the program to residents. Faculty members in behavioral science are recruited to observe and give feedback to residents in all three years of their training. Gradually, the amount of time that residents observe and provide feedback to each other has grown as well. Each resident is observed seven to nine times per year by behavioral science faculty or physicians.

The communications training carried out at the UW reflects the skills identified in the Kalamazoo Consensus Statement and draws on the expertise of UW faculty members who have conducted research in this area (e.g., Back, Arnold, et al. 2009; Mauksch and Roesler 1990; Mauksch, Dugdale, et al. 2008). The effectiveness of the training is evaluated primarily through surveys of clerkship students and directors and through graduation interviews. Respondents reported that there are very few students who are negative regarding their communications training but that the responses of residents have been mixed. Some residents believe that they benefit from being forced to learn these skills, while others are uncomfortable in being observed. Other than student surveys and physician reports, there is no formal evaluation of the UW programs.

Support for training in communication skills is strong among UW leadership, but financial constraints affect how training can be carried out. In the future, UW plans to continue to strengthen both education in communication skills during the students' clinical training in the third and fourth years and (through grant funds) training in communication with patients around end-of-life issues.

University of Minnesota Medical School

The University of Minnesota Medical School (UM) requires courses in the first and second year of medical school that teach skills in interviewing and physician communication. Beginning in January of the first year, students participate in six tutorials of three hours each to learn "patient-centered" interviewing. There are approximately 10 students per faculty member in these tutorials. Over the last three years, training has incorporated "standardized patients." There are between 60 and 70 individuals recruited and trained each year for this role. The UM moved to this approach because it found that it was too difficult to do communication training with real patients in a busy clinic environment. Students practice interviewing using the standardized patient, with interviews videotaped and reviewed by the student and instructor as well as by other students in the group. At the end of six weeks, students conduct a 10-minute interview with a standardized patient, and their progress is assessed. In the second year of medical school, there is a ten-week course on interviewing patients and conducting physical examinations, which is taught by experienced patient educators. Students conduct six practice interviews, which are not videotaped, and are quizzed on their experience and what they have learned. They also attend large group workshops on communication skills. At the end of the program, students conduct another short patient interview that is graded by patient educators.

The curriculum is guided by "competencies" that students must acquire. At the end of the second year, there is a summative evaluation that includes communication skills. Respondents reported that students generally felt that their training was good but wished that it could have incorporated real, as opposed to standardized, patients. It is difficult to remediate students who perform poorly with respect to physician communication, but only 2 or 3 out of 180 students each year are identified as needing remediation. They are linked with individual faculty members for one-on-one coaching.

At present, the UM is undergoing a major change in its curriculum. Standardized patients still will be used in communications training, but students will begin by interviewing each other and will be placed in a clinic environment in March of their first year. In the past, UM used doc.com for communication training (in collaboration with the American Academy on Communication in Healthcare, discussed later in this chapter). This web-based learning tool is used by many medical schools and must be "purchased" each year. Different modules can be accessed online in different settings. As part of the training, students critique videos of physician-patient interactions. Because of the expense involved, the UM no longer makes this tool available to students, but it does purchase faculty access.

Within the UM, there is leadership support for communication training, but the budget is tight, and effective training in communication skills can be resource intensive. Time constraints faced by faculty can make it difficult to recruit them to this effort. Thus, the program depends heavily on the continued involvement of a small core group of faculty members who are passionate about the need to improve physician communication. There is concern that students' skills may deteriorate when students move to busy clinic environments for their residencies, where practicing physicians may not be good "models" of effective communication. In the UM residency programs, voluntary courses are offered that address communication, and mentoring is provided by faculty interested and trained in the topic. The nature of the training varies considerably depending on the faculty member's approach, but skill-building workshops with feedback are typically involved. The residents provide assessments of the effectiveness of the training they receive, but no other physician or patient-related outcomes are measured.

Integrated Delivery Systems

In the United States, organizations other than medical schools have undertaken to improve physician communication skills. One notable example is the work of the Kaiser Permanente medical groups to teach their physicians the Four Habits Model for communicating with patients (Stein, Frankel, et al. 2005), as described in chapter 5. Other organizations have developed their own, typically less intensive programs, frequently with the involvement of external bodies such as the American Academy on Communication in Health Care and the Institute for Healthcare Communication.

We interviewed representatives from Group Health of Puget Sound, located in Seattle, Washington, and HealthPartners Health Plan, located in Minneapolis–St. Paul. Both are not-for-profit IDSs that own and operate large regional health plans. Group Health has a close affiliation with the Kaiser health care system, and its approach to physician communication training has been influenced by the Kaiser Four Habits Model. HealthPartners has recently refocused and somewhat reduced its training program in communication skills for physicians, in response to financial pressures that are a relatively common part of the operational environment for IDSs at present. Both IDSs are consumer governed, suggesting that their approaches to building skills in physician communication could be both more aggressive and possibly more nuanced than those of other IDSs.

Group Health of Puget Sound

Group Health of Puget Sound (GH), founded in 1947, serves primarily residents in the Puget Sound area of Washington State. It currently enrolls approximately 580,000 people in its various health benefits products. About two-thirds of the services received by its members are provided by GH-operated medical clinics.

During their first six months, all new physicians at GH participate in a daylong skills-building program on physician communication. In the morning, they are taught the Kaiser Four Habits Model (see chapter 5) and the use of the computer in the examining room. The importance of being effective communicators in their interactions with patients is explained as well. In the afternoon, small groups (three to four physicians) meet with coaches and actors for role-playing exercises. GH trains about 120 new physicians per year in these sessions. Measures of patient satisfaction are not collected for new physicians until after one year of employment, so all physicians go through the program before satisfaction data are collected from their patients.

In addition to this general program, GH offers several programs for physicians who wish to improve their communication skills or are asked to do so by GH. Patient satisfaction scores for physicians are reviewed within GH, and physicians receive feedback that includes comparisons with their colleagues. Also, as-needed one- or two-hour programs, provided at medical centers, address such issues as how to work with patients to accomplish behavioral change. Practicing physicians, sometimes with the encouragement of their section chiefs, contact GH if they want to take action to improve their scores. These physicians are sent a questionnaire designed to identify problem areas. A coach meets with each physician to assess willingness to explore new approaches. The physician then typically is offered a program consisting of six days per year in which the physician is observed in meetings with patients, with feedback offered on how to improve communication skills. At the end of the year, the physician is asked if she or he wants to continue in the program.

A third level of assistance in improving communication skills consists of a three-and-a-half-day intensive program conducted in a retreat-like setting. There have been about 100 physicians who have participated in this program over a four-year period (there are currently about 900 GH physicians), and the program recently has been expanded to include non-physician clinicians as well. It is offered twice a year, with 18 to 20 people attending each session. The program is conducted using small groups of physicians (three or four) and a faculty coach. Typically, didactic learning occurs in the morning, with role playing involving actors in the afternoon. The entire program is intended to be low-key and nonthreatening. The goal is for participants to feel respected and supported in their efforts to improve their skills. On completion of the program, participants typically enter into the coaching program already described. All graduates of the residential, intensive training program are invited to gather once a year for a review session.

GH has two major motivations for sponsoring these efforts. First, it wants its members to be satisfied with their experience in the GH system, as measured by patient satisfaction scores on standard instruments. GH faced a financial crisis in 1995–99, which increased its "market awareness." One of GH's goals now is to be better than its competitors along a variety of dimensions, including service. Second, it wants to avoid letting physicians go, as replacing a physician is costly. GH believes that improved physician communication with patients can improve job satisfaction on the part of physicians as well as the quality of the work environment. GH monitors the impact of its programs by tracking patient satisfaction scores. To this point, it has not attempted to measure program impacts on patient compliance with treatment guidelines or other patient outcomes in addition to satisfaction, nor has it attempted to calculate a return on investment in these programs. However, support within GH for skills-building programs in physician communication remains strong. It has just inaugurated an initiative to train each physician in its medical group on how to give patients bad news and conduct end-of-life conversations more generally. It also is incorporating its physician communications training into its effort to create "medical homes" within GH.

HealthPartners

HealthPartners (HP), founded in 1957 and located in the Twin Cities of Minneapolis and St. Paul, Minnesota, serves 1.25 million members through its various health plan products and sees 350,000 patients annually at its clinics. HP has 720 employed physicians, who are part of a total workforce of approximately 9,600. HP provides patient care services at 50 different locations and owns one large teaching-affiliated hospital and two smaller hospitals. Orientation for new physicians includes information on the importance that the organization places on patient satisfaction. They also are told how they will receive their quarterly patient satisfaction scores, with a portion of pay tied to their achievement on these scores. (Currently, about 2 percent of a physician's compensation is linked to patient satisfaction, but this is likely to increase in the future.) Physicians have a checklist of recommended actions thought to be related to patient-reported physician satisfaction. Newly hired physicians are trained in the use of the electronic health record (EHR) and are asked to encourage patients to register to receive information online. During their first three months of employment, physicians are assessed for their competency with the EHR by an EHR specialist and receive feedback from their physician leader on their interactions with patients.

Patient satisfaction scores and HP's patient complaint system are reviewed continuously to identify physicians who may be having problems. Physicians with low satisfaction scores have discussions with their physician leaders on expectations, and they are given suggestions for improvement. Physicians may request assistance in improving their patient satisfaction scores. Several methods are used to help physicians improve, including reviewing literature on patient satisfaction and discussing how to implement improvements in practice. Physicians also can be linked with a physician who has high satisfaction scores and can "shadow" this physician for about half a day. An additional option is to have the physician who has low scores be shadowed by a nonphysician reviewer using a checklist of recommended actions. While all physicians receive regular reports on patient satisfaction, approximately 10 to 15 physicians per year are involved in a more intensive improvement process. Webinars on improving patient satisfaction and communication skills also are available to all interested physicians. To resolve other difficult issues, such as timeliness and productivity, physician leaders work directly with a physician. Internal and external resources are available to assist physicians and their leaders. Occasionally, one-on-one coaching (with outside coaches) is offered where performance warrants this intensive intervention. Physicians who do not improve can be terminated from employment. The majority of HP physicians are "at-will" employees who do not have employment contracts. Physicians care about their patients' satisfaction, but a physician with low scores may have no idea what actions to take to improve those scores. These physicians are quite willing and interested in new communication approaches provided by HP that could raise their scores.

In the past, HP utilized programs delivered by internal physicians who were certified by the Institute for Healthcare Communication. Physicians who participated in these programs generally covered 75 percent of the cost using their allowance for continuing medical education, with 25 percent of the cost contributed by the organization. These programs, which were approximately three days in length including a follow-up session, were discontinued due to cost considerations. Actual program cost was one factor, but the cost embodied in lost work time for the physicians and their trainers was also important in making this decision. HP has adopted a philosophy of "just-in-time," rather than "just-in-case," training. Organizational leaders believe that a focus at the direct local level has a bigger impact on improving patient satisfaction scores than physician participation in more formal didactic programs.

The key motivation for physician training in communication at HP is a desire to improve patient satisfaction scores (reflecting a better patient experience in the care system) and to increase patient loyalty. HP is working to make a "great patient experience" a stronger part of its organizational culture. Irrespective of this organizational goal, interview respondents also suggested that physicians with low scores often express a strong desire to improve simply because they want their patients to be satisfied with the care they are providing. For the future, HP is considering a more structured approach to mentoring new physicians with respect to patient communication. It may provide greater financial incentives as well. Interview respondents noted that a difficult challenge in structuring programs to improve physician communication skills is balancing the production demands placed on physicians with the time needed to improve communication skills. HP also is learning that many different elements of the patient visit can affect a patient satisfaction score. For example, physicians walking their patients from the examining room to the checkout area has a positive effect on patient satisfaction.

Supporting Organizations

The content for the skill-building programs in physician communication offered by medical schools, residency programs, and medical care delivery systems such as IDSs can be developed internally or in collaboration with external organizations. The two organizations that are the most active in this arena are the American Academy on Communication in Healthcare and the Institute for Healthcare Communication.

American Academy on Communication in Healthcare

The American Academy on Communication in Healthcare, formerly the American Academy on Physician and Patient, is an interdisciplinary group of physicians, nurses, other clinicians, and communications researchers, both academic and community-based. It states that its mission is to improve health care "through education, research, and practice that focuses on communication and relationships with patients, families and healthcare teams" (http://www.aachonline.org/?page=MissionVision). The Academy sponsors national and international meetings on this topic and produces two journals (*Medical Encounter* and *Patient Education and Counseling*) that include teaching and research on communication in healthcare and news about Academy activities. It also offers to customize programs to meet the needs of specific institutions, delivering them on-site or through other means. For instance, it provided support to the Mayo Clinic for six years in physician communication training efforts. Recently, the Academy expanded the scope of its activities to include the teaching of team-building skills. It is particularly known for its programs to improve the knowledge and skills of medical school faculty charged with teaching and mentoring undergraduates and residents in communication skill building.

A nonprofit entity headquartered in St. Louis, Missouri, the Academy is funded primarily through conference fees and fees generated through programs offered to health care systems. It has few paid staff, relying instead on partnerships and donated time to carry out its work. In its programs, the Academy places emphasis on physician self-awareness, which it believes is fundamental to helping and healing relationships. It also regards relationship building and communications as dependent on skills that can be learned and taught. In general, the demand for its programs to improve physician communication seems to be growing. The Academy notes several reasons for this. Currently, organizations are particularly interested in the impact of improved physician communication on patient satisfaction scores, given that it is becoming more common for these scores to be compared publicly to the scores of competitors. Another source of demand comes from individual physicians within organizations who are unhappy in their practices and searching for a more meaningful relationship with their patients, in the face of intensifying pressures to control the length of a patient visit. That improved communication with patients might reduce the probability of malpractice lawsuits also can be a motivating factor, but one that appears somewhat less important. The Academy uses a standardized approach to evaluating the impact of its programs on participants, but it sees a need for more research that addresses the link between skill-building efforts in physician communication and patient health outcomes.

The Institute for Healthcare Communication

The Institute for Healthcare Communication (IHC), founded in 1987, is a nonprofit organization with an independent board of directors. Located in New Haven, Connecticut, the IHC was called the Bayer Institute for Healthcare Communication until 2005, with the Bayer Corporation providing the majority of its funding; its current name reflects a reduced funding role for Bayer. The IHC defines its mission as advancing "the quality of healthcare by optimizing the experience and process of healthcare communication through four activities: education, advocacy, research and partnerships" (http://healthcarecomm.org). Since its founding, the IHC has conducted more than 9,000 workshops for more than 120,000 clinicians and other health care workers. It counts Kaiser Permanente, Geisinger Health System, and Affinity Health System among its IDS clients.

IHC offers a broad array of programs, and it has recently expanded into the area of veterinary medicine. It offers continuing education workshops on a wide range of medical topics (under such titles as "Connecting Communicating and Computing," "Difficult Clinician-Patient Relationships," and "Beyond Informed Consent"). Programs can be tailored to meet the needs of partnering organizations. One interview respondent distinguished the American Academy on Communication in Healthcare from IHC by observing that the IHC places more emphasis on skill building and the development of communication techniques, while the Academy pays more attention to internal motivation, although there clearly is considerable overlap between the approaches of the two groups.

Conclusions

While the research literature reviewed in previous chapters emphasizes the connection between better physician communication and improved patient outcomes along a variety of dimensions, organizational objectives for physician skill-building programs are more narrowly focused. Medical schools, the primary source of skill-building programs, emphasize knowledge and skill-building for physicians in training as a goal in itself and focus measurement of program success on these outcomes. This measurement takes place proximate to course completion, raising concerns among some program educators about possible deterioration in knowledge and skills by the time physicians enter practice. They fear that conditions in real-world practices will accelerate this process, with the result that skills learned as part of a physician's education will be forgotten or may never be applied, for other reasons. In the best case, favorable impacts on patients of these training programs are assumed but not directly measured.

In contrast, the IDSs we focused on in this chapter place primary emphasis on the potential impact of physician communication training programs on a specific patient outcome: satisfaction with the physician-patient encounter. This focus is driven by a changing culture within medicine that places greater emphasis on "service" as an important dimension of the "product" of the medical care delivery system. One of our interview respondents argued that it was a logical consequence of the "commodification" of medical care. Improving patient health behaviors and health status was a "hoped-for" consequence of improved communication, but it was not measured, nor was it central to the decisions of these organizations in supporting skill-building programs in physician communication.

Given these considerations, it seems reasonable to expect that the content of physician skill-building programs may well evolve over time to better align with the needs of program sponsors. (In this vein, one IDS respondent suggested that researchers need to "get real" in their design of skill-building programs for their studies, implying that many of these research interventions would not be practical for an IDS to implement.) Should this occur, the content of these programs may become increasingly oriented toward building physician communication skills needed to create satisfied patients, possibly (but not inevitably) at the expense of skills required to, for example, gain patient commitment to care plans, medication adherence, or healthy behaviors that could lead to improved patient health status. If "real-world" skill-building programs on communication are tailored to achieve this objective, relying on existing research findings as the basis for an assumed link between skill-building programs and improvement in longer-term patient health outcomes would become more problematic than currently is the case.

7 | Looking to the Future: Opportunities and Challenges

Issues relating to physician communication have received growing attention over the last 30 years, and their visibility and importance likely will continue to increase over the next decade. Supporting this expectation are a variety of changes, anticipated or already under way, relating to the financing and delivery of care. They include evolution in the role patients will be expected to play in managing their own care, new expectations about interactions between primary care physicians and patients in the context of "medical home" models of care, changes in the illness profile of primary care physicians' practices, the impact of a growing shortage of primary care physicians, the introduction of new communication technologies in physician practices, and the increasing competition for scarce resources within health care organizations (see table 7.1).

The Evolving Role of Patients

The term *patient-centered health care* has assumed a variety of meanings in discussions of a reformed future health care system. At its core, it has been defined by the Institute of Medicine as "health care that establishes a partnership among practitioners, patients and their families (when appropriate) to ensure that decisions respect patients' wants, needs, and preferences and that patients have the education and support they need to make decisions and participate in their own care" (Hurtado, Swift, et al. 2001). According to Lin and Dudley (2009), the concept of patient-centered care implies that "medical care providers should respect patients' preferences, wants, and needs; solicit patients' input into decisions; and customize treatment recommendations" (1551). The federal Agency for Healthcare Research and Quality (AHRQ 2008) notes that patient-centered care involves "improving communication techniques" and can "reduce the chance of misdiagnosis due to poor communication" (154).

The concept of patient-centered care already has contributed to an expansion of the measurement effort around health care quality. AHRQ's *National Health Quality Report* tracks four different concepts relating to the patient's care experience, including "patient assessments of how often their provider listened carefully to them, explained things clearly, respected what they had to say, and spent enough time with them" (AHRQ 2008, chap. 5). If "patient-centered care" encompassing these dimensions moves from concept to reality in increasing numbers of physician practices, it seems likely that physicians will be under growing pressure to improve the quality of their communication with patients, especially as it relates to patient self-management of their illnesses (Coleman and Newton 2005). With respect to the latter, physicians "who want to provide increased support of their patients' self-management are advised to address ... structuring patient-physician interactions to include goal setting and problem solving strategies" (Coleman and Newton 2005, 1505). While goal-setting conversations for patients with chronic illnesses are common, teaching patients problem-solving skills is not necessarily part of physi-

TABLE 7.1. Assumptions about Future Demands for Improved Physician Communication

The medical care system, and the patients that physicians care for, are changing in ways that will create new, sometimes greater, pressures on physician communication

- Increased involvement of patients in decision making regarding health care issues will increase the need for physician communication skills in gathering information, negotiating over care plans, defining roles, and selecting of treatment options.
- The medical home model of primary care will increase the importance of physician communication with patients in the context of parallel communications between other care team members and patients, as well as communication with patients through other team members.
- The aging of the baby boom segment of primary care and specialty practices, and the resulting growing numbers of patients with multiple chronic conditions, will increase pressure on physicians to communicate effectively within the time limits of standard primary care practices.
- Lagging payment for primary care will exacerbate the growing physician shortage, which will in turn place pressure on physicians to spend less time with patients, challenging them to apply their communication skills training effectively.
- The use of new electronic modes of communication with patients, especially the more widespread acceptance of "virtual office visits," will require a reassessment of the physician communication skills needed for effective treatment.
- The increasing amount of comparative data on physician performance could alter the focus of patient communication training, placing greater emphasis on communication skills that improve patient satisfaction scores.
- The increasing competition within organizations for care improvement resources will challenge physician communication skill building programs to demonstrate their effectiveness compared to other quality improvement interventions.

cians' communication skills training at present. This raises the important question of which elements of communication with patients should be the responsibility solely of physicians rather than shared by other clinicians in the physician practices.

The Vision of the Medical Home

Separate from, but related to, the concept of patient-centered care is the current movement to establish "medical homes" for patients. Like *patient-centered care,* the term *medical home* has been used in a variety of ways. According to the American Academy of Family Physicians (2009), "A patient-centered medical home integrates patients as active participants in their own health and well-being. Patients are cared for by a physician who leads the medical team that coordinates all aspects of preventive, acute and chronic needs of patients using the best available evidence and appropriate technology." The American College of Physicians defines it as "a team-based model of care led by a personal physician who provides continuous and coordinated care throughout a patient's lifetime to maximize health outcomes . . . It is a model of practice in which a team of health professionals, coordinated by a personal physician, works collaboratively to provide high levels of care, access and communication, care coordination and integration, and care quality and safety" (ACP 2009, 4). In 2007, the National Committee for Quality Assurance launched a pilot program to test a set of measures that would qualify physician practices to be designated as "medical homes" (Backer 2007). These measures were subsequently refined and have received support from payers and from the National Quality Forum (O'Malley, Peikes, et al. 2008). Currently, various medical home models are being tested by state governments in the context of their Medicaid programs, and many large insurers are developing medical home initiatives (Rosenthal 2008; O'Malley, Peikes, et al. 2008).

While definitions of the medical home vary slightly (O'Malley, Peikes, et al. 2008) and while methods of payment for medical homes are still being developed and tested (Pham, Peikes, et al. 2008), the vision of the medical home is that people have a primary care physician where they go first to seek care and that care is provided by the primary care physician in a coordinated way, with the involvement of other providers as needed and with an integral role for the patient. The hope is that primary care will become more effective and more satisfying for patients and for health care providers as well. For the medical home model to function effectively in achieving its goals, primary care physicians and other clinicians will need to have clearly defined responsibilities for communication with patients.

For example, in their discussion of "teamlet models" for primary care, Bodenheimer and Laing (2007) suggest that physicians "focus on cognitive work . . . and on building relationships with patients" (459), while "health coaches" work with patients to solicit their concerns, to recap what was said during the physician visit, to set goals, and to develop action plans. These are communication activities that physicians are expected to carry out in some earlier models of physician-patient communication. While the medical home model is expected to encourage increased communication with patients, it may restructure the nature of that communication as well (Ginsburg, Maxfield, et al. 2008).

The Time Demands on Physician Practices

Primary care physicians, especially, cite pressures to generate practice revenues under a fee-for-service reimbursement system as constraining the time they have available to spend with patients. Time pressures can lead to lower levels of physician satisfaction and, in the view of some, contribute to poor or incomplete physician communication with patients. Recent studies (Yarnall, Pollak, et al. 2003; Ostbye, Yarnall, et al. 2005) support these concerns. They suggest that a primary care physician with a (typical) panel size of 2,500 patients would need to spend 7.4 hours per day to deliver all recommended preventive treatments and 10.6 hours to meet chronic care guidelines (Laing, Ward, et al. 2008). Furthermore, it appears that physicians are spending considerable time related to patient care outside of the office visit—6.7 minutes for every 30 minutes of time scheduled with ambulatory patients (Farber, Siu, et al. 2007). Recent research suggests that the time spent per patient visit has not declined over the past decade and may have risen (Commonwealth Fund 2009; Chen, Farwell, et al. 2009).

This result may reflect the aging of the baby boom generation. With the leading edge of the baby boomers nearing 65, an increasing share of the patients in primary care and specialty practices suffer from chronic illnesses and, in many cases, have multiple conditions. According to an analysis conducted by Yawn, Goodwin et al. (2003), visits to manage chronic illnesses take longer and involve "a greater percentage of time spent in history taking, assessing compliance, negotiating, providing or discussing preventive services and providing evidence regarding exercise, nutrition and health promotion" (476). Also, it seems likely that difficult end-of-life discussions with patients will become more frequent as the age profile in primary care practices increases. All of these changes mean that increased demands will be placed on physicians to be effective communicators and that there will be a growing number of opportunities for ineffective physician communication to harm patients.

While increasing time pressures on primary care physicians, caused by a reimbursement system that rewards throughput and by a patient population that increasingly suffers from complex medical conditions, could lead to a deterioration of physician communication, some authors argue that this does not have to be the case. Experts suggest that limitations on the time physicians have to spend with patients will pressure physicians to improve their communication skills (Gabriel 2008). Mauksch, Dugdale, et al. (2008) argue that effective communication skills are essential if physicians are to use their limited time with patients effectively.

The Impact of the Shortage in Primary Care Physicians

Primary care fees have lagged behind medical practice costs and the growth in specialist fees, while the costs of medical school and debts incurred by medical school graduates have continued to rise. Financial considerations likely constitute one reason that fewer medical school graduates choose to enter primary care (Tisdale, Ranji, et al. 2009). It seems unlikely that payers will increase primary care fees substantially in the near future, in light of the financial burden imposed on payers by continuing increases in medical care costs. As a result, an expanding shortage of primary care physicians has been predicted. This prediction is one motivation for the interest of policy makers in the medical home model, which they hope will encourage the delegation of some physician tasks to other clinicians, alleviating the need for large expenditures aimed at increasing future physician supply (Arvantes 2007). Also, if new reimbursement arrangements for primary care become part of the medical home model, more physicians may be attracted to primary care. However, even if these efforts are successful, they likely would require many years to fully implement. Until then, the growing shortage of primary care physicians could intensify the time pressures on physician practices described in the preceding section, creating challenges for effective physician communication (Lloyd 2009).

New Technologies for Interacting with Patients

To this point, research and educational interventions regarding physician communication have focused on the in-person physician-patient encounter. However, it seems likely that an increasing number of future physician-patient interactions will occur through other means. Several large insurers already have adopted policies that compensate physicians who make "virtual house calls" through secure Internet sites (CNN 2008). In Hawaii, the state's Blue Cross and Blue Shield insurer has made online, face-to-face consultations with doctors available to its members. A recent study (Dixon and Stahl 2009) found that patients were highly satisfied with "virtual visits," as were physicians. A medical care director of a large integrated delivery system in the United States has observed that "primary care physicians are under pressure from technologies such as the Internet" and that "redesigning the way they practice so they can accommodate these technologies and communicate with patients in a secure and appropriate way is a big challenge" (Cross 2007). Communicating effectively with patients using these technologies will likely be challenging for some physicians and require a new type of training in communication skills.

The Growing Presence of Comparative Physician
Performance Measures

Spurred by the efforts of large employers and health plans to create more direct competition among providers for patients, there is a growing amount of comparative data on the performance of medical groups. In some communities, these measures are being disaggregated to the physician practice level. In the reports prepared by health plans and by community or employer coalitions to date, measures of physician performance have focused on compliance with chronic illness and preventive treatment guidelines. Recently, some reports have begun to add data on patient satisfaction with visits to their physicians, in response to research that suggests this is the type of information about physicians that consumers value most (Harris and Buntin, 2008). Less formal reports of patient experience with respect to physician visits are now emerging as well, patterned after consumer rankings in service industries such as dining and lodging. The growing presence of comparative physician performance data could increase the demand on the part of integrated delivery systems and medical groups for skill-building programs in physician communication, to the extent that these programs are seen as a cost-effective means of improving performance scores. As suggested in chapter 6, improving patient satisfaction scores may be of primary concern to physician organizations, and this could affect the practical content of skill-building efforts in physician communication.

Health care organizations have finite organizational resources to allocate across different programmatic options for improving the quality of care they provide to their patients. In allocating their resources, it is reasonable to expect that they will favor programs that deliver the most patient benefits per dollar spent. Looking beyond patient satisfaction scores, skill-building programs in physician communication will need to compete for funding with other initiatives in quality improvement. In the appendix, we summarize the findings from review studies regarding the effectiveness of physician skill-building programs versus other types of quality improvement efforts. (We focused on the "effectiveness" part of the cost-effectiveness ratio, as we found no review studies that compared cost-effectiveness.) As might be expected, differences in study approaches and outcome measures made it difficult to draw definitive conclusions from this literature. However, there is no clear evidence in these comparisons that physician communication training programs should be preferred by organizations over other initiatives in quality improvement. At the least, the review suggests that advocates for investing in skill-building programs in physician communication will need to collect both cost and outcomes data to make their case, with greater attention given to measuring impacts on intermediate and longer-term patient outcomes.

Conclusions

The US health care system seems poised to undergo significant changes in the next decade that will affect physician-patient communication. Clearly, we could not address all of these potential changes in this chapter. We focused our discussion on changes that we think both have the greatest likelihood to occur in the relatively near future and have significant implications for the paradigm of physician-patient communication as it now exists. An important question is how quickly and effectively organizations that employ physicians, third-party payers, and academic institutions that provide physician communication training can adapt to these changes and meet the need for new or enhanced physician communication skills. If the medical home model becomes widely accepted, for example, the communication skills needed by physicians could change, with patient communication responsibilities shared more broadly with other clinicians. If reimbursement for primary care does not improve and if the shortage of primary care physicians is worse than currently projected, a quite different emphasis in physician communication training might be required. Past research on physician-patient communications and physician communication training necessarily reflects the traditional physician-patient encounter. The changing practice environment for primary care physicians, irrespective of the ultimate course it takes, will require a critical reevaluation of the applicability of past findings to possibly quite different modes of practice. There will be a growing need for new, carefully executed research studies that reflect the new physician practice environment, as well as the reality of more aggressive, activated patient participants in the physician-patient encounter.

Appendix: How Do Physician Communication Initiatives Compare to Other Efforts to Improve Patient Outcomes through Changing Physician Behaviors?

In relation to changing physician behaviors, improving physician communication skills is only one of many strategies that potentially could affect resource use and improve patient outcomes. In this appendix, we compare the evidence regarding the impact of physician communication training on resource use and patient outcomes with the research evidence regarding the impact of other strategies. The purpose of our analysis is to provide guidance, where possible, to policy makers and organizational decision makers concerning the allocation of resources toward different strategies aimed at changing physician behaviors, all of which have potential to affect resource use and patient health outcomes. Specifically, we address whether there is a case to be made for preferring interventions to improve physician communications (relative to other strategies involving behavioral change), based on relative impact on resource use and patient outcomes.

In the first part of the appendix, we summarize the findings from review articles that assess the effectiveness of different types of intervention involving physician behavioral change, drawing from the findings of structured literature reviews. In the second part, we compare the findings from these reviews to the results of selected individual studies of physician communication interventions. We conclude our analysis with a discussion of the shortcomings in the published research literature that limit its usefulness in informing real-world decisions on resource allocation.

Review Studies on the Effectiveness of Different Strategies to Change Physician Behavior

In this section, we group our summaries of findings from review studies into two categories: Cochrane reviews and other reviews. The reviews, which were published between 2000 and 2009, highlight the relatively large number of studies measuring the effect of interventions of various types designed to change physician behavior. Cochrane reviews, which measured change in physician behavior across various types of intervention, found small to moderate effect sizes for all strategies, with little variation across studies in impact on health professional outcomes. Other reviews on interventions to change physician behavior found similar small impacts.

Over 330 measures of health professional outcomes were studied in the Cochrane reviews (see table A.2). These measures primarily addressed quality of care in the management of common chronic diseases, screening for prevention, adherence to clinical guidelines, and prescribing practices. This compares with 100 measures of resource use and patient outcomes in the same studies, primarily condition-specific clinical outcomes. Across these different types of outcome, there is little consistency in measure definition, making it difficult to compare effect sizes in a meaningful way. Small sample sizes also inhibit the estimation and comparison of effect sizes. We found that data on patient outcomes generally were summarized in a descriptive fashion in the reviews because, as O'Brien, Rogers, et al. (2007) point out in their assessment of the literature, "it was difficult to determine if there was sufficient power to detect an important difference at the patient level" (13).

Cochrane Reviews

The Cochrane Effective Practice and Organisation of Care Group (EPOC) is a collaborative review group of the Cochrane Library whose focus is on standardized, systematic "reviews of interventions designed to improve professional practice and the delivery of effective health services" (Cochrane Collaboration 2009). Their reviews address various strategies, such as "continuing education, quality improvement, informatics, financial incentives, and organizational and regulatory interventions, aimed at improving the ability of health care professionals to deliver services more effectively and efficiently" (Cochrane Collaboration 2009). From 2007 to 2009, EPOC published systematic reviews related to the effects on physician behavior and patient outcomes of audit and feedback (Jamtvedt, Young, et al. 2006), local opinion leaders (Doumit, Gattellari, et al. 2007), educational outreach visits (O'Brien, Rogers, et al. 2007), printed educational materials (Farmer, Legare, et al. 2008), meetings and workshops for continuing education (Forsetlund, Bjorndal, et al. 2009), and on-screen, point-of-care computer reminders (Shojania, Jennings, et al. 2009) (see table A.1). All of these strategies could be viewed as alternatives to physician communication interventions for improving patient outcomes (see chapter 5). (However, some of the reviews do include results from selected physician communication interventions, as we discuss.)

Using primarily randomized controlled studies and excluding studies with a high risk of bias, the Cochrane reviews calculate the absolute or median risk difference with interquartile range (IQR) for both dichotomous and continuous health professional and health care outcomes, analyzed separately. The focus on median effects across studies is "to avoid spurious precision due to heterogeneity and clustering effects that could not be taken into account in many studies" (Shojania, Jennings, et al. 2009, 14). When there was insufficient data for meta-analysis, researchers presented findings from individual studies as reported by their authors. In the first part of this appendix, we summarize findings from the Cochrane reviews related to both health professional and health care outcomes of different behavioral change strategies, where meta-analysis was used in the reviews.

Audit and Feedback   Jamtvedt, Young, et al. (2006) synthesized the results from 118 randomized controlled trials (RCTs) where interventions included audit and feedback as a component, audit and feedback alone, audit and feedback combined with educational meetings, or multifaceted interventions that included audit and feedback. All studies compared intervention outcomes to no intervention (see table A.1). Results of comparisons for health professional outcomes showed a small and consistent effect on compliance with desired practice, with relative risk (RR) ranging from 1.06 for audit and feedback with educational meetings to 1.10 for audit and feedback as part of a multifaceted intervention (see table A.1). Low baseline compliance and higher intensity of audit and feedback were identified as significant predictors of positive outcomes. Median adjusted risk difference (ARD) ranged from 1.5 percent to 5.7 percent among the four comparisons, with a 5 percent median ARD for audit and feedback of any intervention compared to no intervention (IQR range 3% to 11%) (see table A.1). Analysis of continuous outcomes found a 16 percent increase in desired practice when comparing any audit and feedback intervention to no intervention (see table A.1). Only 10 of 118 studies included in the review reported patient outcomes (see table A.2), so meta-analysis of findings in this area was not possible. Similarly, there were no meta-analyses on health care resource outcomes. There were three studies of physician communication interventions included in the Jamtvedt, Young, et al. (2006) review (see table A.1).

Use of Opinion Leaders   Doumit, Gattellari, et al. (2007) assessed the effectiveness of use of opinion leaders to promote evidence-based care in patients with various health conditions compared to no intervention, a single comparison intervention (e.g., opinion leaders vs. standard lecture), opinion leaders and an additional intervention versus additional intervention only, and opinion leaders as part of a multifaceted intervention versus no intervention. The number of trials included in the four types of comparison was small, ranging from two to five. Median ARD for health professional outcomes in these four types of intervention ranged from .06 to .14 (see table A.1). For the use of opinion leaders compared to controls, the overall median ARD was 10 percent (range –.06 to +.25), representing a 10 percent absolute decrease in noncompliance with evidence-based practice with the use of opinion leaders (see table A.1). The authors noted the wide variation between and within studies, as well as the difficulty in defining and identifying opinion leaders in a reliable way, as these individuals may differ substantially in their approaches to teaching and in their personal and professional characteristics. Five of seven studies included in the review reported patient clinical outcomes (see table A.2), and no analysis was completed on the effectiveness of opinion leaders in improving patient outcomes. There was one study of a physician communication intervention included in this review article (see table A.1).

Educational Outreach Visits   In a 2007 review of 69 RCTs, O'Brien, Rogers, et al. (2007) studied the effectiveness of educational outreach visits (defined as personal visits by trained persons to health care professionals) on desired practice behaviors. In comparing any intervention in which educational outreach visits was a component to no intervention (28 studies), the median ARD for health professional adherence to desired practice was 5.6 percent (IQR range 3% to 9%) (see table A.1). The overall effect was the same, but with greater variation, when comparing educational outreach visits alone to no intervention (median ARD 5%; IQR range 1% to 20%). When examined by prescribing behavior versus other behaviors, the educational outreach visits had, on average, less variation and a smaller effect on prescribing (median ARD 4.8%; IQR range 3% to 6.5%) than on other behaviors (median ARD 6%; IQR range 3.6% to 16%). In studies where continuous health professional outcomes were measured, there was at least a 20 percent relative improvement with educational outreach visits (see table A.1).

Twenty-four of 68 studies in the review reported measures reflecting patient quality-of-life, clinical, or satisfaction outcomes (see table A.2). There were no meta-analyses of patient health outcomes. Results for 15 of the studies that addressed patient outcomes were described, but their interpretation was limited because "for most studies, it was difficult to determine if there was sufficient power to detect an important difference at the patient level" (O'Brien, Rogers, et al. 2007, 13). No studies of physician communication interventions were included in this review (see table A.1).

Printed Educational Materials   The effectiveness of printed educational materials on professional health practice was reviewed by Farmer, Legare, et al. (2008). The number of RCTs used in their calculations ranged from three to six studies. They found that printed educational materials when used alone may have a small desired effect on health professional outcomes with respect to process of care. On categorical process outcomes (e.g., X-ray requests, prescribing and smoking cessation activities), median RD was 4.3 percent (range –8% to +9.6%). On continuous process outcomes (e.g., medication changes, X-ray requests per practice), relative RD was 13.6 percent (range –5% to +26.6%). When printed educational materials were compared to a single intervention (e.g., mailed printed materials vs. personal office visit) in three RCTs, median RD for categorical process outcomes was 5 percent (see table A.1). In their review, the authors addressed three categorical measures of patient outcome (general health, return to work after low back pain, and smoking cessation; see table A.2), finding a median absolute risk reduction of –4.3 percent (range –.4% to –4.6%). Overall, the evidence provided in the Farmer, Legare, et al. (2008) review suggests that interventions based on printed educational materials have a small, favorable effect on physician practice and resource use outcomes (see table A.1). The review included no articles that assessed the impact of physician communication interventions.

Educational Meetings   Forsetlund, Bjorndal, et al. (2009) included 30 RCTs in their analyses of the effects of educational meetings on compliance with professional practice. When interventions with educational meetings as a component were compared to no intervention, the overall median ARD in adherence to desired practice was 6 percent (IQR range 1.8% to 15.9%; see table A.1). Meta-regression analysis found that a higher level of attendance at the educational meetings was significantly associated with larger ARDs, that mixed interactive and didactic education meetings (median ARD 13.6%) were more effective than didactic meetings (ARD 6.9%), and that interactive meetings appeared to be less effective (ARD 3%). The effect was similar when 19 trials with educational meetings alone were compared to no intervention (ARD 6%; IQR range 2.9% to 15.3%). For both comparisons, continuous variable analyses found a 10 percent relative change in professional practice (see table A.1).

Meta-analyses are reported on patient data for the same two comparisons. In five trials that compared dichotomous outcomes for any intervention in which educational meetings were a component to no intervention, the median ARD in the achievement of treatment goals improved by 3 percent (IQR –.9% to 4.0%). For eight studies involving continuous outcomes, the median adjusted relative percentage change in the patient health indicator was 4 percent (IQR 0% to 11%). In three trials where educational meetings alone were compared to no intervention using dichotomous outcome measures, median achievement of treatment goals improved (median ARD 3%; IQR .9% to 4.0%). For continuous patient outcomes (six trials) the median adjusted relative percentage change was 8 percent (IQR 0% to 12.0%). There were eight studies of the effect of physician communication interventions in this review (see table A.1).

On-Screen Computer Reminders   Shojania, Jennings, et al. (2009) reviewed the effects of computer reminders, delivered to clinicians at the point of care, on processes of care (prescribing, vaccinations, test ordering, documentation, and [one] physician communication). Across 32 process outcomes, computer reminders achieved an overall median improvement of 4.2 percent (IQR .8% to 18.8%); for prescribing, 3.3 percent (IQR .5% to 10.6%); for vaccination, 3.8 percent (IQR .5% to 6.6%); for test ordering, 3.8 percent (IQR .4% to 16.3%); and for recommended documentation, 0 percent (IQR 1.0% to 1.3%) (see table A.1). Comparisons of computer reminders alone versus usual care showed a median improvement in care process adherence of 5.7 percent, with wide variation (IQR 2.0% to 24.0%), whereas multifaceted interventions versus those additional interventions alone showed a median improvement in adherence of 1.9 percent (IQR .0% to 6.2%) (see table A.1).

Patient outcomes were reported in 10 studies of the effects of on-screen computer reminders, and resource use was reported in 5 studies. With respect to clinical outcomes, meta-analysis on eight comparisons indicated that intervention patients experienced a median absolute improvement of 2.5 percent (IQR 1.3% to 4.2%). There were improvements in intermediate outcomes, such as blood pressure and serum cholesterol targets, and in longer-term outcomes, such as pulmonary embolism and death.

Other Reviews

We identified three additional structured reviews that assessed impacts of interventions on physician and patient outcomes. These reviews addressed guideline dissemination, continuing medical education, and prompting physicians about preventive care measures. In some cases, these reviews included articles that were also part of the Cochrane reviews already discussed. For instance, among the 68 studies on audit and feedback in Grimshaw, Thomas, et al. 2004, 25 are included in the analyses of RCTs by Jamtvedt, Young, et al. (2006). Grimshaw and colleagues also included 4 studies on local opinion leaders found in Doumit, Gattellari, et al. 2007; 10 studies on educational outreach visits in O'Brien, Rogers, et al. 2007; 6 studies on printed educational materials in Farmer, Legare, et al. 2008; 7 studies on education meetings in Forsetlund, Bjorndal, et al. 2009; and 3 studies on computer reminders in Shojania, Jennings, et al. 2009. Additionally, 3 studies included in the review by Mansouri and Lockyer (2007) on continuing medical education effectiveness also are included in the Cochrane review by Forsetlund, Bjorndal, et al. (2009). The Dexheimer, Talbot, et al. (2008) review contains 1 study found in Shojania, Jennings, et al. 2009 and 3 RCTs in Jamtvedt, Young, et al. 2006.

Guideline Dissemination   Using Cochrane EPOC methods, Grimshaw, Thomas, et al. (2004) reviewed 235 studies on the effectiveness and costs of different strategies in guideline development, dissemination, and implementation. While there were no meta-analyses undertaken—because of the "extreme heterogeneity within the review and the number of studies with potential unit of analysis errors" (9)—the authors report the absolute median effect (the absolute difference across post-intervention measures) for several comparisons. The number of comparisons used across these analyses is small, as results are reported by study design (e.g., RCT, cluster RCT, controlled clinical trial, controlled before and after study), with most outcomes lacking sufficient comparisons for meta-analyses. Main findings include the median absolute improvement in performance across interventions: 14.1 percent (range −1% to 34%) in 14 cluster RCT comparisons of reminders, 8.1 percent (range 3.6% to 17%) in 4 cluster RCTs comparisons of dissemination of educational materials, 7.0 percent (range 1.3% to 16%) in 5 cluster RCT comparisons of audit and feedback, and 6.0 percent (range −4% to 17.4%) in 13 cluster RCT comparisons of multifaceted interventions involving educational outreach (see table A.1).

With respect to patient outcomes, for multifaceted interventions with educational outreach, the median effect size of absolute difference based on five RCT comparisons was 1.0 percent (range −7.0% to 3.0%) for dichotomous outcomes and 0 percent (range −1.4% to 2.7%) relative improvement for continuous outcomes. With respect to reminders, the median effect sizes were small: 1.9 percent (range 1.0% to 6.8%) based on three clinical controlled trials comparisons (dichotomous outcomes) and

1.9 percent (range, −2.0% to 7.2%) for three clinical controlled trials comparisons where continuous outcomes were measured (see table A.1).

Continuing Medical Education Mansouri and Lockyer (2007) reviewed 31 studies that addressed the effect of continuing medical education (CME) on physician performance, conducting meta-analyses for findings related to physician knowledge, physician performance, and patient outcomes. The overall mean effect size (weighted by sample size) across 61 interventions was $r = .28$ (95% CI .20–.39). The overall mean effect size in 19 studies addressing the impact of CME on physician performance was small ($r = .18$; see table A.1). Results for individual interventions demonstrated a consistently small effect size, with auditing and peer group discussion ($r = .24$) and individual training ($r = .32$), each based on one study, having a moderate effect size (see table A.1).

When considering the relationship between CME and patient outcomes (eight studies), the mean effect size also was small: $r = .14$ (95% CI .31–.63). The types of patient outcome were not reported, but results from studies of two CME programs directed at improving physician communication were included in the analyses.

Computerized and Paper-Based Support for Prompting Physicians Dexheimer, Talbot, et al. (2008) reviewed the effects of paper- and computer-based interventions using 16 measures of preventive care. They calculated effect as the unweighted mean percent difference between control or baseline data and the largest increase in effect of compliance to preventive care guidelines. Paper-based methods (e.g., a reminder sheet attached on the front of the patient chart) and computer-generated and computerized prompting methods were similar in their effects, which ranged from 12 to 14 percent (see table A.1). With respect to the prompting strategy, clinician reminders were more effective (14%) compared to clinician and patient reminders (10%; see table A.1). Notably, both the prompting method and the reminder strategy showed wide variation in their effects. Where a prevention measure had three or more studies, prompting clinicians was most effective for smoking cessation (23%), cardiac care (20%), and blood pressure screening (16%), followed by vaccinations, diabetes management, and cholesterol (15%). Mammography reminders had the smallest average effect (10%; see table A.1). The authors cautioned that the effectiveness of prompts may differ based on the existing workflow in physician practices and the organizational support infrastructure, such as available personnel or the information technology used to implement the reminder system. The authors included no studies on physician communication in their review, and they did not analyze patient outcomes.

Effects of Physician Communication Strategies on Patient Outcomes

In this section, to the extent possible, we compare the impact of physician communication training programs on resource use and patient outcomes to effect sizes reported in the review articles previously described, which were calculated for general categories of strategies for physician behavioral change. We were not able to find comparisons of this type in the literature, despite their potential value for decision makers in allocating public or organizational resources. We selected studies in physician communication intervention for inclusion in these comparisons based on three considerations: presence of information on effects on patient outcomes (beyond satisfaction), number of observations large enough to calculate effect sizes, and sufficient information in the article to facilitate calculating effect size. Based on these criteria, we included 8 articles already included in the Cochrane review (Smith, Shaw, et al. 1995; Guadagnoli, Soumerai, et al. 2000; Fallowfield, Jenkins, et al. 2002; Levinson and Roter 1993; Roter, Hall, et al. 1995; Clark, Gong, et al. 1998; Brown, Boles, et al. 1999; Harmsen, Bernsen, et al. 2005). We calculated effect sizes individually for 2 of these studies (Roter, Hall, et al. 1995; Clark, Gong, et al. 1998). We also included 2 studies from our review of the literature in chapter 5 (see table 5.2), for which we calculated effect sizes (Hobma, Ram, et al. 2006; Welschen, Kuyvenhoven, et al. 2004). When comparisons are possible, we here contrast individual study results with the overall effect sizes reported in review articles.

Effects on Patients of Interventions to Improve Physician Communication: Cochrane Review Studies

In their review on the effect of audit and feedback in changing physician behavior, Jamtvedt, Young, et al. (2006) report (http://epoc.cochrane .org/sites/epoc.cochrane.org/files/uploads/A&F-Table2B.pdf) a greater effect for audit and feedback with educational meetings, compared to a control group, in a study of an intervention to improve obstetricians' ($n = 9$) and midwives' ($n = 26$) explanations to patients of a routine prenatal screening test (Smith, Shaw, et al. 1995). They found a 32 percent improvement for the communication intervention versus a 23.8 percent improvement in professional practice (e.g., prescribing or test ordering; see table A.1) for the meta-analysis of multifaceted interventions including audit and feedback. The communications study was conducted in six British hospitals, with an intervention consisting of a one-hour video-based training and discussion. The sample size was small, but statistically significant changes in communication skills were observed immediately after intervention; these skills declined to baseline levels after a three-month period. There were no patient outcomes measured in this study.

In a second study on the effects of physician communication (cited in Jamtvedt, Young, et al. 2006 and Doumit, Gattellari, et al. 2007), Guadagnoli, Soumerai, et al. (2000) compare audit and feedback in multifaceted interventions versus audit and feedback alone, using a sample of surgeons from 28 hospitals. In this study, medical opinion leaders and performance feedback were used to reduce the proportion of women who reported that surgeons did not discuss treatment options prior to surgery for early-stage breast cancer. The study reported hospital-level patient outcomes (see table 5.2). In addition to hospital-specific performance feedback to both groups, the intervention consisted of slide presentations at grand rounds or tumor board meetings, personal or mail contact with surgeons on graphical materials that summarized surgical options, and other strategies as individual opinion leaders desired. The number of surgeons trained is not reported. Outcomes included the proportion of women who said their surgeons did not discuss surgical treatment alternatives and the proportion of patients who underwent breast-conserving surgery. Jamtvedt, Young, et al. (2006) calculated an effect size for this study and reported an adjusted RR of .98—essentially no effect (see http://epoc.cochrane.org/sites/epoc.cochrane.org/files/uploads/A&F-Table4.pdf)—on patients reporting that their surgeon did not discuss both breast-conserving surgery and mastectomy. A second effect size comparison for the Guadagnoli, Soumerai, et al. (2000) study is found in the Doumit, Gattellari, et al. (2007) meta-analysis of the effect of opinion leader plus one additional intervention versus additional intervention only. They calculated a median ARD of .02 for the communication study, less than the meta-analysis ARD of .09. Guadagnoli, Soumerai, et al. (2000) also found there was no effect over time of the intervention on patient outcomes. While the rate of breast-conserving surgery increased over time ($p = <.05$), there was no statistically significant change between the intervention hospitals and the comparison hospitals (the change was from 34% to 43% for intervention hospitals and from 41% to 46% for control hospitals).

While these two studies examined the effect of brief interventions designed to improve physician communication and patient outcomes and accompanied by audit and feedback, a third study focused on a comprehensive intervention to improve physician communication. This prospective study involved 80 oncologists (Fallowfield, Jenkins, et al. 2002) who received a three-day intensive training course on communication skills. Participants were assigned to four groups: 1) comprehensive written feedback followed by the training course; 2) training course only; 3) written feedback only, following a consultation; and 4) control. Physician feedback included a summary of patient satisfaction scores and comments made by patients following their interviews, a summary of the congruency of the doctor's own ratings of patient distress and understanding of information with patients' self-reports and brief exit interviews with researchers, a glossary of communication skills words and phrases, and key references about effective communication skills. Analyses compared 1) training groups versus feedback-only groups and controls and 2) feedback groups versus course-only groups plus controls. Effect sizes were estimated for the feedback groups for six desired communication outcomes: 1) uses focused questions (RR = 1.07), 2) uses focused and open questions (RR = 1.06), 3) expresses empathy (RR = 1.06, (4) summarizes information (RR = .93), 5) checks understanding (RR = 1.03), and 6) responds appropriately (RR = 1.16). With the exception of the last two outcomes, the effect sizes are similar to the median adjusted RR (1.08) for any intervention in which audit and feedback is a component, as described in the Jamtvedt, Young, et al. (2006) review. Fallowfield and Jenkins (2002) found that physicians who attended the course (with and without feedback) had a significantly greater number of focused questions (RR = 1.34), expressions of empathy (RR = 1.69), and appropriate responses to patients' cues (RR = 1.38) than the combined feedback-only and control groups.

While this study provides useful information on effect sizes for a comprehensive intervention aimed at oncologists, the effect of the intervention on patient outcomes beyond patient satisfaction is not clear. Aggregated patient satisfaction data on 1,816 patients gathered from baseline and 3-month patient questionnaires used for feedback to physicians (Shilling, Jenkins, et al. 2003) found no significant effect of the skills training (see table 5.2). When intervention effects were measured again at 12 months (Fallowfield, Jenkins, et al. 2003), researchers found maintenance of physician skills pertaining to asking more focused and open questions and fewer leading questions, as well as improvement in summarizing and fewer interruptions, but there was a decline in expressions of empathy. There were no patient clinical outcomes measured at follow-up.

Five additional studies on improving physician communication skills through CME meetings and workshops were included in the Forsetlund, Bjorndal, et al. (2009) Cochrane review. A randomized controlled study of a four-and-a-half-hour workshop with 31 physicians (Levinson and Roter 1993) found no effect on physician communication using analysis of audiotapes. There also was no effect of the intervention on patient communication patterns (biomedical information-giving and psychosocial talk).

Using a longer-term intervention, Roter, Hall, et al. (1995) found large effect sizes (33% to 132%) associated with two training sessions of four hours each. These effect sizes compare to an effect size of 10 percent found in the review on CME workshops for changing physician behavior (Forsetlund, Bjorndal, et al. 2009). In the Roter, Hall, et al. (1995) study, physicians were randomized into three groups: a control group, a group that received training on handling emotions, and a group that was trained in problem solving. Outcomes were captured using audiotape analysis with both actual and simulated patients. For physicians attending the training in emotion handling, the effect size was 132 percent for targeted emotion handling with actual patients. For physicians attending the training in problem identification, the effect size was 97 percent for targeted problem defining with actual patients. Additionally, for the latter physician group, effect sizes were calculated for patients experiencing emotional distress: for recognizing emotional problems, 33 percent; for recognizing emotional distress, 43 percent; and for using any strategy to manage emotional distress, 61 percent. For the two intervention groups combined, the effect size for counseling emotionally distressed patients was 45 percent. Emotionally distressed patients of the physicians trained on problem defining showed a significant reduction in emotional distress for up to six months, as compared to patients of the control group and of the physicians trained in emotion handling. The number of visits and visit length did not differ across physician groups.

Patient and physician process outcomes were reported in a study with pediatricians (Clark, Gong, et al. 1998) found in Forsetlund, Bjorndal, et al. (2009). While Forsetlund, Bjorndal, et al. report a 10 percent effect size for physician outcomes (continuing medical education vs. none), comparatively larger effect sizes were found for the Clark and Gong RCT using two interactive seminars of two and a half hours each. The study was based on the theory of self-regulation (guiding physicians to develop partnerships with their patients), with a convenience sample of 74 community-based, general pediatricians. This study examined both change in physician communication behaviors for asthma and patient outcomes. Effect sizes, based on physician self-assessment, ranged from 9.8 percent to 24 percent for six communication behaviors: address specific fears about new medication (10%), give written instructions (16%), go over instructions for the new medication (14%), write down for family how to adjust the medicine when symptoms change (24%), provide guidelines for patients to use (23%); and time spent on a visit for newly diagnosed child with asthma (−16%). Effect sizes for parents' perceptions of physician communication ranged from 2 percent to 20 percent on six factors: physician was reassuring and encouraging (5%), looked into how the family managed from day to day (8%), described how the child should be fully active (20%), described at least one of three goals (17%), gave information to relieve specific worries (5%), and enabled family to know how to make decisions on asthma management (2%). These are all measures of the effectiveness of communication between physicians and patients. No patient health status measures were reported. There was no effect on number of emergency department visits or hospitalizations, but effect sizes for reduction in office visits were large, for number of scheduled doctor office visits 44.9%) and number of scheduled office visits after an episode of symptoms (41.6%).

Two studies evaluated communication skills training programs in a not-for-profit group-model health maintenance organization. In a program consisting of two four-hour interactive workshops for 69 primary care and specialty clinicians, Brown, Boles, et al. (1999) found no effect on patient satisfaction. In the second intensive communication skills training study, Harmsen, Bernsen, et al. (2005) examined the effects of a two-and-a-half-day training program for 38 Dutch general practitioners on intercultural communication, aimed at decreasing inequalities in care provided between Western and non-Western patients. Patients also received an intervention, consisting of a 12-minute videotaped instruction on communicating directly and expressing freely any misunderstanding and disagreement. The outcome measures were mutual understanding, patient satisfaction, and perceived quality of care. The effect size for mutual understanding, determined by scaling answers from the physician and patient about different aspects of the consultation, was 11 percent for non-Western patients, compared to 10 percent in the Forsetlund, Bjorndal, et al. (2009) review. There was no effect of the intervention on patient satisfaction, but an effect size of 7 percent was found for perceived quality of care with consultation or whether the physician was considerate, similar to the 8 percent effect size for patient outcomes reported by Forsetlund, Bjorndal, et al. (2009).

Effects on Patients of Interventions to Improve Physician Communication: Additional Studies

Of the two additional studies (not found in Cochrane reviews) included in our discussion, the first evaluated an intervention that identified individual communication skills deficiencies of 76 Dutch general practitioners (Hobma, Ram, et al. 2006), who then received six to eight hours of small-group meetings with a tutor. Outcomes were measured using videotaped consultations relating to aspects of the patient visit: introduction, request for help, evaluation of the consultation, explorations, emotions, empathy, summarization, and structuring. Participants reported eight items as personal improvement goals, and improvement was seen on five, with a corresponding overall effect size (*d*-value) of .66, indicating a moderate to large effect. There was no attempt to measure impact on resource use.

The second study, by Welschen, Kuyvenhoven, et al. (2004), used a multifaceted intervention directed at 89 Dutch general practitioners, with the goal of reducing antibiotic prescription rates for symptoms of the respiratory tract in primary care. The intervention included group education meetings, with a consensus procedure on indication for and type of antibiotics and with training in communication skills; monitoring and feedback on prescribing behavior; group education for assistants of general practitioners and pharmacists; and education material for patients. Antibiotic prescription rates in the intervention group fell by 4 percent, and those in the control group rose by 8 percent, with a mean difference in change of –12% (range –18.9% to –4.0%). This effect size is similar to that reported by Forsetlund, Bjorndal, et al. (2009) for multifaceted interventions with a medical education component (10%).

Summary of Individual Studies

Continuing education programs in communication skills training were the most common interventions evaluated in the 10 individual studies. Evaluation methods included using actual or video observation with simulated or real patients, scoring physician utterances, or physician self-evaluation. Of the 10 studies reviewed, six interventions used intensive educational efforts, two used brief interventions, and two used multifaceted interventions. Intensive communication skills training carried out over two or more days produced the largest effects on physician behavior. Measures used in these studies addressed common communication problems identified by researchers and displayed in table 2.3 (e.g., recognize emotional distress; show empathy; give counseling; discuss medication purpose, use, adverse effects, or adherence to medication therapy). Use of multiple different measures across studies makes it difficult to identify the specific impacts of communication skills training on individual physician behavior.

Two studies made no attempt to evaluate patient outcomes, while five studies included patient satisfaction but no other patient outcomes. The single exception is the well-designed study of Clark, Gong, et al. (1998), which found a significant impact of the educational intervention on the prescribing and communications behavior of physicians. The theory-driven approach to skills training described in this study focused on educating parents about a treatment for asthma, a common and costly pediatric disease. While this study, as others, did not demonstrate an effect on parent satisfaction, there were large effects on aspects of parents' disease understanding and management and on office-based health care utilization.

Discussion and Conclusions

Both reviews of interventions intended to change physician behavior and specific studies of the impact of interventions intended to improve physician communication suggest that CME meetings and workshops have the greatest potential to affect physician behaviors, where behaviors are measured using change scores, quality-of-care measures, and compliance with standards or desired practice (e.g., disease management and prevention). The measures used for evaluation of effectiveness in these different interventions varied widely. Where studies used different outcome measures to assess effectiveness, it was not possible to reach conclusions regarding relative effectiveness.

There is more similarity, conceptually, in measures of the impact on resource use and patient health, but most studies do not address these measures. Therefore, we found it almost impossible to judge whether training interventions in physician communication are more or less effective at improving these patient outcomes as compared to other strategies employed to effect change in physician behavior. The Forsetlund, Bjorndal, et al. (2009) Cochrane review provides some, but limited, evidence on patient outcomes. Patient outcome meta-analyses in this review were based on a small number of studies (5 to 8 trials), and the effect sizes were modest (3% to 8%). Similarly, findings from the analysis of patient outcomes in individual studies on the effectiveness of communication skills training are based on small sample sizes and measures that are difficult to compare.

Given the present state of the literature, we believe a reasonable conclusion is that while there have been many efforts to improve physician communication, there is no strong case that those efforts have been any more effective at improving patient health outcomes than other interventions for physician change. This conclusion reflects primarily a lack of research on the impact of communication training on patient health outcomes or resource use.

In this appendix, we set out to compare the impact of physician communication training on patient outcomes and resource use, relative to other strategies designed to change physician behavior. There is an extensive literature relating to the impact of behavioral change interventions directed at physicians, and there are several strong meta-analyses of impacts. However, because outcome measures used in these studies vary widely, it is difficult to reach conclusions about relative effectiveness of different intervention strategies, including physician communication interventions. Therefore, the literature as it now exists provides little guidance concerning how to invest scarce resources to accomplish physician behavioral change that improves patient health outcomes. It is not clear whether physician communications interventions should be given preference in decisions on resource allocation, relative to other behavioral change interventions, such as audit and feedback. Decision makers presumably also would desire data on the relative costs of different interventions, but cost data are generally not reported in evaluations of intervention impacts. With respect to studies of physician communication interventions, there is the further limitation that longer-term patient outcomes associated with the interventions are assessed only infrequently.

TABLE A.1.   Main Effects of Interventions to Change Physician Behavior

Reference	Number of Studies/ Physician Behavioral Change Targeted	Meta-Analysis (Y/N)	Studies Assessed Patient Outcomes (Y/N/outcomes)	Main Effects
Cochrane Systematic Reviews				
Jamtvedt, Young, et al. 2006 Audit and feedback: effects on professional practice and health care outcomes	118 RCTs (audit and feedback alone, audit and feedback with educational meetings, or multifaceted interventions that included audit and feedback): 21 preventive care; 14 test ordering; 20 prescribing practice; 3 communication skills; 43 other studies focused on general management of a variety of clinical problems	Y	Y/smoking cessation; blood pressure control; quality of care to nursing home patients	Health professional outcomes, ARD adjusted by baseline compliance. Compared to no intervention: (1) any intervention in which audit and feedback is a component: dichotomous outcomes, median ARD = 5% (IQR = 3%–11%), median adjusted RR = 1.08 (IQR = .99–1.30), continuous outcomes, adjusted % change = 16% (IQR = 5%–37%); (2) audit and feedback alone: dichotomous outcomes, median ARD = 4% (IQR = −.8%–9.0%), median adjusted RR = 1.07 (IQR = .98–1.18), continuous outcomes, adjusted % change = 11.9% (IQR = 5.1%–22%); (3) audit and feedback plus educational meetings: dichotomous outcomes, median ARD = 1.5% (IQR = 1.0%–5.5%), median adjusted RR = 1.06 (IQR = 1.03–1.09), continuous outcomes, adjusted % change = 28.7% (IQR = 14.3%–36.5%); (4) multifaceted interventions including audit and feedback: dichotomous outcomes, median ARD = 5.7% (IQR = .85%–13.6%), median ad-

Reference	Number of Studies/ Physician Behavioral Change Targeted	Meta-Analysis (Y/N)	Studies Assessed Patient Outcomes (Y/N/outcomes)	Main Effects
				justed RR = 1.10 (IQR = 1.03–1.36), continuous outcomes, adjusted % change = 23.8% (IQR = 5.3%–49%). No meta-analyses on health care outcomes.
Doumit, Gattellari, et al. 2007 Local opinion leaders: effects on professional practice and health care outcomes	12 RCTs: MDs targeted in 10 trials on general management of a clinical problem. One study on physician communication.	N	Y/pain intensity and pain prevalence; received breast conserving surgery; received epidural anesthesia; received a trial of labor and vaginal birth; mothers' intention to breast feed	Health professional outcomes, ARD adjusted by baseline noncompliance: (1) opinion leader vs. no intervention: ARD = .07 (range −.06 to +.12); (2) opinion leader vs. single intervention: ARD = .14 (range .12–.17); (3) opinion leader plus 1 additional intervention vs. additional intervention only: ARD .09 (range .02–.25); (4) opinion leader as part of multiple interventions vs. no intervention: ARD = .06 (range .01–.14). No meta-analyses on health care outcomes.
O'Brien, Rogers et al. 2007 Educational outreach visits (EOV): effects on professional practice and health care outcomes	69 RCTs: 29 prescribing practice; 29 general medical management; 11 preventive care	Y	Y/functional status; patient satisfaction; mortality; fall rate; asthma care; lipid control; colorectal cancer screening; number of drugs taken; nosocomial events; cardiac care; discharge home; resource use; blood pressure; vaccina-	Health professional outcomes, ARD adjusted by baseline compliance: (1) any intervention in which EOV is a component: dichotomous outcomes, median ARD = 5.6% (IQR = 3%–9%); prescribing behavior, median ARD = 4.8% (IQR = 3%–6.5%); vs. other behaviors, median ARD = 6% (IQR = .3.6%–16%); continuous outcomes, median adjusted % change = 21% (IQR = 11%–41%); (2) EOV vs. no intervention: dichotomous outcomes,

Reference	Number of Studies/ Physician Behavioral Change Targeted	Meta-Analysis (Y/N)	Studies Assessed Patient Outcomes (Y/N/outcomes)	Main Effects
			tion status; blood glucose level	median ARD = .05 (IQR = .01–.20); continuous outcomes, median adjusted % change = .23 (IQR = .12–.39). No meta-analyses on health care outcomes.
Farmer, Legare et al. 2008 Printed educational materials: effects on professional practice and health care outcomes	23 studies: 12 prescribing; 6 prevention and general medical management; 3 test ordering; 2 surgical rates	Y	General health; smoking cessation; return to work	Health professional outcomes: (1) printed educational materials vs. no intervention: RCTs (n = 6): categorical process outcomes, median RD = 4.3% (range –8% to +9.6%); continuous process outcomes, RCTs (n = 4), relative RD = 13.6% (range –5% to +26.6%); (2) printed educational materials vs. single interventions: categorical process outcomes RCTs (n = 3), median RD = .05 (range not given). Patient outcomes: (1) categorical outcomes RCTs (n = 3), median ARD = –4.3% (range –.4% to –4.6%).
Forsetlund, Bjorndal et al. 2009 Continuing education meetings and workshops: effects on professional practice and health care outcomes	81 RCTs: 34 general medical management; 13 prescribing practices; 11 preventive care; 8 communication skills; 3 test ordering; 6 screening for cancer; 6 other	Y	Y/quality of life and functional status; patient satisfaction; depression score; smoking cessation; blood glucose control; successful TB treatment completion;	Health professional outcomes, ARD adjusted by baseline compliance: (1) any intervention in which educational meetings were a component vs. no intervention, dichotomous outcomes: median ARD = 6% (IQR = 1.8%–15.9%); continuous outcomes, adjusted % change = 10% (IQR = 9%–24%); (2) educa-

Reference	Number of Studies/ Physician Behavioral Change Targeted	Meta- Analysis (Y/N)	Studies As- sessed Patient Outcomes (Y/N/outcomes)	Main Effects
			neonatal mortality; psychiatric symptoms; distress and anxiety; vaccination; drug use; care use for asthma	tional meetings alone compared to no intervention, dichotomous outcomes: ARD = 6% (IQR = 2.9%–15.3%); continuous outcomes, adjusted % change = 10% (IQR = 8%–32%). Patient outcomes: (1) any intervention in which educational meetings were a component vs. no intervention, dichotomous outcomes: for achievement of treatment goals, median ARD = 3% (IQR = 1%–4%); continuous outcomes, adjusted % change in patient health indicator = 4% (IQR = 0%–11%); (2) educational meetings alone compared to no intervention, dichotomous outcomes: median ARD = 3% (IQR = −.9%–4%); continuous outcomes, adjusted % change = 8% (IQR = 0%–12%).
Shojania, Jennings et al. 2009 The effects of on-screen, point of care computer reminders on processes and outcomes of care	28 studies (study may have targeted more than one behavior): 17 prescribing practices; 9 test ordering; 6 adherence to recommended vaccinations; 5 resource use; 2 documentation	Y	Y/blood pressure and cholesterol targets; clinical outcomes, such as development of pulmonary embolism and mortality	Median effect size, % improvements in MD care process adherence: (1) all process outcomes, 4.2 % (IQR = .8%–18.8%); (2) prescribing, 3.3% (IQR = .5%–10.6%); (3) vaccination, 3.8% (IQR = .5%–6.6%); (4) test ordering, 3.8% (IQR = .4%–16.3%); (5) documentation, 0% (IQR = −1.0%–1.3%); (6) interventions targeting inpatient settings (based on 2 computer-mature aca-

Reference	Number of Studies/ Physician Behavioral Change Targeted	Meta- Analysis (Y/N)	Studies Assessed Patient Outcomes (Y/N/outcomes)	Main Effects
				demic centers) showed a trend toward larger improvements in processes of care 8.7% (IQR = 2.7%– 22.7%) vs. outpatient 3.0% (.6%–11.5%), $p = .34$; (7) single interventions 5.7% (IQR = 2.0%– 24.0%) vs. multifaceted interventions 1.9% (IQR = 0.0%–6.2%), $p = .04$. Patient outcomes: (1) dichotomous clinical endpoints: median absolute improvement of 2.5% (IQR = 1.3%–4.2%).

Other Reviews

Dissemination of Clinical Guidelines

Reference	Number of Studies/ Physician Behavioral Change Targeted	Meta- Analysis (Y/N)	Studies Assessed Patient Outcomes (Y/N/outcomes)	Main Effects
Grimshaw, Thomas et al. 2004 Effectiveness and efficiency of guideline dissemination and implementation strategies	235 studies on general management, prescribing, test ordering, prevention, diagnosis, discharge planning, financial, procedures, professional to patient communication, record keeping and referrals	N	Y / not specified	Median effect size (range) % absolute or relative improvements in MD care process adherence. Provider performance: (1) educational materials vs. no intervention dichotomous process outcomes: 8.1% (3.6%–17%); (2) audit and feedback vs. no intervention dichotomous process outcomes: 7% (1.3%–16%); (3) reminders vs. no intervention dichotomous process outcomes: 14.1% (−1%–34%); (4) multifaceted interventions with educational outreach vs. no intervention dichotomous process

Reference	Number of Studies/ Physician Behavioral Change Targeted	Meta- Analysis (Y/N)	Studies As- sessed Patient Outcomes (Y/N/outcomes)	Main Effects
				outcomes: 6% (−4%−17.4%); (5) multifaceted interventions with educational outreach vs. no intervention continuous process outcomes: 15% (1.7%−24%); (6) multifaceted interventions with educational materials and outreach vs. no intervention dichotomous process outcomes: 1.2% (−5.6%−13.1%); (7) combinations of educational materials and meetings vs. no intervention dichotomous process outcomes: 1.9% (−3%−5%); (8) multifaceted interventions with educational outreach vs. other interventions dichotomous process outcomes: 4.5% (−5.2%−24.3%); (9) educational meetings and reminders vs. outreach vs. educational meetings dichotomous process outcomes: 7.9% (3.9%−32%). Patient outcomes: (1) multifaceted interventions with educational outreach vs. no intervention, dichotomous outcomes: 1.0% (range −7.0%−3.0%); (2) multifaceted interventions with educational outreach vs. no intervention, continuous outcomes: 0% (range −1.4

Reference	Number of Studies/ Physician Behavioral Change Targeted	Meta-Analysis (Y/N)	Studies Assessed Patient Outcomes (Y/N/outcomes)	Main Effects
				to 2.7%); (3) reminders vs. no intervention dichotomous outcomes: 1.9% (range 1.0%–6.8%); (4) reminders vs. no intervention continuous outcomes: 1.9% (range −2.0%–7.2%)

Continuing Medical Education

Reference	Number of Studies/ Physician Behavioral Change Targeted	Meta-Analysis (Y/N)	Studies Assessed Patient Outcomes (Y/N/outcomes)	Main Effects
Mansouri and Lockyer 2007 A meta-analysis of continuing medical education effectiveness	31 studies (61 interventions; 27 on MD performance); MD behaviors not identified	Y	Y/ outcomes not described	Provider performance: (1) overall mean effect size between CME and physician performance ($n = 19$ studies): $r = .18$ (.21); (95% CI, .08–.28); (2) conference and lecture ($n = 5$): $r = .06$ (.15); (3) interactive small group ($n = 2$): $r = .13$ (.15); (4) multidisciplinary educational outreach visits ($n = 2$): $r = .02$ (.06); (5) multifaceted educational program ($n = 3$): $r = .04$ (.11); (6) online education ($n = 2$): $r = .18$ (.13). Patient outcomes ($n = 8$ studies): (1) mean effect size: $r = .14$

Computerized and Paper-Based Support for Prompting and Clinical Decisions

Reference	Number of Studies/ Physician Behavioral Change Targeted	Meta-Analysis (Y/N)	Studies Assessed Patient Outcomes (Y/N/outcomes)	Main Effects
Dexheimer, Talbot et al. 2008 Prompting clinicians about preventive care mea-	61 studies (34 combined paper and computer generated, 19 paper based, 8 computer based) examined 264 preventive care interventions, with 110	N	N	Effect = mean % difference between control or baseline data and largest increase in effect of preventive care compliance: (1) prompting methods: paper-based 14% (range

TABLE A.1—*Continued*

Reference	Number of Studies/ Physician Behavioral Change Targeted	Meta- Analysis (Y/N)	Studies As- sessed Patient Outcomes (Y/N/outcomes)	Main Effects
sures: a systematic review of randomized controlled trials	studies addressing cancer screening be- havior			–18%–46%); computer- generated 12% (range –24%–59%); computer- ized 13% (range –8%–60%); (2) reminder strategy: clinician only 14% (range –18%–60%); clinician and patient 10% (range –24%–45%); (3) reminder types: vaccina- tion 15% (range –15%–50%); fecal occult blood testing 12% (range –11%–37%); Papanico- laou smear 12% (range –24%–48%); mammo- gram 10% (range –18%–49%); blood pres- sure 16% (range –8%–59%); cholesterol 15% (range –1%–54%); diabetes management 15% (range 5%–51%); smoking cessation 23% (range 3%–44%); cardiac care 20% (range –8%–59%). No analysis of patient out- comes.

ARD = adjusted risk difference
CME = continuing medical education
COPD = chronic obstructive
   pulmonary disease
EOV = educational outreach
   visit(s)

N = no
Median improvement = the
   median improvement in the
   intervention group minus
   the improvement in the control group
MD = physician

r = mean effect size, where
   0.10 = small, 0.24 =
   medium, and 0.37 = large
RD = risk difference
RR = relative risk
Y = yes

TABLE A.2. Changing Physician Behavior: Type and Number of Outcomes Addressed in Six Cochrane Review Articles

Reference/Intervention	Health Professionals	Patients
Jamtvedt, Young, et al. 2006 Audit and feedback	Studies with physicians: 29 measures for compliance with guidelines or clinical criteria (e.g., use of benzodiazepines; polypharmacy; intensive care, hand washing and drug use; MRI use; test for lipids; referrals for x-rays of knee and spine; preventive and wellness care; management of asthma, angina, diabetes, cardiovascular disease, hypertension, depression, low back pain, anemia, burns, cystitis and vaginitis, and domestic violence) 25 patients screened or offered preventive care (e.g., vaccination, mammography, clinical breast examination, skin cancer prevention counseling, colorectal cancer, detection of psychological distress, AIDS counseling, prophylactic aspirin) 20 quality of care measures for the management of, e.g., diabetes, depression, cardiovascular disease, asthma, obstetrics, pediatric mental health, and burn care 20 resource use (e.g., lab tests per admission; prescriptions per patient; inappropriate tests; generic prescriptions; length of stay and cost of episode; number of services; consultation time; cost of anesthetics, lab tests, and managing depression) 17 quality of care measures for prescribing (e.g., analgesics, hypnotics, sedatives, antibiotics, H2 blockers, benzodiazepines) 3 communication (e.g., explain to patients a routine prenatal screening test; discuss options prior to surgery for early stage breast cancer; communication skills) 4 MD practice management measures	7 clinical outcomes: smoking cessation, blood pressure control, blood glucose control, weight control 1 patient satisfaction 2 recall discussion about exercise, smoking status
Doumit, Gattellari, et al. 2007 Local opinion leaders	Studies with physicians or physicians and nurses: 7 quality of care measures: knowledge and attitudes about pain management; trial of labor; antenatal corticosteroids for fetal maturation; drugs for treatment of acute myocardial infarction; and management of rheumatoid arthritis, COPD, and osteoarthritis and total hip arthroplasty 1 measure for guideline compliance with angina 1 physician communication: discuss options prior to surgery for early stage breast cancer	5 clinical outcomes: pain intensity and pain prevalence; received breast conserving surgery; received epidural anesthesia; received a trial of labor and vaginal birth; mothers' intention to breastfeed

Reference/Intervention	Health Professionals	Patients
O'Brien, Rogers, et al. 2007 Educational outreach visits	26 quality of care measures for prescribing (e.g., antibiotics, NSAIDS, benzodiazepines, psychotropics, lipid lowering drugs, cerebral and peripheral vasodilators, thiazides, proton pump inhibitors, antidepressants; antifungal dispensing) 16 patients screened or offered preventive care (e.g., smoking cessation counseling; implementation of "drink less" program; index of preventive care performance, hemoglobinopathy testing for at-risk patients; STD counseling; vaccination; cholesterol, prostate-specific antigen cervical cancer, mammography, and colorectal cancer testing; stroke and atrial fibrillation) 11 measures for compliance with guidelines, criteria, or targets (e.g., urinary incontinence, asthma, diabetes, prescribing practice, cardiovascular risk, management of Helicobacter pylori, mechanically ventilated patients in ICUs, blood transfusion) 8 quality of care measures for the management of, e.g., acid-peptic disease, acute diarrhea, obesity, obstetrics/cesarean section, low back pain 3 resource use (e.g., prescription cost, fills, and inappropriate prescribing) 4 MD practice management (e.g., documentation)	5 quality of life, functional status 17 clinical outcomes (e.g., reached treatment goals, or overall improvement; vaccination status; blood pressure; lipid, and blood glucose control; number of drugs taken, colorectal cancer screening; mortality, falls, nosocomial events; unscheduled asthma care; discharge to home; self-reported exercise and social contact) 2 patient satisfaction
Farmer, Legare, et al. 2008 Printed educational materials	13 quality of care measures for prescribing (e.g., medications for management of hypertension and cholesterol; antibiotics, antispasmodics, analgesics, angiotensin-converting enzyme [ACE] inhibitors, antidepressants) 7 measures of compliance with guidelines or criteria for, e.g., cesarean delivery; vaginal delivery after cesarean section; referral for chest radiography; angina; prevention of stroke in atrial fibrillation 5 quality of care measures for clinical outcomes (e.g., surgical rates for pediatric ear disease; medications based on evidence-based drug therapy; medication and psychotherapy for treatment of major depression; and detection of mental disorder) 1 patients screened or offered preventive care, smoking cessation counseling 1 resource use: national promotional expenditures for hormone replacement therapy for women	1 functional status i.e., return to work clinical outcomes, i.e., general health, smoking quit attempts
Forsetlund, Bjorndal, et al. 2009 Continuing education meetings and work-	27 quality of care measures for the management of, e.g., pulmonary disease; low back pain; heart failure; urinary tract infections in women; sore throat; depression; obstetric care; asthma; diabetes;	5 quality of life, functional status 16 measures of clinical outcomes (e.g.,

Reference/Intervention	Health Professionals	Patients
shops	neonatal respiratory distress; osteoporosis; hypertension; respiratory tract infection; diarrhea/vomiting; appropriate testing 19 patients screened or offered preventive care (e.g., breast, cervical, skin, colorectal, and prostate cancer; sexually transmitted disease; health promotion for elderly; smoking cessation counseling; cardiovascular disease; breast-feeding; exercise and nutrition counseling; domestic violence; pulmonary disease) 13 measures of compliance with guidelines, targets, or criteria for, e.g., angina; low back pain; hypercholesterolemia; epilepsy; depression; infertility testing; acute myocardial infarction; otitis media; arthritis in elderly patients 8 physician communication 6 quality of care measures for prescribing (e.g., antibiotics, inappropriate drug use for non-prescription analgesics, NSAIDS; reducing injection use and dispensing of illegal steroids) 2 resource use: referral rates to specialists, number of out-of-hours service contacts	depression score; smoking cessation; blood glucose and weight control; successful TB treatment completion; neonatal mortality; psychiatric symptoms, distress, and anxiety; vaccination, drug use) 10 patient report and observational measures of MD communication skills (e.g., mutual understanding, survey scores, patient satisfaction, behavior counts). 1 patient satisfaction
Shojania, Jennings, et al. 2009 Reminders, alerts, presenting guideline-based suggestions, prompting, identifying at-risk patients, and decision support on processes and outcomes of care	17 prescribing practices for, e.g., antibiotics for otitis media in children and surgery patients; cardiovascular risk and disease; suspected urinary tract infection or sore throat; hypertension; diabetes; adverse drug events; aspirin for cardiovascular risk; patient at risk for thromboembolism; asthma and chronic obstructive pulmonary disease; hemoglobinopathy 9 test ordering for, e.g., suspected urinary tract infection or sore throat; preventive care; asthma and chronic obstructive pulmonary disease; cardiovascular disease; glucose and cholesterol control 6 adherence to recommended vaccinations (e.g., for hospitalized patients; outpatient screening and preventive care; cardiovascular disease) 5 resource use (e.g., reduce redundant tests) 2 recommended documentation (e.g., angina, asthma, preventive care)	1 resource use, care use for asthma 8 clinical outcomes, (e.g., blood pressure and cholesterol targets; development of pulmonary embolism and mortality)

Note: There may be more than one assessed outcome per study.

References

Abdulhadi, N., M. Al Shafaee, et al. 2007. "Patient-provider interaction from the perspectives of type 2 diabetes patients in Muscat, Oman: a qualitative study." *BMC Health Serv Res* 7: 162.

ACP. 2009. *Statement to the Senate Finance Committee, Recommendations for Health Care Delivery System Reform*, April 21, American College of Physicians. Available at http://www.acponline.org/advocacy/events/testimony/hcd_reform.pdf (accessed November 23, 2011).

Adams, R. J., B. J. Smith, et al. 2001. "Impact of the physician's participatory style in asthma outcomes and patient satisfaction." *Ann Allergy Asthma Immunol* 86(3): 263–71.

AHRQ. 2008. "Patient centeredness." Chap. 5 in *National Healthcare Quality Report, 2007*. AHRQ Publication No. 08–0040. Rockville, MD: Agency for Healthcare Research and Quality.

Aiarzaguena, J. M., G. Grandes, et al. 2007. "A randomized controlled clinical trial of a psychosocial and communication intervention carried out by GPs for patients with medically unexplained symptoms." *Psychol Med* 37(2): 283–94.

Alexander, S. C., S. A. Keitz, et al. 2006. "A controlled trial of a short course to improve residents' communication with patients at the end of life." *Acad Med* 81(11): 1008–12.

American Academy of Family Physicians. 2008. "Patient-centered medical home, definition of." Available at http://www.aafp.org/online/en/home/policy/policies/p/patientcenteredmedhome.html (accessed October 11, 2009).

Amiel, G. E., L. Ungar, et al. 2006. "Ability of primary care physician's to break bad news: a performance based assessment of an educational intervention." *Patient Educ Couns* 60(1): 10–15.

Arber, S., J. McKinlay, et al. 2004. "Influence of patient characteristics on doctors' questioning and lifestyle advice for coronary heart disease: a UK/US video experiment." *Br J Gen Pract* 54(506): 673–78.

Armstrong-Coben, A. 2009. "The computer will see you now." *New York Times*, March 6.

Arora, N. K. 2003. "Interacting with cancer patients: the significance of physicians' communication behavior." *Soc Sci Med* 57(5): 791–806.

Arvantes, J. 2007. "Primary care physician shortage creates medically disenfranchised population." *AAFP News Now*, March 22. Available at http://www.aafp.org (accessed October 11, 2009).

Ashton, C. M., P. Haidet, et al. 2003. "Racial and ethnic disparities in the use of health services: bias, preferences, or poor communication?" *JGIM* 18(2): 146–52.

Audrey, S., J. Abel, et al. 2008. "What oncologists tell patients about survival benefits of palliative chemotherapy and implications for informed consent: qualitative study." *Bmj* **337**: a752.

Azoulay, E., S. Chevret, et al. 2000. "Half the families of intensive care unit patients experience inadequate communication with physicians." *Crit Care Med* **28**(8): 3044–49.

Back, A. 2006. "Patient-physician communication in oncology: what does the evidence show?" *Oncology (Williston Park)* **20**(1): 67–74; discussion 77–78, 83.

Back, A. L., R. M. Arnold, et al. 2003. "Teaching communication skills to medical oncology fellows." *J Clin Oncol* **21**(12): 2433–36.

Back, A. L., R. M. Arnold, et al. 2005. "Approaching difficult communication tasks in oncology." *CA Cancer J Clin* **55**(3): 164–77.

Back, A. L., R. M. Arnold, et. al. 2007. "Efficacy of communication skills training for giving bad news and discussing transitions to palliative care." *Arch Intern Med* **167**(5): 453–60.

Back, A. L., R. M. Arnold, et al. 2009. "Faculty development to change the paradigm of communication skills teaching in oncology." *J Clin Oncol* **27**(7): 1137–41.

Back, A. L., S. M. Bauer-Wu, et al. 2009. "Compassionate silence in the patient-clinician encounter: a contemplative approach." *J Palliat Med* **12**(12):1113–17.

Backer, L. A. 2007. "The medical home: an idea whose time has come . . . again." *Fam Pract Manag* **14**(8): 38–41.

Baile, W. F., and J. Aaron. 2005. "Patient-physician communication in oncology: past, present, and future." *Curr Opin Oncol* **17**(4): 331–35.

Barfod, T. S., F. M. Hecht, et al. 2006. "Physicians' communication with patients about adherence to HIV medication in San Francisco and Copenhagen: a qualitative study using grounded theory." *BMC Health Serv Res* **6**: 154.

Barnhart, J., V. Lewis, et al. 2007. "Physician knowledge levels and barriers to coronary risk prevention in women: survey results from the Women and Heart Disease Physician Education Initiative." *Women's Health Issues* **17**(2): 93–100.

Barry, C. A., C. P. Bradley, et al. 2000. "Patients' unvoiced agendas in general practice consultations: qualitative study." *Bmj* **320**(7244): 1246–50.

Baumal, R., and J. Benbassat. 2008. "Current trends in the educational approach for teaching interviewing skills to medical students." *Isr Med Assoc J* **10**(7): 552–55.

Beach, M. C., E. G. Price, et al. 2005. "Cultural competence: a systematic review of health care provider educational interventions." *Med Care* **43**(4): 356–73.

Beck, R. S., R. Daughtridge, et al. 2002. "Physician-patient communication in the primary care office: a systematic review." *J Am Board Fam Pract* **15**(1): 25–38.

Bell, R. A., R. L. Kravitz, et al. 2002. "Unmet expectations for care and the patient-physician relationship." *J Gen Intern Med* **17**(11): 817–24.

Bennett, I., J. Switzer, et al. 2006. "'Breaking it down': patient-clinician communication and prenatal care among African American women of low and higher literacy." *Ann Fam Med* **4**(4): 334–40.

Bensing, J., S. van Dulmen, et al. 2003. "Communication in context: new directions in communication research." *Patient Educ Couns* **50**(1): 27–32.

Bikker, A. P., S. W. Mercer, et al. 2005. "A pilot prospective study on the consultation and relational empathy, patient enablement, and health changes over 12 months in patients going to the Glasgow Homoeopathic Hospital." *J Altern Complement Med* **11**(4): 591–600.

Blendon, R. J., T. Buhr, et al. 2008. "Disparities in physician care: experiences and perceptions of a multi-ethnic America." *Health Aff (Millwood)* 27(2): 507–17.

Bodenheimer, T., and B. Y. Laing. 2007. "The teamlet model of primary care." *Ann Fam Med* 5(5): 457–61.

Bokhour, B. G., D. R. Berlowitz, et al. 2006. "How do providers assess antihypertensive medication adherence in medical encounters?" *J Gen Intern Med* 21(6): 577–83.

Boodman, S. G. 2007. "New doctors develop an old skill: they call it empathy, previously known as bedside manner." *Washington Post,* May 15.

Boyles, S. 2008. "Misdiagnoses caused in part by overconfidence." *WebMD Health News,* April 30. Available at http://www.Medscape.com (accessed December 29, 2008).

Brinkman, W. B., S. R. Geraghty, et al. 2007. "Effect of multisource feedback on resident communication skills and professionalism: a randomized controlled trial." *Arch Pediatr Adolesc Med* 161(1): 44–49.

British Medical Association. 2004. *Communication skills education for doctors: an update.* London, UK.

Britten, N., F. A. Stevenson, et al. 2000. "Misunderstandings in prescribing decisions in general practice: qualitative study." *Bmj* 320(7233): 484–88.

Brown, J. B., M. Boles, et al. 1999. "Effect of clinician communication skills training on patient satisfaction: a randomized, controlled trial." *Ann Intern Med* 131(11): 822–29.

Burd, I. D., N. Nevadunsky, et al. 2006. "Impact of physician gender on sexual history taking in a multispecialty practice." *J Sex Med* 3(2): 194–200.

Butler, L., L. Degner, et al. 2005. "Developing communication competency in the context of cancer: a critical interpretive analysis of provider training programs." *Psychooncology* 14(10): 861–72; discussion 873–74.

Bylund, C. L., and G. Makoul. 2002. "Empathic communication and gender in the physician-patient encounter." *Patient Educ Couns* 48(3): 207–16.

Calam, B., S. Far, et al. 2000. "Discussions of 'code status' on a family practice teaching ward: what barriers do family physicians face?" *Cmaj* 163(10): 1255–59.

Calkins, D. R., R. B. Davis, et al. 1997. "Patient-physician communication at hospital discharge and patients' understanding of the postdischarge treatment plan." *Arch Intern Med* 157(9): 1026–30.

Cals, J. W., N. A. Scheppers, et al. 2007. "Evidence based management of acute bronchitis; sustained competence of enhanced communication skills acquisition in general practice." *Patient Educ Couns* 68(3): 270–78.

Carter, M. M., E. L. Lewis, et al. 2006. "Cultural competency training for third-year clerkship students: effects of an interactive workshop on student attitudes." *J Natl Med Assoc* 98(11): 1772–78.

Cegala, D. J. 2003. "Patient communication skills training: a review with implications for cancer patients." *Patient Educ Couns* 50(1): 91–94.

Cegala, D. J., and S. Lenzmeier Broz. 2002. "Physician communication skills training: a review of theoretical backgrounds, objectives, and skills." *Med Educ* 36(11): 1004–16.

Cegala, D. J., R. L. Street, Jr., et al. 2007. "The impact of patient participation on physicians' information provision during a primary care medical interview." *Health Commun* 21(2): 177–85.

Chen, L. M., W. R. Farwell, et al. 2009. "Primary care visit duration and quality." *Arch Intern Med* 169(20): 1866–72.

Chen, P. W. 2008. "Taking time for empathy." *New York Times,* September 25.

Cheraghi-Sohi, S., and P. Bower. 2008. "Can the feedback of patient assessments, brief training, or their combination, improve the interpersonal skills of primary care physicians? A systematic review." *BMC Health Serv Res* 8: 179.

Chibnall, J. T., M. L. Bennett, et al. 2004. "Identifying barriers to psychosocial spiritual care at the end of life: a physician group study." *Am J Hosp Palliat Care* 21(6): 419–26.

Claramita, M., and G. Majoor. 2006. "Comparison of communication skills in medical residents with and without undergraduate communication skills training as provided by the Faculty of Medicine of Gadjah Mada University." *Educ Health (Abingdon)* 19(3): 308–20.

Clark, N. M., M. Gong, et al. 1998. "Impact of education for physicians on patient outcomes." *Pediatrics* 101(5): 831–36.

CNN. 2008. "No LOL: Doctors don't answer e-mails." *CNN.com,* April 22 (accessed December 29, 2008).

Cochrane Collaboration. 2009. "Scope of our work." Cochrane Effective Practice and Organisation of Care Group. Available at http://epoc.cochrane.org/scope-our-work (accessed November 23, 2011).

Coleman, M. T., and K. S. Newton. 2005. "Supporting self-management in patients with chronic illness." *Am Fam Physician* 72(8): 1503–10.

Collins, T. C., J. A. Clark, et al. 2002. "Racial differences in how patients perceive physician communication regarding cardiac testing." *Med Care* 40(1 Suppl): I27–34.

Commonwealth Fund. 2009. "Time spent with physician." Performance Snapshots. Available at http://www.commonwealthfund.org (accessed November 22, 2009).

Cooper, V., and A. Hassell. 2002. "Teaching consultation skills in higher specialist training: experience of a workshop for specialist registrars in rheumatology." *Rheumatology (Oxford)* 41(10): 1168–71.

Corke, C. F., P. J. Stowe, et al. 2005. "How doctors discuss major interventions with high risk patients: an observational study." *BMJ* 330(7484): 182.

Cox, E. D., M. A. Smith, et al. 2007. "Effect of gender and visit length on participation in pediatric visits." *Patient Educ Couns* 65(3): 320–28.

Cross, M. A. 2007. "What the primary care physician shortage means for health plans." *Managed Care Magazine,* June 2007. Available at http://www.managed caremag.com (accessed October 11, 2009).

Curtis, J. R., R. A. Engelberg, et al. 2005. "Communication about palliative care for patients with chronic obstructive pulmonary disease." *J Palliat Care* 21(3): 157–64.

Curtis, J. R., D. L. Patrick, et al. 2000. "Why don't patients and physicians talk about end-of-life care? Barriers to communication for patients with acquired immunodeficiency syndrome and their primary care clinicians." *Arch Intern Med* 160(11): 1690–96.

Davidson, B., V. Vogel, et al. 2007. "Oncologist-patient discussion of adjuvant hormonal therapy in breast cancer: results of a linguistic study focusing on adherence and persistence to therapy." *J Support Oncol* 5(3): 139–43.

Davis, K., S. C. Schoenbaum, et al. 2002. *Room for improvement: patients report on the quality of their health care.* New York: Commonwealth Fund.

Deep, K. S., C. H. Griffith, et al. 2008. "Discussing preferences for cardiopulmonary resuscitation: what do resident physicians and their hospitalized patients think was decided?" *Patient Educ Couns* 72(1): 20–25.

de Ridder, D. T., N. C. Theunissen, et al. 2007. "Does training general practitioners to elicit patients' illness representations and action plans influence their communication as a whole?" *Patient Educ Couns* 66(3): 327–36.

Detmar, S. B., M. J. Muller, et al. 2001. "The patient-physician relationship: patient-physician communication during outpatient palliative treatment visits; an observational study." *Jama* 285(10): 1351–57.

Deveugele, M., A. Derese, et al. 2002. "Is GP-patient communication related to their perceptions of illness severity, coping, and social support?" *Soc Sci Med* 55(7): 1245–53.

Deveugele, M., A. Derese, et al. 2004. "Consultation in general practice: a standard operating procedure?" *Patient Educ Couns* 54(2): 227–33.

Dexheimer, J. W., T. R. Talbot, et al. 2008. "Prompting clinicians about preventive care measures: a systematic review of randomized controlled trials." *J Am Med Inform Assoc* 15(3): 311–20.

Di Blasi, Z. E., E. Harkness, et al. 2001. "Influence of context effects on health outcomes: a systematic review." *Lancet* 357(9258): 757–62.

Dimoska, A., P. N. Butow, et al. 2008. "An examination of the initial cancer consultation of medical and radiation oncologists using the Cancode interaction analysis system." *Br J Cancer* 98(9): 1508–14.

Dixon, R. F., and J. E. Stahl. 2009. "A randomized trial of virtual visits in a general medicine practice." *J Telemed and Telecare* 15:115–17.

Dosanjh, S., J. Barnes, et al. 2001. "Barriers to breaking bad news among medical and surgical residents." *Med Educ* 35(3): 197–205.

Doumit, G., M. Gattellari, et al. 2007. "Local opinion leaders: effects on professional practice and health care outcomes." *Cochrane Database Syst Rev*(1): CD000125.

Dow, A. W., D. Leong, et al. 2007. "Using theater to teach clinical empathy: a pilot study." *J Gen Intern Med* 22(8): 1114–18.

Dunham, W. 2008. "U.S. doctors offer patients scant empathy in study." *Boston Globe,* September 22.

Elkington, H., P. White, et al. 2001. "GPs' views of discussions of prognosis in severe COPD." *Fam Pract* 18(4): 440–44.

Epstein, R. M., P. Franks, et al. 2005. "Patient-centered communication and diagnostic testing." *Ann Fam Med* 3(5): 415–21.

Fallowfield, L., V. Jenkins, et al. 2002. "Efficacy of a Cancer Research UK communication skills training model for oncologists: a randomised controlled trial." *Lancet* 359(9307): 650–56.

Fallowfield, L., V. Jenkins, et al. 2003. "Enduring impact of communication skills training: results of a 12-month follow-up." *Br J Cancer* 89(8): 1445–49.

Fallowfield, L., and V. Jenkins. 2004. "Communicating sad, bad, and difficult news in medicine." *Lancet* 363(9405): 312–19.

Farber, J., A. Siu, et al. 2007. "How much time do physicians spend providing care outside of office visits?" *Ann Intern Med* 147(10): 693–98.

Farber, N. J., S. Y. Urban, et al. 2004. "Frequency and perceived competence in providing palliative care to terminally ill patients: a survey of primary care physicians." *J Pain Symptom Manage* 28(4): 364–72.

Farmer, A. P., F. Legare, et al. 2008. "Printed educational materials: effects on professional practice and health care outcomes." *Cochrane Database Syst Rev*(3): CD004398.

Farmer, S. A., and I. J. Higginson. 2006. "Chest pain: physician perceptions and decision-making in a London emergency department." *Ann Emerg Med* 48(1): 77–85.

Farmer, S. A., D. L. Roter, et al. 2006. "Chest pain: communication of symptoms and history in a London emergency department." *Patient Educ Couns* 63(1–2): 138–44.

Feldman-Stewart, D., M. D. Brundage, et al. 2005. "A conceptual framework for patient-professional communication: an application to the cancer context." *Psychooncology* 14(10): 801–9; discussion 810–11.

Fischer, G. S., and R. M. Arnold. 2007. "Feasibility of a brief workshop on palliative care communication skills for medical interns." *J Palliat Med* 10(1): 19–23.

Forsetlund, L., A. Bjorndal, et al. 2009. "Continuing education meetings and workshops: effects on professional practice and health care outcomes." *Cochrane Database Syst Rev*(2): CD003030.

Foster, N. L. 2001. "Barriers to treatment: the unique challenges for physicians providing dementia care." *J Geriatr Psychiatry Neurol* 14(4): 188–98.

Frankel, R., A. Altschuler, et al. 2005. "Effects of exam-room computing on clinician-patient communication: a longitudinal qualitative study." *J Gen Intern Med* 20(8): 677–82.

Franks, P., A. F. Jerant, et al. 2006. "Studying physician effects on patient outcomes: physician interactional style and performance on quality of care indicators." *Soc Sci Med* 62(2): 422–32.

Frantsve, L. M., and R. D. Kerns. 2007. "Patient-provider interactions in the management of chronic pain: current findings within the context of shared medical decision making." *Pain Med* 8(1): 25–35.

Frich, J. C., K. Malterud, et al. 2006. "Women at risk of coronary heart disease experience barriers to diagnosis and treatment: a qualitative interview study." *Scand J Prim Health Care* 24(1): 38–43.

Furman, C. D., B. Head, et al. 2006. "Evaluation of an educational intervention to encourage advance directive discussions between medicine residents and patients." *J Palliat Med* 9(4): 964–67.

Gabriel, B. A. 2008. "Your 15 minutes." *New Physician* 57(3). Available at http://www.amsa.org (accessed October 11, 2009).

Gaffan, J., J. Dacre, et al. 2006. "Educating undergraduate medical students about oncology: a literature review." *J Clin Oncol* 24(12): 1932–39.

Ginsburg, P. A., M. Maxfield, et al. 2008. "Making medical homes work: moving from concept to practice." HSC Policy Analysis No. 1, Center for Studying Health Systems Change, December. Available at http://www.hschange.org.

Goncalves, F., A. Marques, et al. 2005. "Breaking bad news: experiences and preferences of advanced cancer patients at a Portuguese oncology centre." *Palliat Med* 19(7): 526–31.

Gordon, G. H. 2003. "Care not cure: dialogues at the transition." *Patient Educ Couns* 50(1): 95–98.

Gott, M., E. Galena, et al. 2004. "'Opening a can of worms': GP and practice nurse barriers to talking about sexual health in primary care." *Fam Pract* 21(5): 528–36.

Grady, D. 2008. "For cancer patients, empathy goes a long way." *New York Times,* January 8.

Greco, M., A. Brownlea, et al. 2001. "Impact of patient feedback on the interpersonal skills of general practice registrars: results of a longitudinal study." *Med Educ* 35(8): 748–56.

Griffin, J. P., J. E. Nelson, et al. 2003. "End-of-life care in patients with lung cancer." *Chest* 123(1 Suppl): 312S–331S.

Grimshaw, J. M., R. E. Thomas, et al. 2004. "Effectiveness and efficiency of guideline dissemination and implementation strategies." *Health Technol Assess* 8(6): iii–iv, 1–72.

Guadagnoli, E., S. B. Soumerai, et al. 2000. "Improving discussion of surgical treatment options for patients with breast cancer: local medical opinion leaders versus audit and performance feedback." *Breast Cancer Res Treat* 61(2): 171–75.

Gulbrandsen, P., E. Krupat, et al. 2008. "'Four Habits' goes abroad: report from a pilot study in Norway." *Patient Educ Couns* 72(3): 388–93.

Gysels, M., A. Richardson, et al. 2004. "Communication training for health professionals who care for patients with cancer: a systematic review of effectiveness." *Support Care Cancer* 12(10): 692–700.

Hack, T. F., L. F. Degner, et al. 2005. "The communication goals and needs of cancer patients: a review." *Psychooncology* 14(10): 831–45; discussion 846–47.

Hagerty, R. G., P. N. Butow, et al. 2005. "Communicating prognosis in cancer care: a systematic review of the literature." *Ann Oncol* 16(7): 1005–53.

Hall, J. A. 2003. "Some observations on provider-patient communication research." *Patient Educ Couns* 50(1): 9–12.

Han, P. K., L. B. Keranen, et al. 2005. "The palliative care clinical evaluation exercise (CEX): an experience-based intervention for teaching end-of-life communication skills." *Acad Med* 80(7): 669–76.

Harding, A. 2009. "Messages often muddled in doctor-patient talks." *Reuters.com,* January 12 (accessed January 13, 2009).

Harding, R., L. Selman, et al. 2008. "Meeting the communication and information needs of chronic heart failure patients." *J Pain Symptom Manage* 36(2): 149–56.

Harms, C., J. R. Young, et al. 2004. "Improving anaesthetists' communication skills." *Anaesthesia* 59(2): 166–72.

Harmsen, H., R. Bernsen, et al. 2005. "The effect of educational intervention on intercultural communication: results of a randomised controlled trial." *Br J Gen Pract* 55(514): 343–50.

Harrington, J., L. M. Noble, et al. 2004. "Improving patients' communication with doctors: a systematic review of intervention studies." *Patient Educ Couns* 52(1): 7–16.

Harrington, N. G., G. R. Norling, et al. 2007. "The effects of communication skills training on pediatricians' and parents' communication during 'sick child' visits." *Health Commun* 21(2): 105–14.

Harris, T., and M. Buntin. 2008. *Choosing a health care provider: the role of quality information.* Research Synthesis Report No. 14. Princeton, NJ: Robert Wood Johnson Foundation.

Hart, C. N., D. Drotar, et al. 2006. "Enhancing patient-provider communication in ambulatory pediatric practice." *Patient Educ Couns* 62(1–2): 38–46.

Haskard, K. B., S. L. Williams, et al. 2008. "Physician and patient communication training in primary care: effects on participation and satisfaction." *Health Psychol* 27(5): 513–22.

Haywood, K., S. Marshall, et al. 2006. "Patient participation in the consultation process: a structured review of intervention strategies." *Patient Educ Couns* 63(1–2): 12–23.

Heisler, M., R. R. Bouknight, et al. 2002. "The relative importance of physician communication, participatory decision making, and patient understanding in diabetes self-management." *J Gen Intern Med* 17(4): 243–52.

Heisler, M., I. Cole, et al. 2007. "Does physician communication influence older patients' diabetes self-management and glycemic control? Results from the Health and Retirement Study (HRS)." *J Gerontol A Biol Sci Med Sci* 62(12): 1435–42.

Hietanen, P. S., A. R. Aro, et al. 2007. "A short communication course for physicians improves the quality of patient information in a clinical trial." *Acta Oncol* 46(1): 42–48.

Hobma, S., P. Ram, et al. 2006. "Effective improvement of doctor-patient communication: a randomised controlled trial." *Br J Gen Pract* 56(529): 580–86.

Hulsman, R. L., W. J. Ros, et al. 1999. "Teaching clinically experienced physicians communication skills: a review of evaluation studies." *Med Educ* 33(9): 655–68.

Hurtado, M. P., E. K. Swift, et al. 2001. *Envisioning the National Health Care Quality Report.* Washington, DC: Institute of Medicine, National Academy Press.

Irwin, R. S., and N. D. Richardson. 2006. "Patient-focused care: using the right tools." *Chest* 130(1 Suppl): 73S–82S.

Jamtvedt, G., J. M. Young, et al. 2006. "Audit and feedback: effects on professional practice and health care outcomes." *Cochrane Database Syst Rev*(2): CD000259.

Jenkins, L., N. Britten, et al. 2003. "Developing and using quantitative instruments for measuring doctor-patient communication about drugs." *Patient Educ Couns* 50(3): 273–78.

Jerant, A. F., M. M. von Friederichs-Fitzwater, et al. 2005. "Patients' perceived barriers to active self-management of chronic conditions." *Patient Educ Couns* 57(3): 300–307.

Johnson, K. B., J. R. Serwint, et al. 2008. "Computer-based documentation: effects on parent-provider communication during pediatric health maintenance encounters." *Pediatrics* 122(3): 590–98.

Kaduszkiewicz, H., C. Bachmann, et al. 2008. "Telling 'the truth' in dementia—do attitude and approach of general practitioners and specialists differ?" *Patient Educ Couns* 70(2): 220–26.

Kaner, E., B. Heaven, T. Rapley, M. Murtagh, R. Graham, R. Thomson, et al. 2007. "Medical communication and technology: a video-based process study of the use of decision aids in primary care consultations." *BMC Med Inform Decis Mak* 7(2): 1–11.

Keating, N. L., J. C. Weeks, et al. 2003. "Treatment of early stage breast cancer: do surgeons and patients agree regarding whether treatment alternatives were discussed?" *Breast Cancer Res Treat* 79(2): 225–31.

Kelly, P. A., and P. Haidet. 2007. "Physician overestimation of patient literacy: a potential source of health care disparities." *Patient Educ Couns* 66(1): 119–22.

Kennedy, S. 2005. "Communication in oncology care: the effectiveness of skills training workshops for healthcare providers." *Clin J Oncol Nurs* 9(3): 305–12.

Kerr, J., J. Engel, et al. 2003. "Communication, quality of life, and age: results of a 5-year prospective study in breast cancer patients." *Ann Oncol* 14(3): 421–27.

Kim, S. S., S. Kaplowitz, et al. 2004. "The effects of physician empathy on patient satisfaction and compliance." *Eval Health Prof* 27(3): 237–51.

King, J. T., Jr., H. Yonas, et al. 2005. "A failure to communicate: patients with cerebral aneurysms and vascular neurosurgeons." *J Neurol Neurosurg Psychiatry* 76(4): 550–54.

Kinnersley, P., A. Edwards, et al. 2008. "Interventions before consultations to help patients address their information needs by encouraging question asking: systematic review." *Bmj* 337: a485.

Klaristenfeld, D. D., D. T. Harrington, et al. 2007. "Teaching palliative care and end-of-life issues: a core curriculum for surgical residents." *Ann Surg Oncol* 14(6): 1801–6.

Knauft, E., E. L. Nielsen, et al. 2005. "Barriers and facilitators to end-of-life care communication for patients with COPD." *Chest* 127(6): 2188–96.

Koedoot, C. G., F. J. Oort, et al. 2004. "The content and amount of information given by medical oncologists when telling patients with advanced cancer what their treatment options are: palliative chemotherapy and watchful-waiting." *Eur J Cancer* 40(2): 225–35.

Koning, C. J., A. R. Maille, et al. 1995. "Patients' opinions on respiratory care: do doctors fulfill their needs?" *J Asthma* 32(5): 355–63.

Kravitz, R. L., E. J. Callahan, et al. 1996. "Prevalence and sources of patients' unmet expectations for care." *Ann Intern Med* 125(9): 730–37.

Kreps, G. L., D. O'Hair, et al. 1994. "The influences of health communication on health outcomes." *Am Behav Sci* 38(2): 248–56.

Krupat, E., R. Frankel, et al. 2006. "The Four Habits coding scheme: validation of an instrument to assess clinicians' communication behavior." *Patient Educ Couns* 62(1): 38–45.

Laing, B. Y., L. Ward, et al. 2008. "Introducing the 'teamlet': initiating a primary care innovation at San Francisco General Hospital." *Permanente J* 12(2): 4–9.

Laupacis, A., A. M. O'Connor, E. R. Drake, F. D. Rubens, J. A. Robblee, F. C. Grant, et al. 2006. "A decision aid for autologous pre-donation in cardiac surgery: a randomized trial." *Patient Educ Couns* 61(3): 458–66.

Leatherman, S., and L. Warrick. 2008. "Effectiveness of decision aids: a review of the evidence." *Med Care Res Rev* 65(6 Suppl): 79S–116S.

Levin, T. T., Y. Li, et al. 2008. "How do-not-resuscitate orders are utilized in cancer patients: timing relative to death and communication-training implications." *Palliat Support Care* 6(4): 341–48.

Levine, M. 2004. "Tell the doctor all your problems, but keep it to less than a minute." *New York Times,* June 1.

Levinson, W., R. Gorawara-Bhat, et al. 2000. "A study of patient clues and physician responses in primary care and surgical settings." *Jama* 284(8): 1021–27.

Levinson, W., and D. Roter. 1993. "The effects of two continuing medical education programs on communication skills of practicing primary care physicians." *J Gen Intern Med* 8(6): 318–24.

Lewin, S. A., Z. C. Skea, et al. 2001. "Interventions for providers to promote a patient-centred approach in clinical consultations." *Cochrane Database Syst Rev*(4): CD003267.

Li, H. Z., and J. Lundgren. 2005. "Training patients to ask information verifying questions in medical interviews." *Health Education* 105(6): 451–66.

Lienard, A., I. Merckaert, et al. 2008. "Factors that influence cancer patients' and relatives' anxiety following a three-person medical consultation: impact of a communication skills training program for physicians." *Psychooncology* 17(5): 488–96.

Lin, G. A., and R. A. Dudley. 2009. "Patient-centered care: what is the best measuring stick?" *Arch Intern Med* **169**(17): 1551–53.

Ling, B. S., J. M. Trauth, et al. 2008. "Informed decision-making and colorectal cancer screening: is it occurring in primary care?" *Med Care* **46**(9 Suppl 1): S23–29.

Little, P., H. Everitt, et al. 2001. "Observational study of effect of patient centredness and positive approach on outcomes of general practice consultations." *Bmj* **323**(7318): 908–11.

Liu, X., Y. Sawada, et al. 2007. "Doctor-patient communication: a comparison between telemedicine consultation and face-to-face consultation." *Intern Med* **46**(5): 227–32.

Lloyd, J. 2009. "Doctor shortage looms as primary care loses its pull." *USA Today*, August 8. Available at http://www.USAToday.com (accessed August 18, 2009).

Lown, B. A., J. P. Sasson, et al. 2008. "Patients as partners in radiology education: an innovative approach to teaching and assessing patient-centered communication." *Acad Radiol* **15**(4): 425–32.

Lukoschek, P., M. Fazzari, et al. 2003. "Patient and physician factors predict patients' comprehension of health information." *Patient Educ Couns* **50**(2): 201–10.

Maguire, P., and C. Pitceathly. 2002. "Key communication skills and how to acquire them." *Bmj* **325**(7366): 697–700.

Makaryus, A. N., and E. A. Friedman. 2005. "Patients' understanding of their treatment plans and diagnosis at discharge." *Mayo Clin Proc* **80**(8): 991–94.

Makoul, G. 2001. "Essential elements of communication in medical encounters: the Kalamazoo consensus statement." *Acad Med* **76**(4): 390–93.

Makoul, G. 2003. "The interplay between education and research about patient-provider communication." *Patient Educ Couns* **50**(1): 79–84.

Makoul, G., R. H. Curry, et al. 2001. "The use of electronic medical records: communication patterns in outpatient encounters." *J Am Med Inform Assoc* **8**(6): 610–15.

Maly, R. C., B. Leake, et al. 2003. "Health care disparities in older patients with breast carcinoma: informational support from physicians." *Cancer* **97**(6): 1517–27.

Mansouri, M., and J. Lockyer. 2007. "A meta-analysis of continuing medical education effectiveness." *J Contin Educ Health Prof* **27**(1): 6–15.

Marvel, M. K., R. M. Epstein, et al. 1999. "Soliciting the patient's agenda: have we improved?" *Jama* **281**(3): 283–87.

Mauksch, L. B., D. C. Dugdale, et al. 2008. "Relationship, communication, and efficiency in the medical encounter: creating a clinical model from a literature review." *Arch Intern Med* **168**(13): 1387–95.

Mauksch, L. B., and T. Roesler. 1990. "Expanding the context of the patient's explanatory model using circular questioning." *Fam Syst Med* **8**(1): 3–13.

McCauley, J., M. W. Jenckes, et al. 2005. "Spiritual beliefs and barriers among managed care practitioners." *J Relig Health* **44**(2): 137–46.

McCluskey, L., D. Casarett, et al. 2004. "Breaking the news: a survey of ALS patients and their caregivers." *Amyotroph Lateral Scler Other Motor Neuron Disord* **5**(3): 131–35.

McGorty, E. K., and B. H. Bornstein. 2003. "Barriers to physicians' decisions to discuss hospice: insights gained from the United States hospice model." *J Eval Clin Pract* **9**(3): 363–72.

McIntosh, A., and C. F. Shaw. 2003. "Barriers to patient information provision in primary care: patients' and general practitioners' experiences and expectations of information for low back pain." *Health Expect* **6**(1): 19–29.

McLafferty, R. B., R. G. Williams, et al. 2006. "Surgeon communication behaviors that lead patients to not recommend the surgeon to family members or friends: analysis and impact." *Surgery* 140(4): 616–22; discussion 622–24.

McManus, P. L., and K. E. Wheatley. 2003. "Consent and complications: risk disclosure varies widely between individual surgeons." *Ann R Coll Surg Engl* 85(2): 79–82.

Mead, N., and P. Bower. 2002. "Patient-centred consultations and outcomes in primary care: a review of the literature." *Patient Educ Couns* 48(1): 51–61.

Mercer, S. W., D. Reilly, et al. 2002. "The importance of empathy in the enablement of patients attending the Glasgow Homoeopathic Hospital." *Br J Gen Pract* 52(484): 901–5.

Merckaert, I., Y. Libert, et al. 2005a. "Communication skills training in cancer care: where are we and where are we going?" *Curr Opin Oncol* 17(4): 319–30.

Merckaert, I., Y. Libert, et al. 2005b. "Factors that influence physicians' detection of distress in patients with cancer: Can a communication skills training program improve physicians' detection?" *Cancer* 104(2): 411–21.

Merckaert, I., Y. Libert, et al. 2008. "Factors influencing physicians' detection of cancer patients' and relatives' distress: can a communication skills training program improve physicians' detection?" *Psychooncology* 17(3): 260–69.

Michie, S., J. Miles, et al. 2003. "Patient-centredness in chronic illness: what is it and does it matter?" *Patient Educ Couns* 51(3): 197–206.

Montgomery, J. E., J. T. Irish, et al. 2004. "Primary care experiences of medicare beneficiaries, 1998 to 2000." *J Gen Intern Med* 19(10): 991–98.

Moral, R. R., M. M. Alamo, et al. 2001. "Effectiveness of a learner-centred training programme for primary care physicians in using a patient-centred consultation style." *Fam Pract* 18(1): 60–63.

Morita, T., T. Akechi, et al. 2005. "Late referrals to specialized palliative care service in Japan." *J Clin Oncol* 23(12): 2637–44.

Morse, D. S., E. A. Edwardsen, et al. 2008. "Missed opportunities for interval empathy in lung cancer communication." *Arch Intern Med* 168(17): 1853–58.

Mukohara, K., K. Kitamura, et al. 2004. "Evaluation of a communication skills seminar for students in a Japanese medical school: a non-randomized controlled study." *BMC Med Educ* 4: 24.

Murphy, J., H. Chang, et al. 2001. "The quality of physician-patient relationships: patients' experiences 1996–1999." *J Fam Pract* 50(2): 123–29.

Murphy, K. 2007. "Teaching doctors to teach patients about lifestyle." *New York Times,* April 17.

Muthny, F. A., S. Wiedebusch, et al. 2006. "Training for doctors and nurses to deal with bereaved relatives after a sudden death: evaluation of the European Donor Hospital Education Programme (EDHEP) in Germany." *Transplant Proc* 38(9): 2751–55.

Mystakidou, K., E. Tsilika, et al. 2005. "Patterns and barriers in information disclosure between health care professionals and relatives with cancer patients in Greek society." *Eur J Cancer Care (Engl)* 14(2): 175–81.

Nelson, J. E., D. C. Angus, et al. 2006. "End-of-life care for the critically ill: a national intensive care unit survey." *Crit Care Med* 34(10): 2547–53.

Nelson, J. E., A. F. Mercado, et al. 2007. "Communication about chronic critical illness." *Arch Intern Med* 167(22): 2509–15.

Nelson, M., and H. E. Hamilton. 2007. "Improving in-office discussion of chronic obstructive pulmonary disease: results and recommendations from an in-office linguistic study in chronic obstructive pulmonary disease." *Am J Med* **120**(8 Suppl 1): S28–32.

Neumann, M., M. Wirtz, et al. 2007. "Determinants and patient-reported long-term outcomes of physician empathy in oncology: a structural equation modelling approach." *Patient Educ Couns* **69**(1–3): 63–75.

Oates, C. T., R. Sloane, et al. 2007. "Evaluation of agreement between physicians' notation of 'no evidence of disease' (NED) and patients' report of cancer status." *Psychooncology* **16**(7): 668–75.

O'Brien, M. A., S. Rogers, et al. 2007. "Educational outreach visits: effects on professional practice and health care outcomes." *Cochrane Database Syst Rev*(4): CD000409.

Oh, J., R. Segal, et al. 2001. "Retention and use of patient-centered interviewing skills after intensive training." *Acad Med* **76**(6): 647–50.

O'Malley, A., D. Peikes, and P. Ginsburg. 2008. "Qualifying a physician practice as a medical home." *Policy Perspective* **1**: 1, 3–8.

Ong, L. M., J. C. de Haes, et al. 1995. "Doctor-patient communication: a review of the literature." *Soc Sci Med* **40**(7): 903–18.

Ong, L. M., M. R. Visser, et al. 2000. "Doctor-patient communication and cancer patients' quality of life and satisfaction." *Patient Educ Couns* **41**(2): 145–56.

Ostbye, T., K. S. Yarnall, et al. 2005. "Is there time for management of patients with chronic diseases in primary care?" *Ann Fam Med* **3**(3): 209–14.

Ozanne, E. M., C. Annis, et al. 2007. "Pilot trial of a computerized decision aid for breast cancer prevention." *Breast J* **13**(2): 147–54.

Park, E. R., J. R. Betancourt, et al. 2005. "Mixed messages: residents' experiences learning cross-cultural care." *Acad Med* **80**(9): 874–80.

Park, E. R., J. R. Betancourt, et al. 2006. "Internal medicine residents' perceptions of cross-cultural training: barriers, needs, and educational recommendations." *J Gen Intern Med* **21**(5): 476–80.

Parker, P. A., B. J. Davison, et al. 2005. "What do we know about facilitating patient communication in the cancer care setting?" *Psychooncology* **14**(10): 848–58; discussion 859–60.

Pham, H. H., D. Peikes, et al. 2008. "Paying for medical homes: a calculated risk." *Policy Perspective* **1**(1): 15–17.

Pho, K., A. Geller, et al. 2000. "Lack of communication about familial colorectal cancer risk associated with colorectal adenomas (United States)." *Cancer Causes Control* **11**(6): 543–46.

Pollak, K. I., R. M. Arnold, et al. 2007. "Oncologist communication about emotion during visits with patients with advanced cancer." *J Clin Oncol* **25**(36): 5748–52.

Poon, E. G., J. S. Haas, et al. 2004. "Communication factors in the follow-up of abnormal mammograms." *J Gen Intern Med* **19**(4): 316–23.

Post, D. M., D. J. Cegala, et al. 2001. "Teaching patients to communicate with physicians: the impact of race." *J Natl Med Assoc* **93**(1): 6–12.

Post, D. M., D. J. Cegala, et al. 2002. "The other half of the whole: teaching patients to communicate with physicians." *Fam Med* **34**(5): 344–52.

Quinn, G. P., S. T. Vadaparampil, et al. 2008. "Patient-physician communication barriers regarding fertility preservation among newly diagnosed cancer patients." *Soc Sci Med* **66**(3): 784–89.

Rhoades, D. R., K. F. McFarland, et al. 2001. "Speaking and interruptions during primary care office visits." *Fam Med* **33**(7): 528–32.

Robinson, J. D., and J. Heritage. 2006. "Physicians' opening questions and patients' satisfaction." *Patient Educ Couns* **60**(3): 279–85.

Rodriguez, H. P., M. P. Anastario, et al. 2008. "Can teaching agenda-setting skills to physicians improve clinical interaction quality? A controlled intervention." *BMC Med Educ* **8**: 3.

Rosen, J., E. S. Spatz, et al. 2004. "A new approach to developing cross-cultural communication skills." *Med Teach* **26**(2): 126–32.

Rosen, P., and C. K. Kwoh. 2007. "Patient-physician e-mail: an opportunity to transform pediatric health care delivery." *Pediatrics* **120**(4): 701–6.

Rosen, R., D. Kountz, et al. 2006. "Sexual communication skills in residency training: the Robert Wood Johnson model." *J Sex Med* **3**(1): 37–46.

Rosenbaum, M. E., K. J. Ferguson, et al. 2004. "Teaching medical students and residents skills for delivering bad news: a review of strategies." *Acad Med* **79**(2): 107–17.

Rosenberg, E., C. Richard, et al. 2006. "Intercultural communication competence in family medicine: lessons from the field." *Patient Educ Couns* **61**(2): 236–45.

Rosenthal, T. C. 2008. "The medical home: growing evidence to support a new approach to primary care." *Jabfm* **21**(5): 427–40.

Roter, D. L., R. M. Frankel, et al. 2006. "The expression of emotion through nonverbal behavior in medical visits. Mechanisms and outcomes." *J Gen Intern Med* **21**: S28–34.

Roter, D. L., J. A. Hall, et al. 2002. "Physician gender effects in medical communication: a meta-analytic review." *Jama* **288**(6): 756–64.

Roter, D. L., J. A. Hall, et al. 1995. "Improving physicians' interviewing skills and reducing patients' emotional distress: a randomized clinical trial." *Arch Intern Med* **155**(17): 1877–84.

Roter, D. L., S. Larson, et al. 2004. "Use of an innovative video feedback technique to enhance communication skills training." *Med Educ* **38**(2): 145–57.

Rouf, E., J. Whittle, et al. 2007. "Computers in the exam room: differences in physician-patient interaction may be due to physician experience." *J Gen Intern Med* **22**(1): 43–48.

Ruiz-Moral, R., E. Perez Rodriguez, et al. 2006. "Physician-patient communication: a study on the observed behaviours of specialty physicians and the ways their patients perceive them." *Patient Educ Couns* **64**(1–3): 242–48.

Safran, D. G., M. Karp, et al. 2006. "Measuring patients' experiences with individual primary care physicians: results of a statewide demonstration project." *J Gen Intern Med* **21**(1): 13–21.

Safran, D. G., J. E. Montgomery, et al. 2001. "Switching doctors: predictors of voluntary disenrollment from a primary physician's practice." *J Fam Pract* **50**(2): 130–36.

Satterfield, J. M., and E. Hughes. 2007. "Emotion skills training for medical students: a systematic review." *Med Educ* **41**(10): 935–41.

Scanlon, D. P., J. B. Christianson, et al. 2008. "Hospital responses to the leapfrog group in local markets." *Med Care Res Rev* **65**(2): 207–31.

Schmid Mast, M., and J. A. Hall. 2007. "Disentangling physician sex and physician communication style: their effects on patient satisfaction in a virtual medical visit." *Patient Educ Couns* **68**(1): 16–22.

Schneider, J., S. H. Kaplan, et al. 2004. "Better physician-patient relationships are associated with higher reported adherence to antiretroviral therapy in patients with HIV infection." *J Gen Intern Med* **19**(11): 1096–1103.

Schouten, B. C., and L. Meeuwesen. 2006. "Cultural differences in medical communication: a review of the literature." *Patient Educ Couns* 64(1–3): 21–34.

Shapiro, J., J. Hollingshead, et al. 2003. "Self-perceived attitudes and skills of cultural competence: a comparison of family medicine and internal medicine residents." *Med Teach* 25(3): 327–29.

Shaw, W. S., A. Zaia, et al. 2005. "Perceptions of provider communication and patient satisfaction for treatment of acute low back pain." *J Occup Environ Med* 47(10): 1036–43.

Shilling, V., V. Jenkins, et al. 2003. "Factors affecting patient and clinician satisfaction with the clinical consultation: can communication skills training for clinicians improve satisfaction?" *Psychooncology* 12(6): 599–611.

Shojania, K. G., A. Jennings, et al. 2009. "The effects of on-screen, point of care computer reminders on processes and outcomes of care." *Cochrane Database Syst Rev* (3): CD001096.

Siegler, E. L., and B. W. Levin. 2000. "Physician–older patient communication at the end of life." *Clin Geriatr Med* 16(1): 175–204, xi.

Siminoff, L. A., G. C. Graham, et al. 2006. "Cancer communication patterns and the influence of patient characteristics: disparities in information-giving and affective behaviors." *Patient Educ Couns* 62(3): 355–60.

Sliwa, J. A., G. Makoul, et al. 2002. "Rehabilitation-specific communication skills training: improving the physician-patient relationship." *Am J Phys Med Rehabil* 81(2): 126–32.

Slutsman, J., L. Emanuel, et al. 2002. "Managing end-of-life care: comparing the experiences of terminally ill patients in managed care and fee for service." *J Am Geriatr Soc* 50(12): 2077–83.

Smith, D. K., R. W. Shaw, et al. 1995. "Training obstetricians and midwives to present screening tests: evaluation of two brief interventions." *Prenat Diagn* 15(4): 317–24.

Smith, S., J. L. Hanson, et al. 2007. "Teaching patient communication skills to medical students: a review of randomized controlled trials." *Eval Health Prof* 30(1): 3–21.

Stein, T., R. M. Frankel, et al. 2005. "Enhancing clinician communication skills in a large healthcare organization: a longitudinal case study." *Patient Educ Couns* 58(1): 4–12.

Stepien, K. A., and A. Baernstein. 2006. "Educating for empathy: a review." *J Gen Intern Med* 21(5): 524–30.

Stewart, M., L. Meredith, et al. 2000. "The influence of older patient–physician communication on health and health-related outcomes." *Clin Geriatr Med* 16(1): 25–36, vii–viii.

Stewart, M. A. 1995. "Effective physician-patient communication and health outcomes: a review." *Cmaj* 152(9): 1423–33.

Stratos, G. A., S. Katz, et al. 2006. "Faculty development in end-of-life care: evaluation of a national train-the-trainer program." *Acad Med* 81(11): 1000–1007.

Street, R. L., Jr. 2002. "Gender differences in health care provider-patient communication: are they due to style, stereotypes, or accommodation?" *Patient Educ Couns* 48(3): 201–6.

Street, R. L., Jr., H. S. Gordon, et al. 2005. "Patient participation in medical consultations: why some patients are more involved than others." *Med Care* 43(10): 960–69.

Tarkan, L. 2008. "E.R. patients often left confused after visits." *New York Times,* September 16.

Tarn, D. M., J. Heritage, et al. 2006. "Physician communication when prescribing new medications." *Arch Intern Med* 166(17): 1855–62.

Teno, J. M., E. Fisher, et al. 2000. "Decision-making and outcomes of prolonged ICU stays in seriously ill patients." *J Am Geriatr Soc* 48(5 Suppl): S70–74.

Theunissen, N. C., D. T. de Ridder, et al. 2003. "Manipulation of patient-provider interaction: discussing illness representations or action plans concerning adherence." *Patient Educ Couns* 51(3): 247–58.

Thorne, S. E., B. D. Bultz, et al. 2005. "Is there a cost to poor communication in cancer care? A critical review of the literature." *Psychooncology* 14(10): 875–84; discussion 885–86.

Tisdale, R., U. Ranji, et al. 2009. "Primary care shortage." Available at http://www.kaiseredu.org (accessed October 11, 2009).

Travado, L., L. Grassi, et al. 2005. "Physician-patient communication among Southern European cancer physicians: the influence of psychosocial orientation and burnout." *Psychooncology* 14(8): 661–70.

Ulene, V. 2009. "Doctors who deliver bad news should do it better." *Los Angeles Times,* March 9.

van Dam, H. A., F. van der Horst, et al. 2003. "Provider-patient interaction in diabetes care: effects on patient self-care and outcomes; a systematic review." *Patient Educ Couns* 51(1): 17–28.

van Dulmen, A. M. 2000. "Physician reimbursement and the medical encounter: an observational study in Dutch pediatrics." *Clin Pediatr (Phila)* 39(10): 591–601.

van Dulmen, A. M., and J. C. van Weert. 2001. "Effects of gynaecological education on interpersonal communication skills." *Bjog* 108(5): 485–91.

van Os, T. W., R. H. van den Brink, et al. 2005. "Communicative skills of general practitioners augment the effectiveness of guideline-based depression treatment." *J Affect Disord* 84(1): 43–51.

van Ryn, M. 2002. "Research on the provider contribution to race/ethnicity disparities in medical care." *Med Care* 40(1 Suppl): I140–51.

Vegni, E., and E. A. Moja. 2004. "Effects of a course on ophthalmologist communication skills: a pilot study." *Educ Health (Abingdon)* 17(2): 163–71.

Vegni, E., L. Zannini, et al. 2001. "Giving bad news: a GPs' narrative perspective." *Support Care Cancer* 9(5): 390–96.

Verhoeven, V., K. Bovijn, et al. 2003. "Discussing STIs: doctors are from Mars, patients from Venus." *Fam Pract* 20(1): 11–15.

von Gunten, C. F. 2003. "Discussing hospice care." *J Clin Oncol* 21(9 Suppl): 31S–36S.

Wachtler, C., A. Brorsson, et al. 2006. "Meeting and treating cultural difference in primary care: a qualitative interview study." *Fam Pract* 23(1): 111–15.

Weiner, J. S., and S. A. Cole. 2004. "Three principles to improve clinician communication for advance care planning: overcoming emotional, cognitive, and skill barriers." *J Palliat Med* 7(6): 817–29.

Weiner, J. S., and J. Roth. 2006. "Avoiding iatrogenic harm to patient and family while discussing goals of care near the end of life." *J Palliat Med* 9(2): 451–63.

Weiner, S. J., B. Barnet, et al. 2005. "Processes for effective communication in primary care." *Ann Intern Med* 142(8): 709–14.

Welschen, I., M. M. Kuyvenhoven, et al. 2004. "Effectiveness of a multiple intervention to reduce antibiotic prescribing for respiratory tract symptoms in primary care: randomised controlled trial." *Bmj* 329(7463): 431.

Wetzels, R., M. Harmsen, et al. 2007. "Interventions for improving older patients' involvement in primary care episodes." *Cochrane Database Syst Rev*(1): CD004273.

Wetzels, R., M. Wensing, et al. 2005. "A consultation leaflet to improve an older patient's involvement in general practice care: a randomized trial." *Health Expect* 8(4): 286–94.

Whelan, T., C. Sawka, et al. 2003. "Helping patients make informed choices: a randomized trial of a decision aid for adjuvant chemotherapy in lymph node–negative breast cancer." *J Natl Cancer Inst* 95(8): 581–87.

Williams, E. S., and A. C. Skinner. 2003. "Outcomes of physician job satisfaction: a narrative review, implications, and directions for future research." *Health Care Manage Rev* 28(2): 119–39.

Wilson, I. B., C. Schoen, et al. 2007. "Physician-patient communication about prescription medication nonadherence: a 50-state study of America's seniors." *J Gen Intern Med* 22(1): 6–12.

Yarnall, K. S., K. I. Pollak, et al. 2003. "Primary care: is there enough time for prevention?" *Am J Public Health* 93(4): 635–41.

Yawn, B., M. A. Goodwin, et al. 2003. "Time use during acute and chronic illness visits to a family physician." *Fam Pract* 20(4): 474–77.

Yiannakopoulou, E., J. S. Papadopulos, et al. 2005. "Adherence to antihypertensive treatment: a critical factor for blood pressure control." *Eur J Cardiovasc Prev Rehabil* 12(3): 243–49.

Zachariae, R., C. G. Pedersen, et al. 2003. "Association of perceived physician communication style with patient satisfaction, distress, cancer-related self-efficacy, and perceived control over the disease." *Br J Cancer* 88(5): 658–65.

Zickmund, S., S. L. Hillis, et al. 2004. "Hepatitis C virus-infected patients report communication problems with physicians." *Hepatology* 39(4): 999–1007.

Zolnierek, K. B., and M. R. Dimatteo. 2009. "Physician communication and patient adherence to treatment: a meta-analysis." *Med Care* 47(8): 826–34.

Zuger, A. 2006. "Doctors learn how to say what no one wants to hear." *New York Times*, January 10.

Index